AF413024

Clinical Radiology

Clinical Radiology

Clinical Radiology

Fourth Edition

George Simon
MD, FRCP, FFR

Arthur J.A. Wightman
MB BS, FRCR
Consultant Radiologist, City Hospital and Royal Infirmary,
Edinburgh

Butterworths
London   Boston   Durban   Singapore   Sydney   Toronto   Wellington

Second edition 1967
Third edition 1975
Reprinted 1977
Fourth edition 1983

© Butterworth & Co (Publishers) Ltd, 1983

British Library Cataloguing in Publication Data

Simon, George
    Clinical radiology.—4th ed.
    1. Diagnosis, Radioscopic   2. X-rays
    I. Title   II. Wightman, Arthur J.A.
    III. Simon, George. X-ray diagnosis for clinical students
    616.07′572   RC78

    ISBN 0–407–00224–3

Typeset by Scribe Design, Gillingham, Kent
Printed in England by Mackays of Chatham Ltd
Bound by Robert Hartnoll Ltd, Bodmin, Cornwall

Preface

This book is written for clinical students, and for postgraduates engaged in hospital practice or preparing for higher qualifications in medicine or surgery. The principal objectives of the book are to describe and illustrate the radiological appearances of the common and important diseases encountered in practice, and to discuss the logical order of investigation of difficult diagnostic problems, using the various imaging modalities which are now widely available.

Clinical Radiology is a revision of the third edition of Dr George Simon's *X-ray Diagnosis for Clinical Students*. The text has been extensively rewritten to incorporate descriptions of the principles and applications of isotope scanning, ultrasound and computed tomography, imaging methods which have developed rapidly since the publication of the last edition. These changes, together with the wider aim of providing a book for both postgraduate and under-graduate use, have demanded the adoption of a more general title.

Despite the advent of the newer techniques, the bulk of radiological requirements remains satisfied by plain film and simple contrast examinations. This is reflected in the book, the greater part of which concentrates on the description and illustration of diseases shown by routine X-ray examinations.

Dr George Simon's death in 1977 was an incalculable loss to the specialty of radiology. In an exceptionally productive career, he earned an international reputation for his contributions to the radiology of chest diseases, and of emphysema in particular. He was a clinical radiologist in the finest sense, tireless in expounding the fundamental importance of a practice based on close professional collaboration between clinician, radiologist and pathologist. Of his numerous teaching commitments, he is perhaps most widely re-membered for his evening seminars at the Brompton Hospital, at which he unfailingly held a packed audience of doctors of all disciplines captivated by his particular combination of erudition, modesty and wit.

Approximately half of the illustrations reproduced in this book are new. I am exceedingly grateful to Mrs Joanna Simon for her painstaking searches for the originals of those illustrations which have been retained from earlier editions. I am especially indebted to Professor George du Boulay for his continued involvement by contributing again to the authorship of Chapter 5. I am very grateful to my clinical colleague, Dr Andrew Douglas, for his helpful comments on Chapter 4; to Dr Keith Dewbury, for providing me with the illustrations of ultrasound examinations; to Dr Tom Philp for *Figures 3.2, 3.9* and *3.21*; and to Dr Mike Buist for *Figures 3.34, 3.35* and *4.59*.

Finally, I wish to record my special appreciation of the patience and help of my wife and children during the preparation of this edition.

Arthur J.A. Wightman
Edinburgh

Contents

3   Radiology of the Abdomen   100

4   Radiology of the Chest — 178

5   Radiology of the Head and Neck — 274

Index — 301

1 Introduction to diagnostic radiology and imaging

Major developments in the techniques and range of radiological investigations have taken place in recent years. During the past decade these developments have been accompanied by rapid advances in diagnostic uses of isotope scanning, ultrasound and computed tomography. These newer disciplines are referred to as imaging techniques, and they commonly form part of the diagnostic service provided by an X-ray department. This chapter provides a general introduction to the techniques in common usage, to which reference is made in later sections.

Some investigations carry an element of risk to the patient, or to the fetus of a pregnant patient. It is important for the clinician referring patients to be aware of the risks attached to certain examinations. These risks are also discussed in this chapter.

The nature and production of X-rays

X-rays are a form of energy wave, comparable with visible light waves but of much shorter wavelength. X-rays, however, have the particular property of being able to penetrate, and undergo partial absorption by, the tissues of the body. Radiation that passes through the body without being absorbed can be recorded on an X-ray film, and this forms the basis of radiological examination.

X-rays are produced in an evacuated glass tube containing a wire filament at one end and a 'target' of tungsten at the other. The filament releases electrons when it is heated to incandescence by an electric current. These electrons are made to accelerate towards the target by applying a very high voltage between the filament and target.

X-rays are produced as one of the forms of energy released when these high-velocity electrons lose their kinetic energy on striking the target. The X-ray tube is covered by a lead shield containing a small hole that allows the passage of a beam of X-rays. The tube is placed in front of the region for X-ray examination, and an X-ray film—which can be likened to a photographic negative—is placed on the opposite side of the body (*Figure 1.1*). High-density tissues

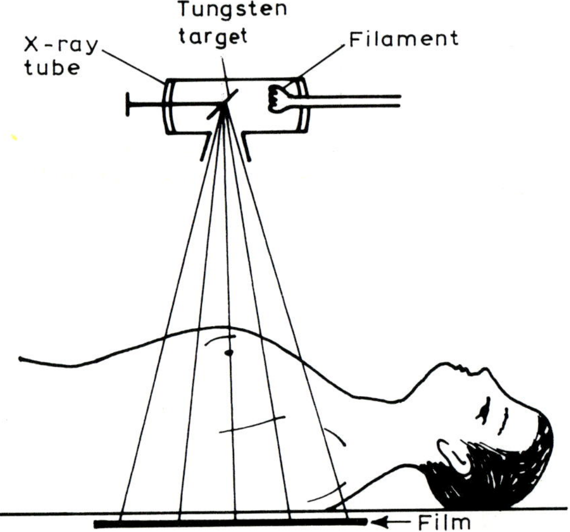

Figure 1.1. Simple X-ray examination

absorb more X-rays than those of low density. Thus absorption is greatest for bone, less for soft tissues of water density, less still for fat, and least of all for structures containing air. When an exposure is made the part of the film lying behind bony structures, in which absorption of X-rays is maximal, will receive very little transmitted radiation, and this part will therefore be represented as an underexposed, light area on the developed film. On the other hand, most of the radiation will pass through structures containing air, such as the lungs, so that the underlying regions of the film will be overexposed and dark. The image produced by soft tissues will be intermediate and grey. In this way the X-ray film produces an image of the body structures.

It is important to realize that an organ will be seen on an X-ray film only when it lies alongside a structure of different density. The lateral borders of the heart are clearly seen on a chest X-ray, for example, because they abut on the much lower density lungs. Only calcium, water (soft tissues), fat and air have sufficient differences in density to be distinguishable from each other on conventional X-ray examination.

Special X-ray techniques

Biplane radiography

A radiograph gives only a two-dimensional image. It is routine practice in all skull radiography, most other skeletal radiography, and in many chest examinations to obtain two films at right angles to each other. If an abnormality is visible on both of these views a three-dimensional image of that abnormality, and its exact position, can be established. A further important reason for obtaining two views routinely is that an abnormality such as a fracture is sometimes visible on only one projection and can therefore be overlooked on a single view (*see Figures 2.3 and 2.4*).

Tomography

Tomography provides a means of obtaining on an X-ray film an image of a selected single layer or thin slice of a region of the body, the parts lying in front of or behind this layer being rendered inconspicuous. In practice, the image on each tomogram produced in the following way corresponds to a layer of tissues a few millimetres thick.

The principle of tomography is illustrated in *Figure 1.2*. If two exposures are made on one film, the first with the X-ray tube at position A and the second with the tube moved to position B, an opacity at the point X in the patient will cast two images on the film at C and D; and an opacity at the point Y, at a different level, will

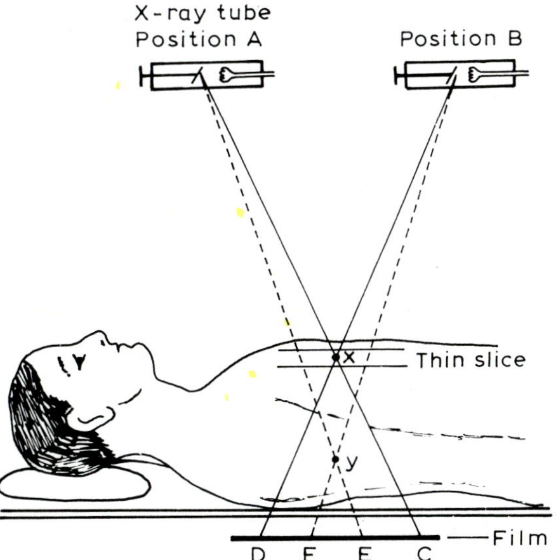

Figure 1.2. The principle of tomography

cast two images at E and F. If the film is also moved between the two exposures, but in a contrary direction to the tube and through a distance equal to CD, the opacity at X will then cast a single image in both exposures, whereas the two images of Y will not be superimposed but will appear twice on the film (since the film has been moved through a distance CD and not EF).

If a continuous exposure is made, instead of the two separate ones, during which the tube is moved from A to B, and the film in a contrary direction from C to D by means of a suitable connecting rod pivoted at the same level as X, then the opacity at X will cast a single shadow throughout the exposure; but opacities at other levels, such as Y, will give a continuous series of shadows so that their images will be blurred out and merged into the general blackening of the radiograph. If the film were moved a distance EF while the tube was moved from A to B, the image of X would be blurred out, while the image of Y would be clear. Thus by adjusting the pivot point of the connecting rod so as to give different ratios of movement between the tube and film, different layers can be examined and unwanted layers eliminated.

With some modern tomography units circular, elliptical and other movements of the X-ray tube and film can be made. This refinement is particularly useful in the examination of small, complex structures such as the anatomy of the ear. As with standard X-ray examination, tomography will provide an image only of that part of the structure which lies adjacent to a structure of different density. The technique, for example, will show in fine detail the outer and inner walls of a cavitating (air-filled) carcinoma in the periphery of the lung (*see Figure 4.63*). Tomography, on the other hand, will not show the presence of a metastasis within the liver, since the tumour and surrounding liver are of similar density.

The main indication for tomography, therefore, is to show the characteristics of a lesion that is poorly visualized on plain radiographs because of superimposed structures. A small lesion behind the hilum of the lung, for example, may be almost completely hidden by the superimposed shadows of the ribs and hilar vessels, and tomography will show the lesion in detail by blurring out these unwanted images.

Tomography has a second role in certain situations in demonstrating the presence of small lesions that are invisible on plain films. Random tomographic cuts through the lungs, for instance, will sometimes reveal the presence of small pulmonary metastases that are not seen on the chest X-ray.

Tomography should always be undertaken for a specific purpose suggested by the plain radiographs and relevant clinical findings. Recent plain radiographs should always be available. Where the decision to use tomography has been based on old films, new ones must be taken to ensure that the need for the examination still exists.

Fluoroscopy

In fluoroscopy the X-ray image is formed on a fluorescent screen instead of on film. The material used in the screen, zinc cadmium sulphide, has the special property of emitting visible light rays when exposed to X-rays. The image formed on the screen can be viewed directly, but nowadays it is customary for this image to be converted electronically for display on a television monitor. This refinement enables the examination to be conducted with a smaller dose of radiation to the patient and, because of the brightness of the image produced on the television monitor, allows the examination to be performed in daylight.

Since a continuous image is produced during the exposure of the patient to X-rays, fluoroscopy is particularly valuable in studying moving structures. Applications include assessment of pulsation of the left ventricle of the heart in suspected aneurysm, study of the movements of the diaphragm in suspected diaphragmatic paralysis, and observation of gastric peristalsis during barium meal examination.

Fluoroscopy is also useful for rapid assessment of positioning during surgical and radiological procedures. Fluoroscopy is sometimes used, for instance, in orthopaedic theatres to confirm satisfactory fracture alignment during operative reduction; it is essential to observe the same stringent precautions as apply in the X-ray department to protect the patient and staff from the dangers of radiation.

A cine or video recording can be made of the image obtained at fluoroscopy when a permanent record of the appearances of moving structures is required.

Contrast studies

Many of the soft-tissue structures of the body are totally or partially invisible on standard X-ray examinations because they merge with other structures of similar density. For example, the only visible segments of intestine are those that contain air, and the abdominal aorta is seen only if calcification is present in its wall.

Many structures can be rendered visible, and seen in great detail, if they can be filled with or outlined by substances of high density (liquid barium or iodine preparations) or low density (air or oxygen). Creation of contrast in this way forms the basis of X-ray contrast examinations. The main applications are as follows.

The alimentary tract

For most alimentary tract examinations a liquid barium sulphate preparation is used. This can be taken by mouth for examination of the oesophagus (barium swallow), stomach and duodenum (barium meal), or small bowel (barium follow-through). It can be run in through a rectal catheter for examination of the colon (barium enema). It is now usual for barium meal and barium enema examinations to be performed using double-contrast techniques. For these, the patient swallows a gas-forming preparation at the start of a barium meal examination, or the colon is insufflated with air during a barium enema study. The barium produces a fine coating on the mucosa of the stomach, duodenum or colon, and this stands out very clearly against the distended, gas-filled lumen.

There are certain situations in which barium is not indicated. In partial obstruction of the bowel the thick barium preparation may render the obstruction complete. Barium should not be used in suspected perforation, since barium in the peritoneal cavity can cause peritonitis, granuloma formation and adhesions.

In these situations in which barium is contraindicated, a water-soluble iodine-containing contrast agent can be given with safety. One such preparation in common use is Gastrografin (sodium methylglucamine diatrizoate). The main disadvantage of Gastrografin is that it is very hypertonic. It must be used with care, therefore, in babies, since it will draw fluid into the gut and cause hypovolaemia. Gastrografin should not be used in a dehydrated baby until the dehydration has been corrected. It is also contraindicated if there is a possibility that the patient will aspirate, since Gastrografin in the lungs can lead to respiratory collapse and death from pulmonary oedema. In this situation barium may be used, since small quantities of barium in the lungs are virtually harmless.

The biliary tract

The contrast investigations that are available for examination of the biliary tract are discussed in Chapter 3. These involve administration, by mouth or intravenous injection, of iodine-containing contrast agents that are excreted in the bile, or injection of iodine preparations directly into the biliary tract.

The renal tract

The standard contrast examination is the intravenous urogram (IVU, excretion urogram or intravenous pyelogram). This entails the intravenous injection of an aqueous iodine-containing contrast agent which is then excreted by the kidneys. Films are taken at intervals after the injection, commonly at 3, 10, and 20 minutes, to show opacification of the renal parenchyma, pelvicalyceal system, ureters and bladder.

Other contrast studies for investigation of the renal tract are described in Chapter 3.

Vascular system

Aqueous iodine preparations can be injected into vessels for examination of arteries (arteriography) or veins (venography). When the vessel supplying the region of interest is superficial (e.g. the carotid artery), the injection can be made through a needle or short cannula inserted directly into the vessel. However, injection into vessels that are not accessible for direct puncture (e.g. the renal arteries) is also often required.

All of the major arteries arising from the aorta, and in turn many of the major branches of these vessels, can be catheterized with appropriately shaped catheters. The catheter is passed percutaneously into a superficial artery, usually the femoral, after arterial puncture with a Seldinger or similar needle of special design: a cut-down on the femoral artery is not required. The catheter is then advanced proximally along the iliac arteries and aorta until the required vessel is reached. Confirmation of correct positioning of the catheter tip is obtained by injecting a small quantity of the contrast agent through the catheter and observing the subsequent vessel opacification on the television monitor.

The venous system is widely accessible for investigation by similar methods from the femoral vein, and the cardiac chambers can be examined by advancing catheters into the heart from accessible veins or arteries in the groin or arm.

There are two main indications for contrast studies of the vascular system. First, intrinsic disease of a vessel, such as atheroma or thrombus formation, can be assessed. Secondly, much information concerning the nature and site of disease within an organ can be obtained by imaging the blood supply. A tumour, for example, will often be revealed by the demonstration of a highly abnormal tumour circulation within it (*see Figure 3.50*), and any space-occupying lesion will commonly displace and distort the adjacent vessels.

Respiratory tract

Bronchography is discussed in Chapter 4.

Central nervous system

Contrast studies are reviewed in Chapter 5.

Miscellaneous

Lymphangiography   The lymphatics of the lower limb and the para-aortic lymphatics and lymph glands can be outlined after the injection of an iodized oil preparation into a lymphatic duct in the foot.

Arthrography   The soft-tissue components of a joint can be outlined by injecting either a water-soluble, iodine-containing preparation or air or oxygen into the joint: in some situations a double-contrast examination can be performed. This procedure is used particularly in the investigation of disorders of the hips, knees and shoulders.

Sialography   Disease of the parotid and submandibular glands can be investigated by opacifying the duct systems by injecting contrast medium into the duct ostia in the mouth.

Hysterosalpingography   Contrast medium is injected through the cervix uteri for visualization of the uterine cavity and Fallopian tubes. The main indication is in the investigation of infertility.

Adverse reactions to intravascular contrast agents

Intravenous or intra-arterial injection of iodine-containing contrast agents carries a certain danger. Patients quite commonly experience minor reactions, but occasionally severe life-threatening reactions occur. It is important for the clinician to be aware of the risks for two reasons. First, he may give the injection of contrast medium himself (for an intravenous urogram, for example) or he may be called upon as a member of a hospital's emergency team to help resuscitate a patient after an intravascular injection. Second, by being aware of an element of risk, the clinician should particularly avoid requesting investigations of this type if the results are unlikely to affect his management of the patient.

Reactions most commonly occur at the time of injection or within the following 10 minutes. Mild reactions include nausea, vomiting, sneezing, a feeling of heat and urticaria. These usually require no treatment. In serious reactions profound hypotension, cardiac arrest, bronchospasm or laryngeal oedema may develop. In these situations urgent resuscitation is needed.

The likelihood of a patient reacting to an intravascular contrast injection is influenced by the following factors.

1. There is a 35 per cent risk of a reaction occurring if the patient has experienced a reaction to an intravascular contrast agent during a previous examination. In this event, therefore, serious consideration should be given to whether the examination is essential, or whether an investigation that does not involve contrast medium could be used instead, e.g. isotope studies of the renal tract instead of an IVU. If it is considered essential to proceed with the investigation the patient should receive a substantial covering dose of steroids beforehand; an appropriate dose is 200 mg hydrocortisone intravenously 1 hour before the injection of contrast. It is also a sound precaution to set up an intravenous drip in case rapid drug treatment of a reaction is required.
2. Patients with a history of asthma or allergies (e.g. to penicillin) have a greater risk of reacting to intravascular contrast media, and steroid cover may again be considered advisable.
3. Since contrast agents are hypertonic, their injection for IVU and other examinations may precipitate pulmonary oedema in patients with incipient cardiac failure.

Apart from reactions to contrast agents, there are other risks attached to intravascular studies, such as thrombus formation at the site of catheterization in arteriography. The clinician should be aware that complications from invasive procedures occasionally arise, but it is the responsibility of the radiologist carrying out the procedure to ensure that full precautions are taken to avoid such complications.

Treatment of severe reactions

In general, standard methods of emergency treatment and resuscitation are used, based on assessment of the patient's life-threatening complications. In all severe reactions to contrast media, however, it is advisable to give 200 mg of intravenous hydrocortisone immediately and to repeat this as necessary.

Immediate action necessitates administration of oxygen, intravenous injection of hydrocortisone, checking that the airways are clear, external cardiac massage and artificial respiration if required, and establishing a venous line for drug treatment. Assistance should be called for from the hospital's emergency resuscitation team or other supporting medical staff.

Severe bronchospasm should be treated as in general medical practice with subcutaneous or intramuscular injection of 0.5 ml of 1:1000 adrenaline (epinephrine) or slow intravenous injection of 250 mg aminophylline in 10 ml, the latter repeated if necessary after a few minutes. If laryngeal oedema is present and has not responded to hydrocortisone, a subcutaneous or intramuscular injection of 0.5 ml 1:1000 adrenaline, and also intravenous antihistamines, should be given, and very occasionally emergency tracheotomy is required. For cardiovascular problems, a continuously running electrocardiograph recording should be established as soon as possible and conventional treatment measures instituted to reverse persisting hypotension or arrhythmias.

Radioisotope imaging

Radioisotope imaging (scanning) is an important form of investigation with many applications. Although the method involves radiation the principle is different from X-ray examination. Scanning and X-ray examination are to a large extent complementary. Scanning is often of considerable value in investigating organs on which simple X-ray study provides little information, such as the brain, liver and thyroid.

The principle of radioisotope imaging centres on recording radiation emitted when the atoms of an unstable element disintegrate spontaneously to a stable form. Several unstable elements (radioisotopes) are found naturally, the best known of which is uranium. The radioisotopes used in scanning, however, are prepared artificially. Once prepared, these then break down spontaneously, some rapidly and some slowly, to stable forms. In this process of disintegration several types of radiation are emitted, and one of these, gamma radiation, is the type recorded in radioisotope scanning. The commonly used recording instrument is the gamma camera.

In practice, a suitable non-toxic radioactive substance is injected intravenously. The radioactive substance is commonly prepared in such a way that it will be taken up preferentially by the organ under investigation. The patient is placed with the region of interest in front of the gamma camera. Emitted gamma rays are recorded by the instrument, and from these data the gamma camera builds up and displays on a cathode-ray oscilloscope a two-dimensional image of the spatial distribution of the radioisotope in the organ being investigated. This image can be photographed on Polaroid or X-ray film to provide a permanent record. Alternatively—for dynamic studies of the passage of isotope through structures such as the vascular system, brain or kidneys—the information received by the gamma camera can be transferred to and processed by a computer.

One isotope in common use is technetium. This has the advantage of disintegrating sufficiently rapidly to avoid undue irradiation of the patient, while remaining in radioactive form long enough for the investigation to be carried out.

The basic principles and commonly used techniques for four frequently requested radioisotope scans are as follows.

Lung scans   For lung perfusion scans technetium can be bound onto albumin aggregates of a slightly larger diameter than the lung capillaries. After intravenous injection these will pass through the right side of the heart and then lodge in the peripheral pulmonary vessels. If the pulmonary vasculature is normal the gamma camera will show these particles distributed uniformly throughout the lungs, but if the patient has had pulmonary emboli the scan will show defects in the radioisotope distribution corresponding with the areas of deficient perfusion (*see Figure 4.58*).

Liver scans   Technetium is commonly bound to sulphur colloid for liver scans. The colloid particles are removed from the circulation by the reticuloendothelial cells of the liver and spleen. A scan of a normal liver will show a uniform distribution of radioisotope. Hepatic metastases or abscesses, devoid of reticuloendothelial cells, will on the other hand show as 'holes' on the scan (*Figure 1.3*).

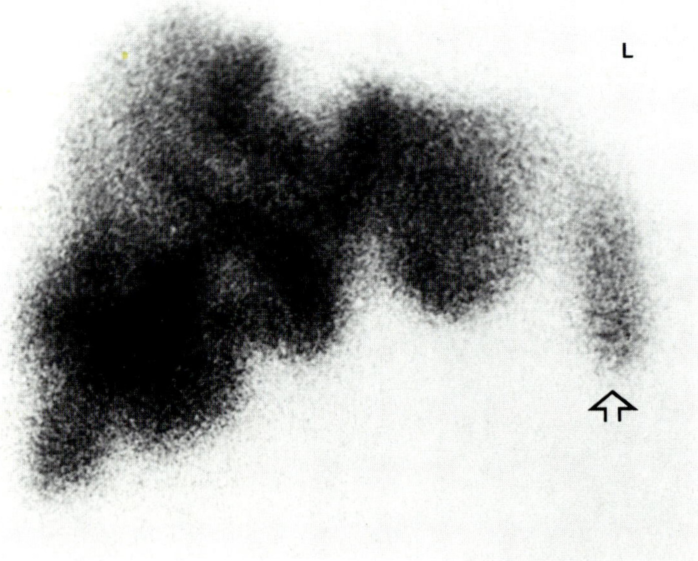

Figure 1.3. Isotope liver scan (technetium–sulphur colloid: anterior projection gamma-camera recording). There are numerous areas of deficient isotope uptake (white areas) in the enlarged liver. These were due to metastases from breast carcinoma. Normal spleen (arrow) on patient's left

Brain scans   Substances that normally do not enter the brain from the blood stream may do so in the presence of disease. In such conditions as cerebral tumours, infarcts or abscesses, technetium injected into the circulation will seep from the blood into the damaged area of the brain. The gamma-camera image will then show a region of high radiation emission corresponding with the area of disease, surrounded by very low activity in the normal brain tissue (*see Figure 5.9*).

Bone scans   Bone is in a constant state of chemical turnover, absorption and deposition occurring concurrently. The isotopes used for scanning are those that will exchange with the mineral components of bone. Technetium-labelled phosphates are commonly used. These will be taken up in the skeleton in the process of normal bone turnover within a few hours of injection. The distribution can then be recorded with the gamma camera.

Concentration of isotope will take place in regions of the skeleton showing increased mineral turnover, as occurs in the presence of such conditions as metastases, fractures, bone infections, or Paget's disease. These sites of high concentration will be shown on the scan (*see Figure 2.87*).

Radioisotope bone scanning is more sensitive than X-ray examination in detecting metastases. The scan, however, is non-specific, and a region of the skeleton showing an abnormal isotope uptake must be examined further with conventional X-rays, which may reveal that a primary or secondary tumour, a fracture, Paget's disease, or other condition of characteristic radiological appearance is present.

Ultrasound

Ultrasound is a form of energy occurring in waves similar to, but of much higher frequency than, audible sound waves. Ultrasound has the properties of penetrating soft tissues, and of being partially reflected at tissue interfaces. The reflected signals can be recorded, and from the information received a spatial reconstruction of the deep tissues can be built up and displayed on a viewing monitor. This forms the basis of ultrasound examination, the principles and method of which are summarized as follows.

Certain substances have the properties of generating waves of ultrasound when a voltage is applied across them and, conversely, of generating a voltage when they receive a beam of ultrasound. A disc of one such substance is used to produce a narrow beam of ultrasound, and this disc, called a transducer, is mounted in a tube-shaped probe, the end of which is held against the patient's skin.

Pulses of ultrasound are generated electrically, and the probe is either rocked to and fro or moved over the skin to obtain echoes from the underlying region of interest. The echoes are detected by the transducer. This incoming information is processed and commonly viewed on the monitor as a grey scale two-dimensional reconstruction of the echoes from the deep tissues (real-time ultrasonography, *Figures 1.4 and 1.5*). The display is called grey scale because the image shows a gradation of shade from near white to near black depending on the relative strengths of the echoes returning from the different tissues.

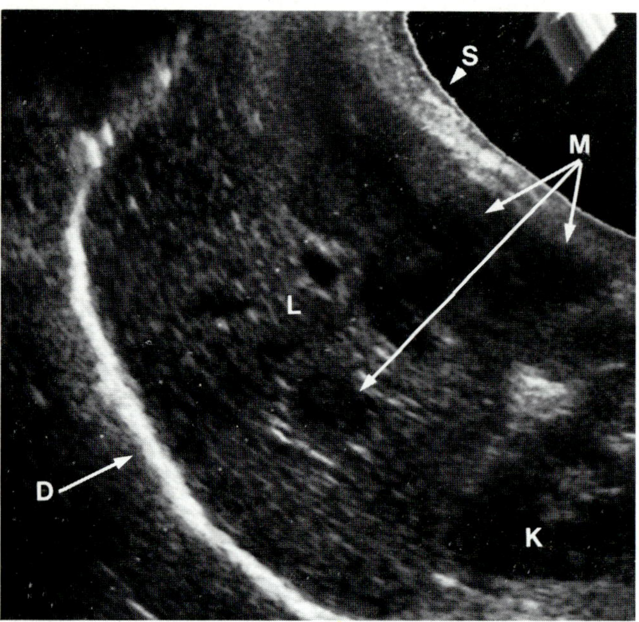

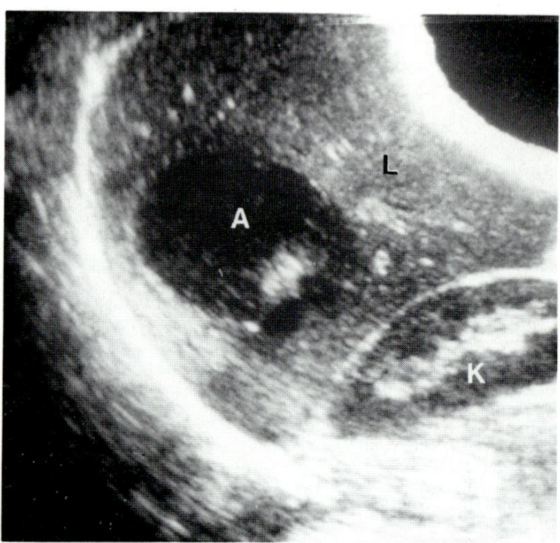

Figure 1.4. Hepatic metastases. Longitudinal ultrasound scan of liver (patient's head to left, feet to right). Liver metastases may generate more or fewer echoes than the normal hepatic parenchyma. In this example of breast metastases, echo-poor metastases (dark areas) are demonstrated within the right lobe of the liver. D, diaphragm; K, upper pole of right kidney; L, liver; M, metastases; S, skin line

Figure 1.5. Hepatic abscess. Longitudinal ultrasound scan of liver. Smooth-walled abscess, mainly transonic but with echoes from areas of contained debris. Cystic nature confirmed by enhanced echoes from tissues behind the abscess. A, abscess; K, upper pole of right kidney; L, liver

Ultrasound has acquired a vitally important role in obstetrics, since images of the fetus and placenta can be produced and abnormalities detected. The technique is also highly valuable in investigating many diseases of the abdomen and pelvis, and disorders of the heart. These applications are discussed further in Chapters 3 and 4. A major limitation of the technique is that ultrasound will not pass through air. This, therefore, excludes the use of ultrasound for the study of diseases of the lungs, although pleural abnormalities can be investigated. Air in the bowel can impose a restriction for the same reason on certain abdominal investigations.

The advantages of examination by ultrasound are that the procedure is painless, non-invasive, and causes no harm to the patient or fetus. There are two important aspects to this last factor. First, a fetus can be examined with complete safety, in contrast to the potential radiation danger associated with X-ray examination. Second, examination can be repeated as often as required, for instance to monitor fetal growth or response of a tumour to treatment.

Ultrasound examination is less sensitive than certain other techniques, such as sophisticated contrast studies. It should be regarded as complementary to other methods of investigation, and because of its advantages should be carried out where appropriate at an early stage in the scheme of investigation of a patient. The result obtained may then eliminate the need for examinations that are either more complex or more uncomfortable for the patient.

Computed tomography

Conventional X-ray examination will record only whether a structure has the density of air, fat, water (soft tissue) or bone. Adjacent structures of closely similar density, for example a tumour within the brain, will not be distinguishable by simple X-ray examination. The importance of computed tomography (CT) is that the technique allows discrimination to be made between tissues of only slight density difference. Pictorial display of a CT examination of the brain, for instance, will show the site, size, outline and other characteristics of a cerebral tumour or other intracranial lesion, as well as the displaced normal anatomical structures. This facility has led to CT assuming a role of immense value in the radiological investigation of intracranial lesions as well as other regions of the body.

The principle is that a narrow beam of X-rays is directed at the region of interest, and detectors on the opposite side of the patient record the transmitted radiation. The X-ray source and detectors are mounted on a common frame so that they can rotate around the patient, the detectors always facing, and lying on the opposite side of the patient to, the X-ray source (*Figure 1.6*). During the examination the X-ray beam is rotated round the patient, and many thousands of recordings of transmitted radiation are made during this procedure. These recordings are processed by a computer, and from this an image of the examined transverse section can be constructed and displayed on a television screen. This image can be photographed if required to produce a visual record for reporting sessions and for inclusion in the patient's case notes. The procedure is repeated at selected intervals along the body to provide a comprehensive series of transverse scans embracing the region under investigation. The radiation dose to the patient from CT scanning is comparable with that from conventional X-ray examination.

Transverse sectional images are also obtained with a new imaging technique, nuclear magnetic resonance (NMR). In this, measurement is made with data processing by computer of proton response to an applied magnetic field: this procedure does not involve X-ray production.

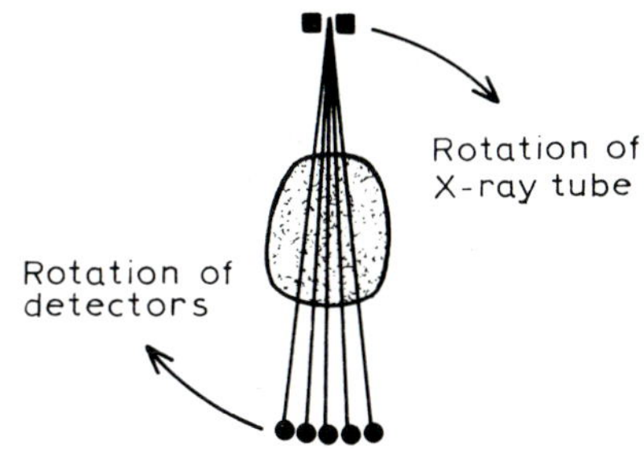

Figure 1.6. Computed tomography. Simplified diagram showing principle of rotation of X-ray tube and detectors round skull during X-ray exposure

Radiation danger and precautions in diagnostic investigation

It is well known that radiation can produce harmful biological effects. This has received widespread documentation, for example, in studies of the victims of the Hiroshima and Nagasaki atomic bomb explosions. Excessive radiation in diagnostic investigation can cause erythema and skin necrosis, and the serious late complications of radiation-induced malignant disease and cataracts. These complications are virtually never encountered nowadays, owing to widespread awareness of the dangers of radiation and the consequent adoption of stringent precautionary measures in the X-ray department.

One particular problem, however, is the need to avoid any unnecessary irradiation of an embryo or fetus. Irradiation *in utero* can cause death of an embryo, or can lead to congenital malformation (most commonly of the brain) or to an increased incidence of malignant disease during childhood. The risk of any one of these complications arising from radiation is greatest in the first 4 months of pregnancy. The danger from radiological investigations is, however, low. It is estimated that the radiation dose for the common X-ray examinations involving the lower abdomen of the mother will increase the likelihood of any abnormality occurring to the fetus by less than 1 in 1000. Compared with this, the overall risk of birth of a child with severe handicap in the general population is greater than 1 in 30.

Since there is a risk, albeit very small, to the fetus from radiological examination it has become the practice in the United Kingdom to observe a policy known as 'the 10-day rule'. This states that women of child-bearing age should have X-ray examinations involving the lower abdomen carried out during the 10 days after the onset of menstruation unless there are overriding reasons for acting otherwise, usually the need for urgent investigation. Pregnancy is least likely during the first 10 days of the menstrual cycle, and the purpose of the rule is to ensure that an unsuspected embryo is not irradiated.

This policy has not been adopted in the United States. The American College of Radiologists stresses that the possibility of pregnancy should always be considered before abdominal radiography of women of child-bearing age is performed but recommends that planned scheduling should be undertaken only for examinations unconnected with the patient's current illness.

Care must also be taken to ensure that staff do not receive excessive radiation. Lead aprons should be worn or lead screens used for the protection of staff in X-ray rooms. X-ray personnel should wear film monitors recording their exposure to radiation. A nurse, medical student or doctor should not repeatedly hold a difficult patient, such as an infant, during X-ray examinations. A student or clinician visiting a properly equipped department is in no danger from radiation, provided that he takes care to avoid direct exposure and wears a lead apron in an examination room.

Full radiological precautions must of course also be observed in orthopaedic and other operating theatres in which fluoroscopy is used. The X-ray beam should be as small as possible, the screening time should be kept to a minimum, and the surgeon should avoid placing his hands within the beam of radiation.

General considerations in investigation and interpretation

Radiology makes its greatest contribution, and the patient benefits most, when there is a close working collaboration between the clinician and radiologist. Sometimes the purpose of a radiological examination, or imaging procedure, is to provide information in connection with a diagnosis that is already known. This is the case, for example, when X-rays are requested to show the position of a fracture that is clinically obvious, or to demonstrate the extent and character of the lesions of pulmonary tuberculosis when tubercle bacilli have been found in the sputum.

In many instances, however, radiological examination is undertaken either alone or in conjunction with other tests to establish a diagnosis. In this situation it is vitally important for two reasons that the radiologist is adequately informed of the relevant clinical and laboratory findings. First, a particular radiological appearance, such as that of fine nodular shadowing throughout the lungs, may be common to many diseases, and a radiologist's report based on his consideration of the individual case is far more valuable than the provision of an encyclopaedic list of possibilities. Second, the radiologist can often provide useful advice on the most appropriate investigations in a difficult diagnostic problem.

As a general principle, the first examinations should be those that involve the patient in the least discomfort and are harmless, quick to perform, and comparatively inexpensive. If these provide insufficient information, investigations appropriate to the problem in hand should be undertaken based on these considerations. In general, investigations are therefore carried out as appropriate in the following order.
1. Standard views.
2. Supplementary views, e.g. obliques.
3. Simple fluoroscopy.
4. Tomography
    and/or simple contrast studies (e.g. barium examination of the intestine, IVU or oral cholecystogram),
    and/or ultrasound,
    and/or isotope scanning.
5. Computed tomography
    and/or sophisticated contrast procedures.

Clearly only a few of these groups are appropriate for any one patient, and in the great majority of cases only the simpler examinations are required. It must be emphasized also that the above is a general scheme of progression, to which exceptions inevitably occur. In those centres where CT is available, for example, this would be used at an early stage in the investigation of patients with head injuries, as investigation by this means has an important, established place in the study of intracranial disease.

It is of mutual educational value for the clinician and radiologist to discuss those patients who present diagnostic problems and, as stated before, this collaboration is of paramount benefit to the patient. The student and clinician will develop a familiarity with the radiological appearances of disease as a result of this collaboration, and with increasing clinical experience. On many occasions the X-ray abnormality will indicate one particular diagnosis or a limited number of possible diseases. In other cases the X-ray is difficult to interpret; it is then helpful to consider what normal anatomical structures occur at the site of the radiographic abnormality, and the various groups of diseases with which these structures can be affected. These can conveniently be considered in the same broad categories as are used in clinical practice:

1. Congenital.
2. Traumatic.
3. Inflammatory. Viral, bacterial, fungal, parasitic, and conditions of unknown cause.
4. Neoplastic.
5. Metabolic, e.g. gout and vitamin deficiencies.
6. Endocrine.
7. Degenerative and infiltrative.
8. Idiopathic.

Further reading

Ansell, G. (1976). *Complications in Diagnostic Radiology*. Oxford: Blackwell Scientific Publications.

Mole, R.H. (1979). Radiation effects on pre-natal development and their radiological significance. *British Journal of Radiology*, **52**, 89–101.

Carmichael, J.H.E. and Warrick, C.K. (1978). The ten day rule—principles and practice. *British Journal of Radiology*, **51**, 843–846.

Radiology of the skeleton and soft tissues

The skeleton

X-ray changes in bone

The radiographic image of a bone is due almost entirely to its calcium content. Pathological lesions will be visible when there are: changes in structural continuity (as in fractures); changes in position (as in dislocations); or changes in shape (as in congenital developmental defects). The bone itself may show a lessening of density (reduced radio-opacity), indicating a low calcium content that may be general in the whole skeleton or confined to a single bone. There may be localized demineralization with disappearance of the trabeculae (bone erosion); increased density from a high calcium content (bone sclerosis); alteration in the trabecular structure (as in Paget's disease); new bone formation (as in periosteal new bone or bony outgrowths); and changes in the width of the space between the ends of two bones (as in arthritis).

The X-ray diagnosis of bone disease often depends on a careful consideration of all these possibilities, and on the relative intensity of any changes that may be present. For instance, much erosion and periostitis will suggest bone infection, while much erosion and minimal periostitis will suggest a neoplasm. It is useful, when studying bone radiographs, to have some such list of possible bone changes in mind.

Therefore, when radiographs of the skeleton are examined, a search should be made for any localized or generalized alteration of bone density or structure. The white cortical line surrounding the bone should be traced in its entirety, and unless this is done a small 'step' in the cortex due to a fracture, or an area of cortical destruction, can be overlooked. When several bones (such as the ribs or vertebrae or small bones of the hand or foot) are shown on the one radiograph, each bone must be carefully examined in turn and any abnormal separation of the articular surfaces or other changes at the joints noted.

The timing of the X-ray examination in bone disease is of great importance, and reference is made to this in the following sections.

Special techniques in orthopaedic radiology

Tomography

Tomography provides excellent demonstration of a bone lesion when this is imperfectly seen on plain films due to overlying bony structures. Applications include examination for a sequestrum (*see Figures 2.43 and 2.44*) and detailed assessment of localized spinal disease.

Myelography

Uses for myelography in orthopaedic conditions include estimation of the extent and direction of prolapse of an intervertebral disc, and determination of the precise level of an acute spinal block due to spinal disease when this information is not clear from plain radiographs. Myelography is discussed further on page 290.

Arthrography

Arthrography is undertaken to outline the non-opaque contents and capsule of a joint. For this purpose an injection is made into the joint of either a water-soluble iodine-containing contrast medium, or air (or oxygen), or a combination of the two. Specific applications for the procedure include examination for a non-opaque intra-articular loose body, assessment of tears in a joint capsule (when contrast medium will spread from the joint into the periarticular soft tissues), and demonstration of tears of the menisci and injuries of the cruciate ligaments of the knee. Arthrography is also carried out in children with failed or unstable reduction of a congenital hip dislocation: in either situation the examination may show soft tissues interposed between the femoral head and acetabulum that prevent satisfactory reduction.

Sinography

Reference to the use of this procedure in chronic infection is made on page 50.

Radioisotope bone scanning

This is described on page 11.

Assessment of skeletal age

Various methods have been devised for estimating skeletal development. One method in common use entails matching an X-ray of the patient's hand and wrist with a published series of illustrations of hand and wrist X-rays of normal male and female children ranging in age from the new-born to 18 years (*Radiographic Atlas of Skeletal Development of the Hand and Wrist*, Greulich and Pyle, Stanford University Press). Features such as the presence, size and shape of individual epiphyses are compared. If the patient's skeletal development is normal his or her radiograph will correspond with the illustration from a child of similar chronological age; if skeletal development is retarded the radiograph will resemble the illustration of a younger child. In the latter situation, follow-up films of the patient can be obtained to assess the effects of specific treatment on skeletal maturation.

Congenital dislocation of the hip

A dislocation may be suspected if the Ortolani 'click' is heard on routine testing of the baby soon after birth. The hips are flexed to a right angle, the knees are also flexed, and the legs are slowly abducted. If a dislocation is present a click is heard when the femoral head slips into the acetabulum. This sign may be positive even if a dislocation is not present, and a radiograph is thus indicated for further assessment. The baby should be radiographed with the legs abducted 45 degrees and internally rotated (Von Rosen's view). In a normal baby, a line drawn along the axis of the centre of the femoral shaft will extend through the acetabulum and cross the midline at the level of the lumbosacral junction. With a dislocated hip such a line will pass above the upper lip of the

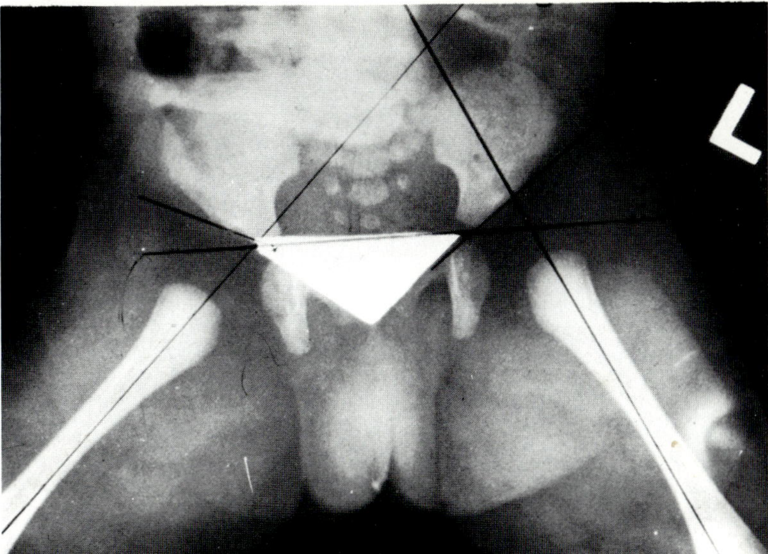

Figure 2.1. Dislocation of left hip (radiograph in Von Rosen's position—legs abducted 45 degrees and internally rotated). Acetabular angle on left side 45 degrees, on normal side 28 degrees. Shaft line crosses acetabulum and midline at L5 on right, much higher on left

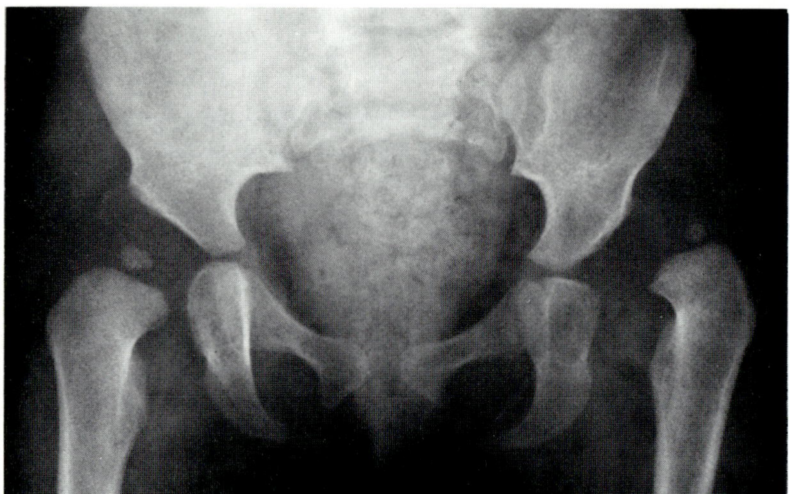

Figure 2.2. Congenital dislocation of the left hip in a baby of 18 months: retarded development of the epiphysis of the femoral head, proximal end of femur displaced upwards and outwards, shallow acetabulum

acetabulum and will cross the midline at a much higher level (*Figure 2.1*). In an older child (*Figure 2.2*) the ossific centre in the femoral head is smaller than normal, the proximal end of the femur is displaced upwards and outwards, and the acetabulum is shallow with a steeply sloping roof.

Further radiographs are taken after reduction to ensure that this is adequate, and later on to see that the reduction is maintained and that development of the femoral head and of the acetabular depression is proceeding satisfactorily.

Trauma

Fractures and dislocations: general principles

Indications for radiology

It is arguable whether all bones suspected of a fracture should be radiographed. For legal purposes this may be wise but for clinical purposes it is not always necessary. A fracture of the clavicle may be so obvious that a radiograph is not needed to prove it, while minor rib injuries are often treated by the same method whether the radiograph does or does not show a fracture. Similarly, the treatment of undisplaced fractures of the nasal bones or injuries of the coccyx or crush fractures of the terminal phalanges is symptomatic and is not influenced by radiological proof of fracture.

For most other regions of the skeleton, radiological demonstration of the presence and position of fractures is contributory to management. The question of skull radiographs in head trauma is discussed on pages 27–31.

Necessity for careful clinical localization

After trauma, whether severe or slight, careful clinical examination should always precede radiological investigation. It may be possible at the former to localize the position of the suspected fracture with some accuracy; or a second lesion may be found, to which the patient did not refer either because he was unconscious or because the pain of one fracture masked that of the other. If this information is acquired in advance it will be possible to produce the most appropriate radiographs with the minimum disturbance to the patient. For example, an X-ray request card on which is written '?fracture of the calcaneum' will be of more help to the radiologist and will lead to better results than one simply asking for 'X-ray of the foot'. Accuracy of clinical localization will often result in special views being taken, which will ensure accuracy in diagnosis.

Timing of X-ray examination

Some judgement is needed when deciding on timing. In many cases radiographs should be taken as soon as the clinical diagnosis has been made, so that the extent of the fractures and the position of the fragments can be shown and treatment started as soon as possible. In other cases, some postponement is indicated. Any urgent measures of resuscitation of shocked and other critically ill patients must, for example, take precedence over skeletal radiography.

After reduction and immobilization further radiographs should be taken (usually within 48 hours) to ensure that the position of the bones is satisfactory. If it is considered that immobilization may not be perfect—for instance, oedema may have subsided and a plaster case may thus have become loose—another radiological examination may be necessary about the end of the first week.

Need for care in examining radiographs

Much of the radiology in trauma work will be carried out in the trauma unit or casualty department without the immediate availability of a radiologist. All radiographs should be inspected under proper conditions with an adequate light from an X-ray viewing box, and when there is any doubt about the X-ray appearances the radiologist should be called in. In some cases further radiographs may be needed. It is sometimes difficult to decide in children whether there is displacement of an unfused epiphysis or other injury in the vicinity of a joint. Provided that the injury is unilateral, it is often most useful in this situation to X-ray the opposite side for comparison. At other times it may be helpful to refer to the skeleton or to the collection of anatomically normal radiographs that should be available in larger departments.

Radiographs should reveal the site and extent of the fracture and (provided that two views are taken at right angles to each other) the position of the fragments.

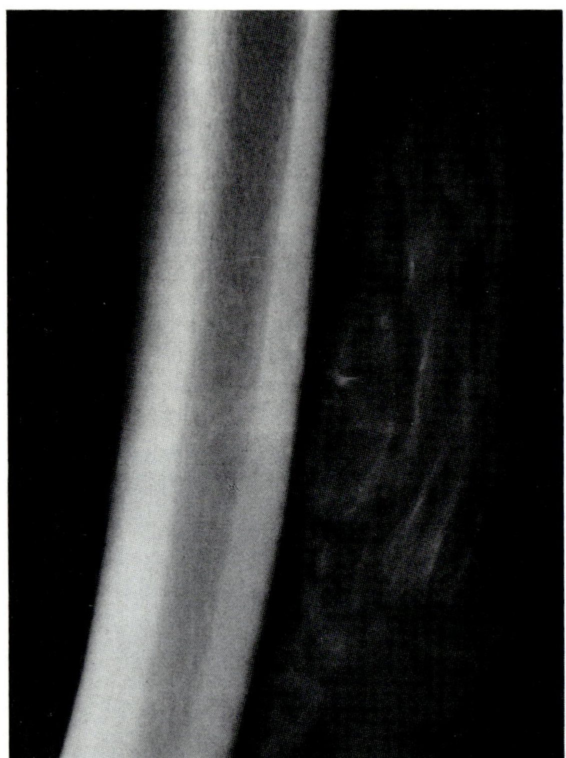

Figure 2.9. Calcified haematoma 3 weeks after an injury to the thigh. The more or less structureless calcification is seen anterior to the shaft of the femur; the latter is normal

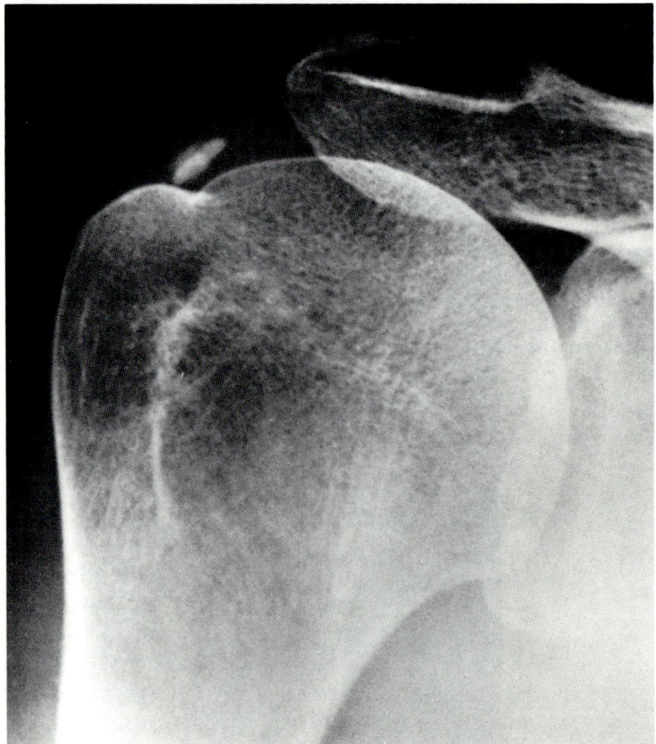

Figure 2.10. Calcification in the supraspinatus tendon in a patient aged 52. No history of injury, but complaint of pain in the shoulder for 3 months

does not develop bone structure may appear in the soft tissues about 2 weeks after an injury (*Figure 2.9*). Such a shadow is usually due to calcification in a haematoma either in or near a muscle, and not to true ectopic bone. It must not be mistaken for a neoplasm. Shrinkage will occur later.

Calcifications may also take place, with or without a previous history of gross trauma, in certain ligaments and tendons, and are often the source of pain. For instance, small opacities indicating calcareous deposits in the supraspinatus tendon may be seen just above the greater tuberosity of the humerus of a patient complaining of a painful shoulder joint (*Figure 2.10*). Another region occasionally affected is the medial ligament of the knee joint and the area just above and around it.

Some special fractures and dislocations

In many fractures the X-ray appearances are obvious and need no describing; but in others difficulties of detection or diagnosis constantly arise, and for this reason special reference is made to them in the following pages.

The vault and base of the skull

X-ray appearances

There are three main types of fracture of the vault and base of the skull: the fissure fracture, the wide gaping type of fracture, and the depressed fracture.

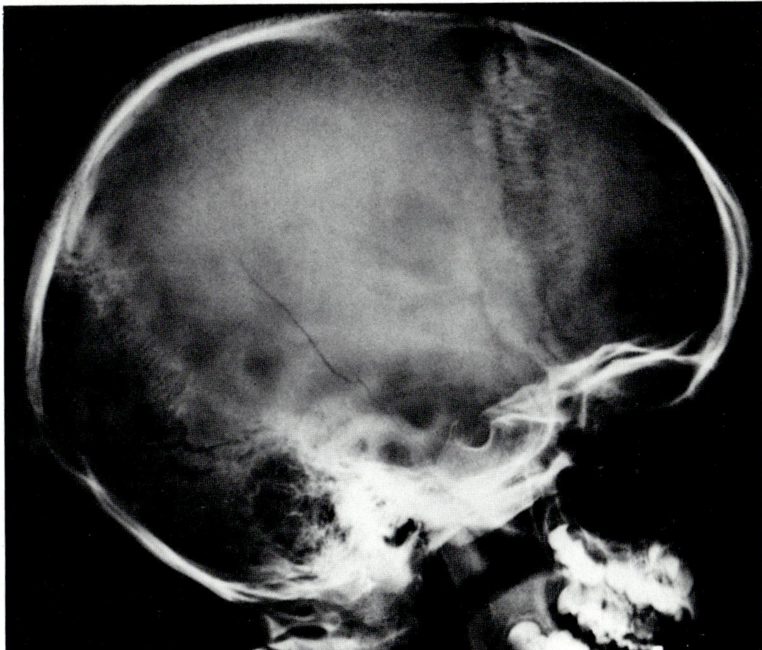

Figure 2.11. Fissure fracture in the parietal area of the skull. The narrow dark line is seen extending downwards and forwards to pass just anterior to the ear region

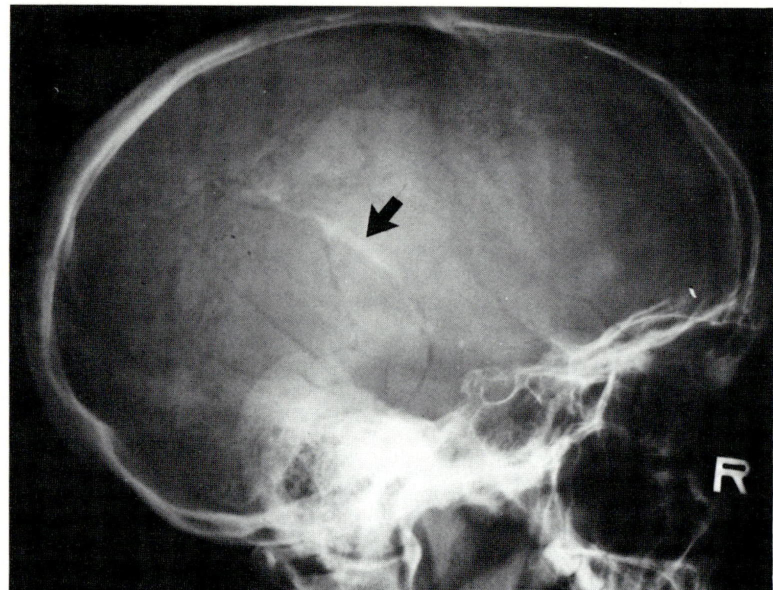

Figure 2.12. Depressed fracture of the skull (lateral view). Owing to slight overlap of the fragments, the fracture appears as a white line (arrow)

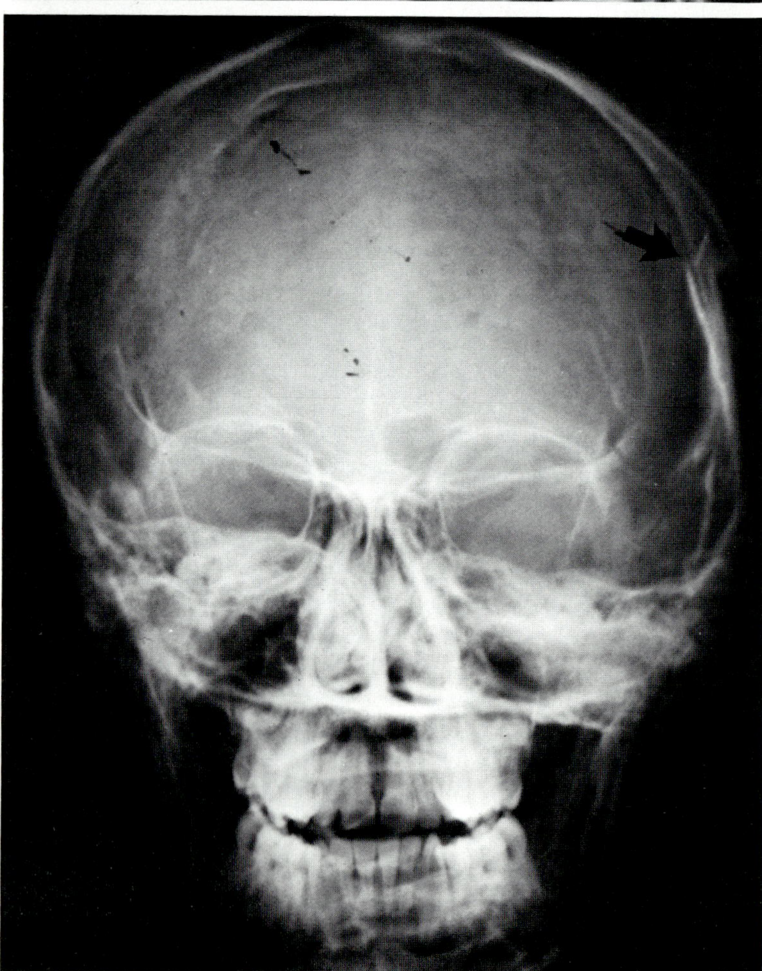

Figure 2.13. The same skull as in *Figure 2.12* (posterior view). The upper end of the depressed fragment is seen opposite arrow. Operative elevation and evacuation of the haematoma was undertaken and recovery followed.

The X-ray appearance of the fissure fracture is a narrow, dark line that can generally be distinguished from the normal vault markings by its position and direction and by the fact that it is not bilaterally symmetrical and is often confined to one side. It is usually clearer and better defined than a skull marking of the same size, and does not show the regular branching pattern of a vascular groove; and if the detail in the radiograph is sufficiently clear, the fracture will be seen to have no white dense bone along its margin. An example of a common parietal fissure fracture, extending down into the middle fossa or ear region, is shown in *Figure 2.11*.

The wide gaping type of fracture and the depressed fracture are usually obvious. In some, however, the fragments may overlap, and the consequent short white line of the superimposed bones (instead of a translucency) may easily be overlooked (*Figure 2.12*). The fracture and the depression may be obvious in a posterior (*Figure 2.13*) or tangential view. Sometimes the trauma causes a slight suture diastasis, particularly in a young person, and the trans-radiant zone of one of the sutures will appear unduly wide. This may be the only sign, or there may be a fissure fracture as well.

Value of radiology

In gross head injuries, radiographs are valuable in showing the extent of the fractures and the positions of the fragments. While

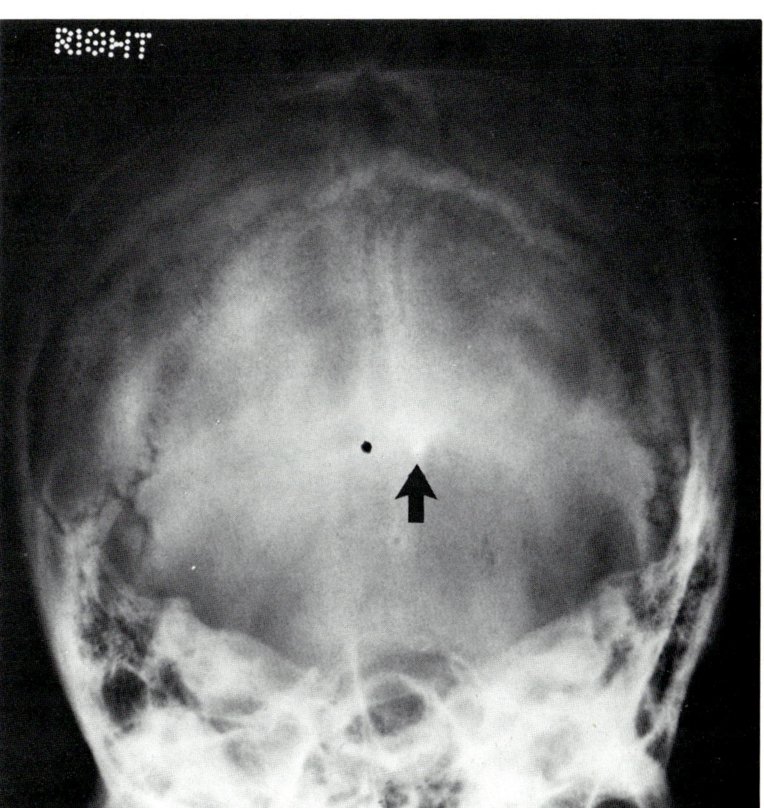

Figure 2.14. Subdural haematoma. Trauma to the skull, with loss of consciousness. Calcified pineal body (opposite arrow) is displaced to the left. The black dot marks the midline

severe cerebral damage is generally found in cases of multiple fracture, a patient can be deeply unconscious with gross neurological deficit after trauma without a fracture being present. Management of head injuries in general, therefore, depends on the clinical state of the patient rather than on the radiographic finding of fractures. However, the X-ray may show a depressed fracture requiring surgical replacement. The radiograph may also indicate a fracture at a site likely to cause haemorrhage or intracranial infection. When, for example, a fracture is found crossing the groove of the middle meningeal artery or one of its branches particular care must be taken to exclude an extradural haemorrhage; and when the fracture extends into the region of the sinuses, postnasal space or ear the possibility of direct spread of infection to the meninges and brain must be kept in mind.

If the pineal is seen to be calcified in the lateral view, attention should be paid to its position in the posterior view. If the symmetry of the two sides is relatively good, indicating that the radiograph was taken with the head straight and not rotated, then displacement of the calcified pineal by 3 mm or more from the midline (*Figure 2.14*) will be significant and may be the only positive evidence of a subdural haematoma requiring immediate surgery.

After the initial dangers have passed, the speed of rehabilitation must depend on the clinical findings and not on the X-ray appearances.

Timing of X-ray examination

In severe head injuries, early X-ray examination should be carried out. In less severe injuries—especially if the patient is restless and uncooperative, often from excessive alcohol—it is often wise to postpone the examination until after a period of clinical observation. It may then not even be necessary.

In trivial injuries without loss of consciousness at any time, radiography is often unnecessary. An exception perhaps is after trauma with a blunt instrument, such as a hammer, which may cause a depressed fracture without loss of consciousness. Many fractures can be shown only with a most careful radiographic technique, while with others special experience is needed for diagnosis—conditions that are not everywhere fulfilled, especially in night emergencies. It may therefore be better in some cases, where there does not appear to be any clinical urgency, to admit the patient for clinical observation and postpone the radiography for a short time until a skilled radiographer and a radiologist are available.

Necessity for clinical localization

Since special views are usually required to show fractures of the ear or facial regions, clinical localization of the lesion before the X-ray examination and provision of appropriate details on the X-ray request form are necessary. If a request is made only for an examination of the skull some special views will probably not be taken and the fracture may be missed, so that whenever clinical evidence, such as bleeding from one ear, makes localization possible, a special request should be made for radiographs of the suspected region.

The face and jaws

Facial bones

Radiological detection of fractures of the facial bones is important, since faciomaxillary surgery may be required to prevent persisting deformity or diplopia. The commonest fractures are those involving the nasal bones and zygoma. Since the latter is a rigid, tripod-shaped bone, fracture separation of one limb cannot occur on its own, and it is usual to find fractures affecting all three limbs. A typical case with fractures involving the roof and lateral wall of the antrum, the zygomatic arch, and the frontozygomatic synchondrosis is illustrated in *Figure 2.15*. Displacement can usually be judged

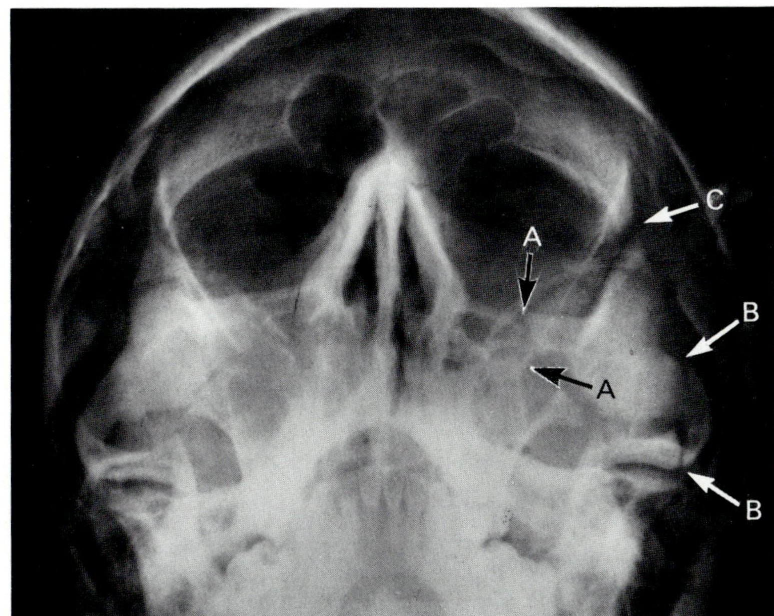

Figure 2.15. Typical tripod fracture of left zygoma. Fractures of (A) roof and lateral wall of antrum, (B) zygomatic arch, and (C) frontozygomatic synchondrosis are present. Fracture in left frontoethmoid region also. Lesser trauma on right side, with opaque antrum and fracture line

from the asymmetry of the two sides. The antrum on the affected side is often opaque, due to blood within it or to oedema of the sinus mucosa.

Blow-out fractures of the orbit are described and illustrated in Chapter 5.

Mandibular fractures

The mandible forms part of a bony ring, and—as in the case of other ring structures (the pelvis, the radius and ulna, and the zygoma)—a fracture separation at one point of the ring is exceptionally rare on its own; almost invariably there is a second fracture or a dislocation.

This second site of injury must therefore be carefully looked for when an obvious fracture is seen.

After reduction and fixation of fractures of the mandible, further radiographs are valuable in confirming that the position of the fragments is satisfactory. Union of a jaw fracture is often found to be firm on clinical examination many months before bony union can be demonstrated in the radiographs, so that radiology is of little value in assessing union.

Severe chest injuries

A radiograph of the chest should be taken as soon as is practicable after severe chest trauma. The chest may show localized or extensive opacification in the lungs (which may be due to lung contusion), a pneumothorax or haemothorax, widening of the mediastinum (due to a haematoma or aortic injury), or air within the mediastinum. If there is any suggestion of aortic injury an arch aortogram should be undertaken without delay (*see Figures 4.82 and 4.83*). The chest X-ray will also define the site and number of rib fractures and will show the extent of any flail segment. An apparent high diaphragm on one side may be due to diaphragmatic rupture: this is an occasional complication of crush injuries, and associated pelvic fractures are often present.

A chest radiograph should be taken if possible before initiating positive pressure respiration, since special care will be needed if air is seen within the pleura or mediastinum.

The vertebral column

Fractures and dislocations of the cervical spine

When a fracture of the cervical spine is suspected, the radiographer should always be warned not to move the patient's head during the

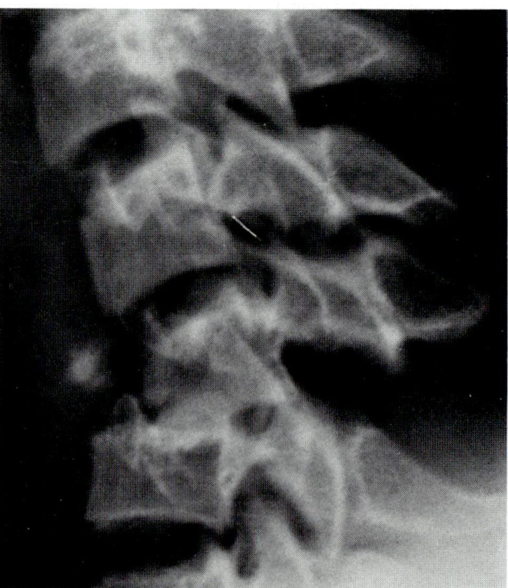

Figure 2.16. Fracture of the body of the fifth cervical vertebra. A small fragment of bone is detached anteriorly, and the body of the fifth cervical vertebra is displaced posteriorly in relation to the sixth

examination so that the danger of causing further injury to the cord can be minimized. If necessary, satisfactory radiographs can occasionally be obtained in the ward. Each vertebra must be carefully examined in turn, and note made of the alignment of the vertebrae. *Figure 2.16* shows an obvious fracture–dislocation involving the body of the fifth cervical vertebra. Special views may be required to demonstrate certain fractures, such as those involving the odontoid peg.

Fractures of the bodies of the vertebrae

A compression fracture often causes the affected vertebral body to be wedge shaped, the compression being most marked anteriorly. A break in the normally continuous white cortical margin is usually

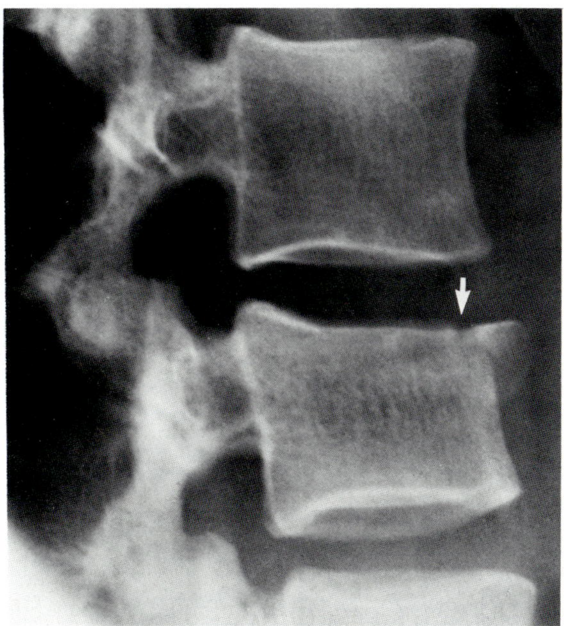

Figure 2.17. Fracture of the antero-superior aspect of the third lumbar vertebra. The small fragment is displaced slightly anteriorly, and a break in the white cortical line can be seen (arrow). There is no reduction of the disc space

clearly visible, and a small fragment, detached from the anterior aspect of the body, may be seen displaced anteriorly (*Figure 2.17*). Except in very severe compression injuries, the adjoining disc spaces are preserved.

Fractures of the transverse processes of the lumbar vertebrae

These are not treated, but the associated muscle trauma generally requires attention. If the outer fragments are seen to be displaced downwards by the pull of the psoas muscle the fracture will be obvious. Congenital non-fusion of the transverse process of the first lumbar vertebra may be mistaken for a fracture, but careful examination will show that the unfused segment has a layer of cortical bone all round it and is not displaced relative to the rest of the transverse process.

Value of radiology in fractures of the vertebrae

Radiographs are of value in substantiating the diagnosis of vertebral fracture. They will show the number of vertebrae involved, the positions of any detached fragments, the degree of compression of the vertebral body, and the displacement, if any, of the vertebrae relative to each other. They should be taken as soon as the patient's clinical state will permit his transport to the X-ray department. In some cases the treatment of haemorrhage, shock or associated injuries will take priority

Radiographs are often of little value in demonstrating the progress of any bone union in vertebral fractures. The fracture is frequently impacted, and during the earlier stages—even after union is firm from the clinical point of view—the narrowness of the fracture line, and the absence of obvious calcification in the callus, make it impossible to judge the degree of union from the X-ray appearances. The fracture line will no longer be visible once bone union is complete, which in adults often takes up to 3 months.

The fracture line will sometimes be more clearly demonstrated in a tomogram than in a routine radiograph, and tomography may be useful in diagnosing doubtful cases or in assessing the degree of union when there is doubt about this after clinical examination.

Fractures of the transverse or spinous processes rarely show any X-ray evidence of bone union, so that radiographs are not indicated for this purpose.

There is a tendency for marked bony lipping to occur between the edges of a fractured vertebra and the vertebrae above or below it. Such lipping is not usually manifest until 3 months after the injury.

The upper extremity

Dislocations of the shoulder

A subcoracoid dislocation of the shoulder is usually obvious both clinically and in the radiograph (*Figure 2.18*); the radiograph is useful chiefly to show the presence or absence of an associated fracture. Radiographs taken after treatment will show whether reduction is complete (*Figure 2.19*).

Elbow injuries in children

Elbow injuries are often difficult to diagnose on clinical examination because of the considerable oedema that commonly develops in the soft tissues around the elbow after trauma. Early diagnosis and reduction of any displacement, particularly of an epiphysis, is essential if future deformity or disability is to be avoided.

A knowledge of the normal positions and appearances of the epiphyses at the various ages of childhood is essential. As already mentioned, radiographs of the opposite side can often be most useful for comparison, provided that the elbow injury is unilateral. *Figures 2.20* and *2.21* show the ossified part of the epiphysis of the medial condyle displaced downwards and into the joint area. The fragment will appear larger on open operation than on the radiograph because of the presence of non-opaque cartilage around the bony nucleus.

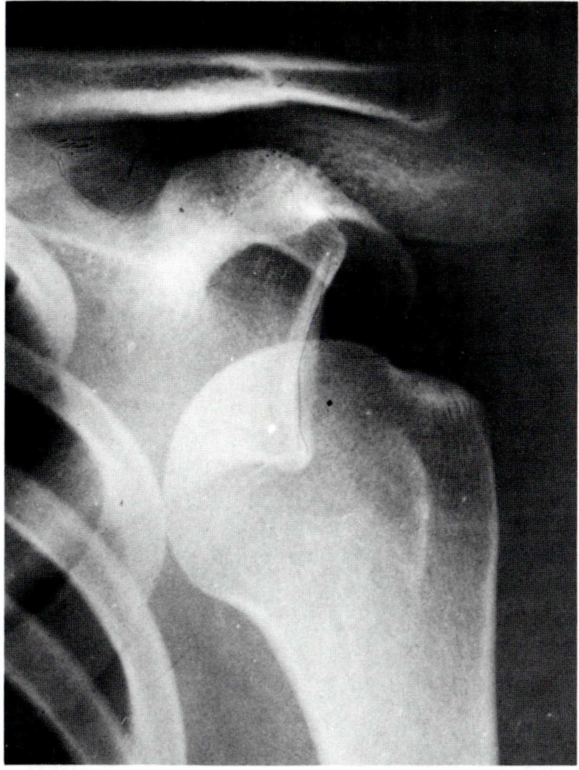

Figure 2.18. Subcoracoid dislocation of the humerus. The head is displaced downwards, and the medial edge is medial to the glenoid

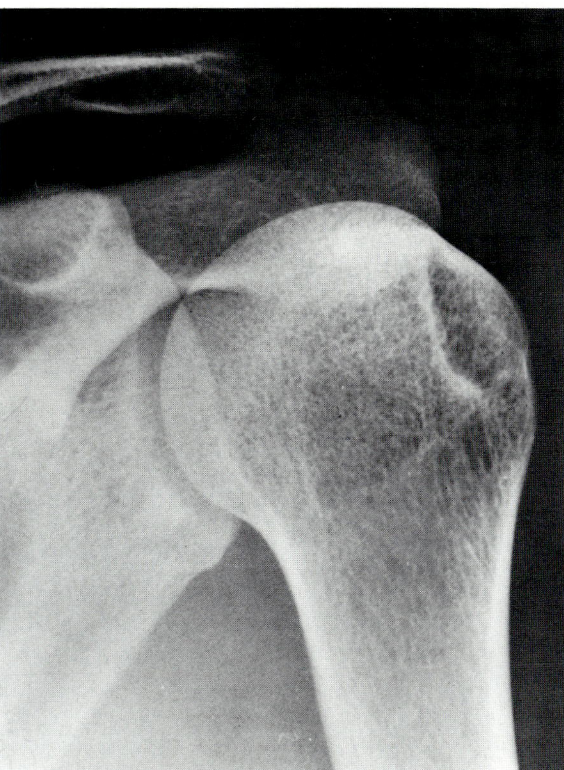

Figure 2.19. The same shoulder as in *Figure 2.18* after reduction. The medial margin of the head is now lateral to the most medial margin of the glenoid

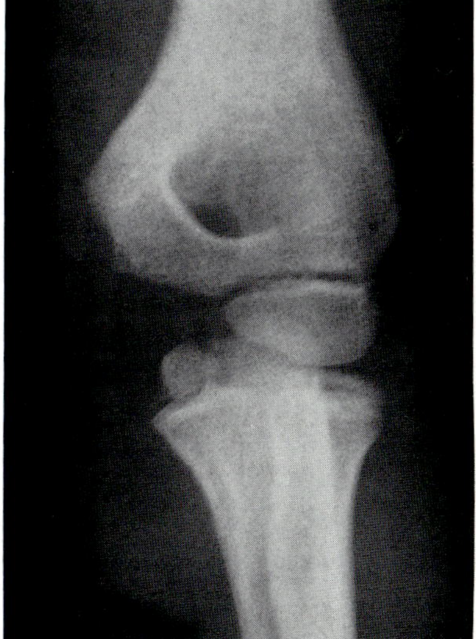

Figure 2.20. Elbow of a child aged 6 years (posterior view). As a result of an injury, the epiphysis of the medial condyle is displaced downwards into the joint and is seen lying just above the ulna

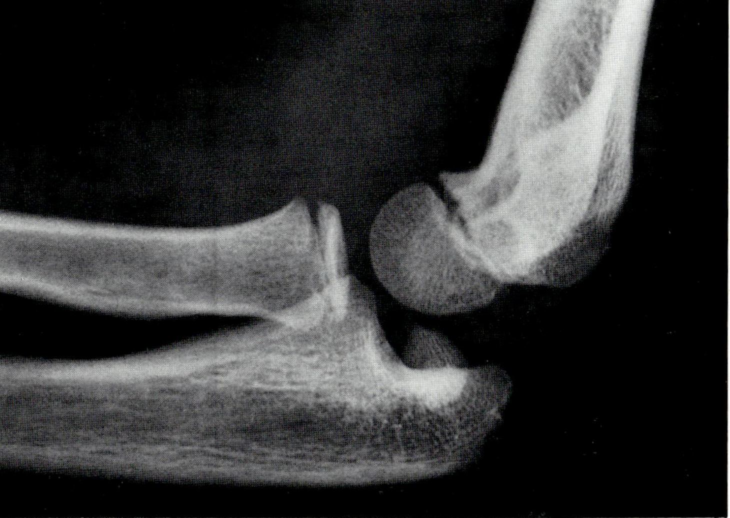

Figure 2.21. The same elbow as in *Figure 2.20* (lateral view). The epiphysis of the medial condyle is seen partly superimposed on the ulna and partly projecting anteriorly into the joint. The head of the radius is opposite the capitulum (normal)

Special attention should be paid to the position of the capitulum if the child is between 2 and 7 years old. If it becomes detached and rotated round and is not reduced, the future growth of the lower end of the humerus may be seriously impaired. In a lateral view the capitulum normally projects anteriorly one third of its thickness beyond the line of the anterior edge of the shaft of the humerus (*Figure 2.21*).

Figure 2.22 shows the classic fracture of the upper third of the shaft of the ulna, with associated forward dislocation of the proximal end of the radius relative to the capitulum. This can be appreciated by comparing *Figure 2.22* with *Figure 2.21*, where the head of the radius is in its normal position opposite the capitulum. It is important not to miss this lesion, since early reduction is easy and satisfactory while late reduction is often the reverse. Try eating, cleaning your teeth, tying your tie and so on without flexing your right elbow more than 90 degrees, which will correspond to the disability if the dislocated radius is untreated.

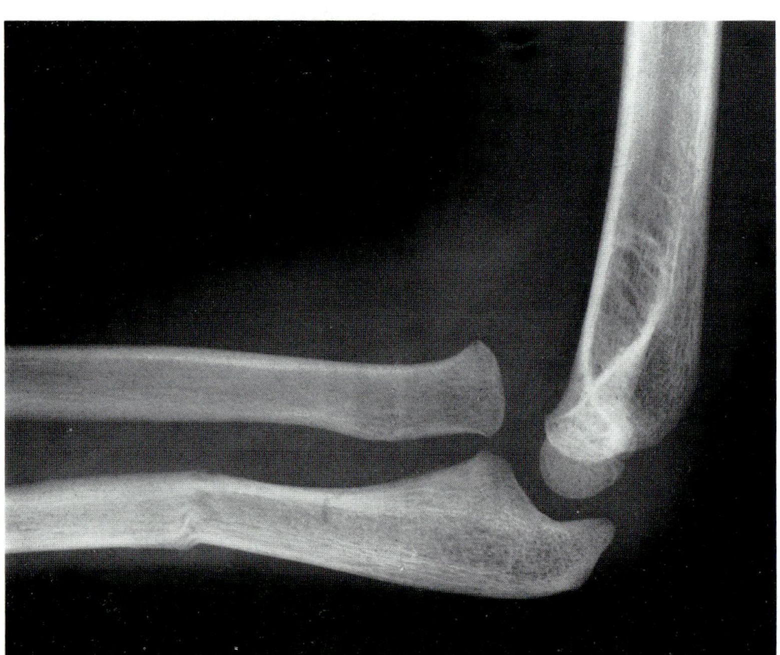

Figure 2.22. Fracture of the shaft of the ulna with forward dislocation of the radius in relation to the capitulum. Flexion was limited to 90 degrees, movement of the head of the radius beyond this being checked by the shaft of the humerus

Another common fracture is the supracondylar fracture with backward displacement of the lower fragment. Again, unless this is reduced, flexion of the elbow will be restricted.

In a fracture of the shaft of the radius with shortening, the posterior and lateral-view radiographs should include the elbow and wrist joints. This is important, since shortening of the radius on its own is anatomically impossible and must be accompanied by either an ulnar fracture or a dislocation at the wrist or elbow.

Elbow injuries in adults

A fissure fracture of the head of the radius (*Figure 2.23*) may be missed radiologically because the patient is often unable to extend

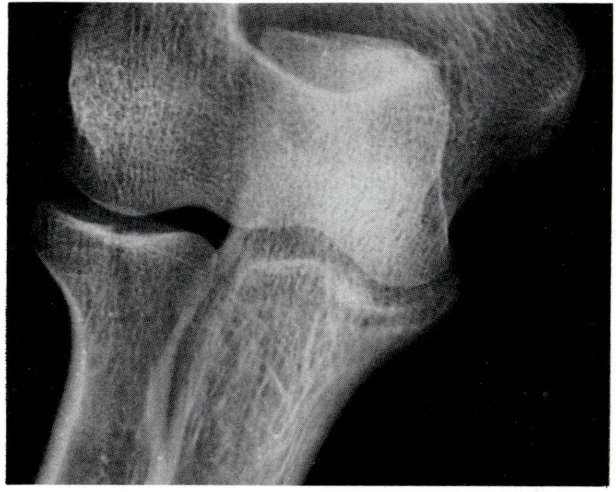

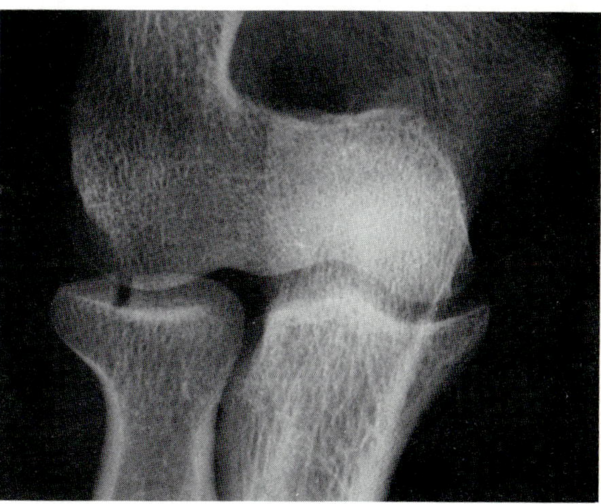

Figure 2.23. Fracture of the head of the radius, poorly shown because the elbow was partly flexed and the head of the radius was not parallel with the film

Figure 2.24. The same elbow as in *Figure 2.23*. The fracture is more clearly shown because the radius is now parallel with the film. The humerus could not be fully extended because of the pain

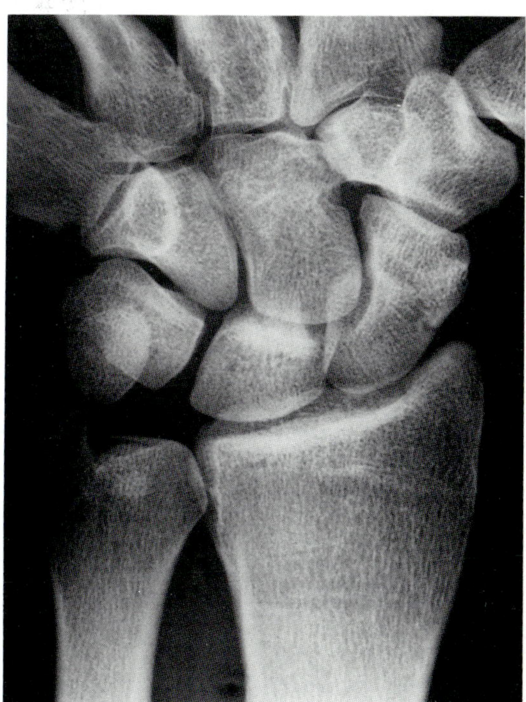

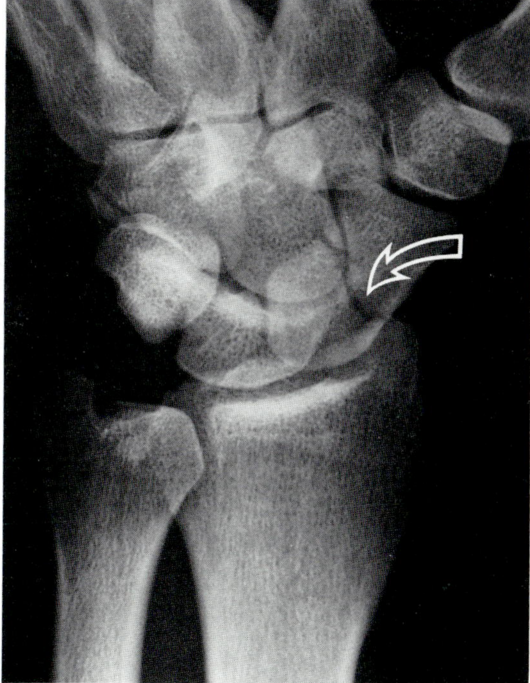

Figure 2.25. Fracture of the body of the scaphoid (anterior view)

Figure 2.26. Oblique view of the same wrist, in which the dark line of the fracture is more clearly seen (arrow)

his elbow fully. Localized tenderness and pain on movements of pronation and supination should suggest this lesion, and special views can then be taken with the radius parallel with the film (*Figure 2.24*).

Wrist injuries

In a fracture of the scaphoid there is often localized tenderness over the bone in the region of the 'anatomical snuff box' to suggest the diagnosis. The fracture may be invisible in the anterior or lateral view (*Figure 2.25*), but clearly seen in an oblique view (*Figure 2.26*) or in an anterior view taken with the wrist in ulnar deviation. The words 'wrist injury' on the X-ray request form will therefore be insufficient, and a careful survey of the carpal area—particularly the scaphoid—must be requested.

If no fracture can be seen but the symptoms and signs of a fracture of the scaphoid persist, further radiographs should be taken a fortnight later. Slight decalcification around the fracture line may render the fracture easier to see after this interval. The proof or exclusion of a fracture is important because unless a fracture is immobilized completely for a long period, non-union is likely, leaving a weak and painful wrist.

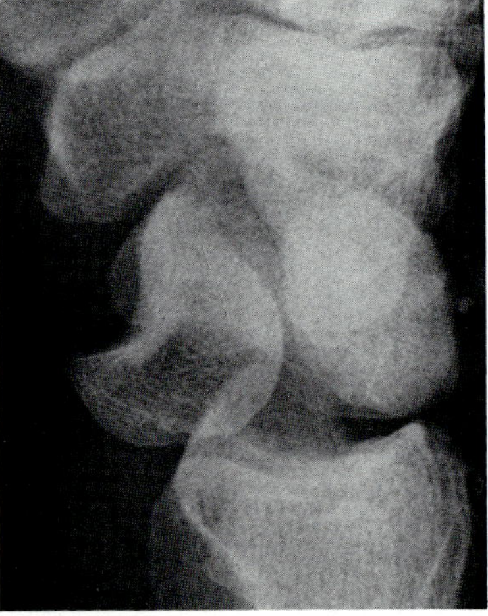

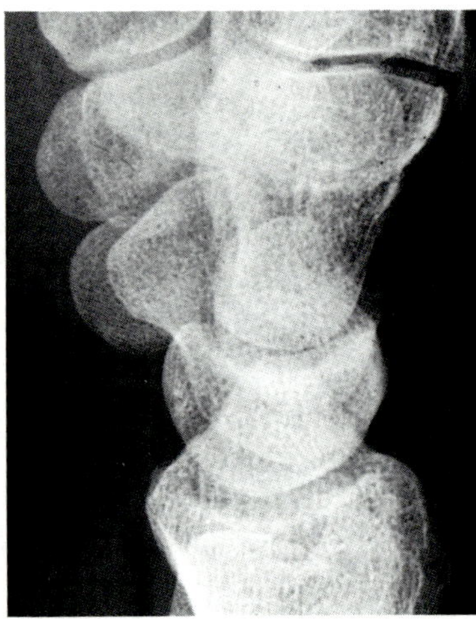

Figure 2.27. Dislocation of the lunate (lateral view). The bone has been rotated so that the distal semilunar surface points anteriorly, and the capitate is displaced proximally

Figure 2.28. Normal wrist. The distal semilunar surface articulates with the proximal end of the capitate

Figure 2.27 shows a dislocation of the lunate, with its concave distal end facing almost anteriorly instead of articulating with the capitate. *Figure 2.28* shows the normal relationship of the bones. Early X-ray diagnosis within 24 hours of the injury should lead to reduction and a successful outcome; late diagnosis may prevent manipulative reduction and lead to a weak and painful wrist that may necessitate later removal of the bone.

A small chip off the dorsum of the cuneiform (*Figure 2.29*) is

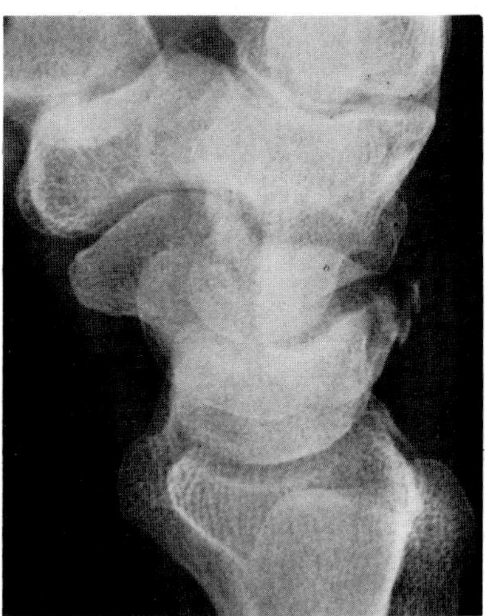

Figure 2.29. A chip off the dorsum of the cuneiform (triquetral)

usually an indication for more rigid immobilization than if the patient were being treated for a sprain.

Finger injuries

A chip off the base of the dorsum of a phalanx indicates a severe tear of the extensor tendon, treatment of which is often unsatisfactory.

The lower extremity

In the hip region, transcervical and transtrochanteric fractures are sometimes difficult to see in radiographs unless there is displacement of the bones. In transcervical fractures, a lateral view may help in diagnosis and is invaluable in judging the position of the fragments.

In the knee area a fracture through the base of the tibial spine, and a depressed fracture of the lateral half of the upper tibial articular surface (*Figure 2.30*), may be easily missed unless the radiographs are examined carefully.

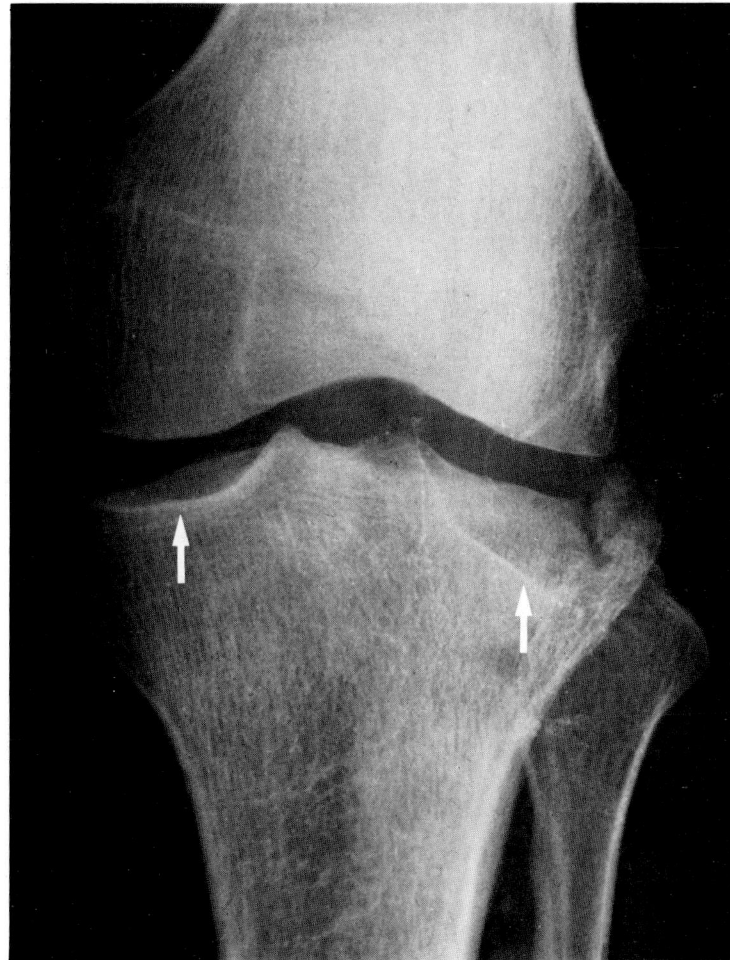

Figure 2.30. Fracture of the lateral half of the upper tibial articular surface, with depression of the fragments. In order to judge the displacement, the level of the lower thin white line of articular cortex should be compared with the line on the medial half (arrows)

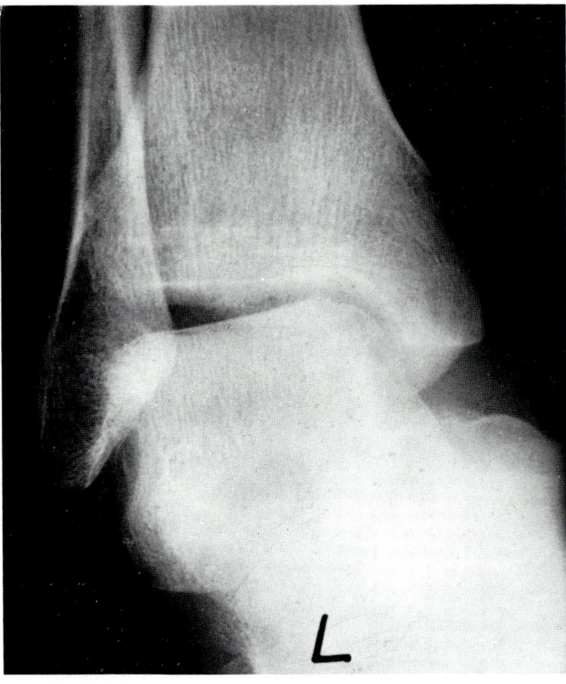
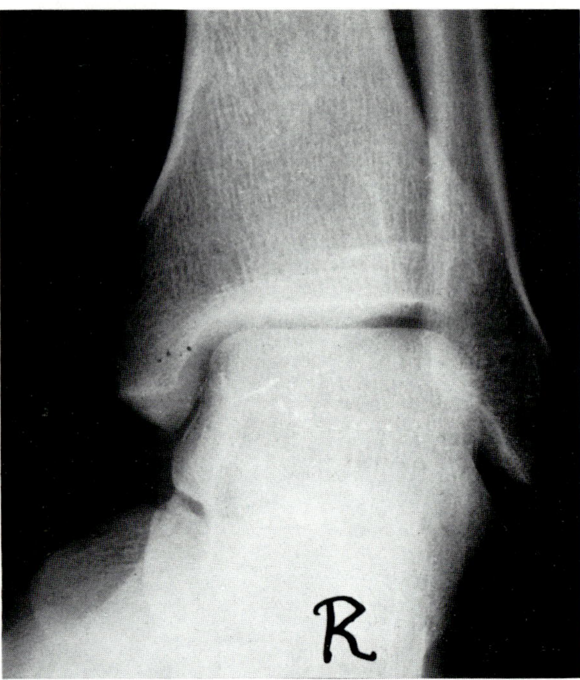

Figure 2.31. Abnormal mobility of the talus on the injured left side. This is demonstrated by holding the feet forcibly inverted, but not to such an extent as to cause pain

In the ankle area a small chip of bone detached from the lower end of the fibula, or from the dorsal aspect of the talus, will indicate considerable ligamentous damage and should therefore be carefully searched for in the radiographs. Should the lateral ligament be severely damaged, there may be an abnormal medial mobility of the talus, which can be demonstrated in a posterior view of the ankle taken with the foot forcibly inverted (*Figure 2.31*). As this is not a routine procedure it will be undertaken only if the radiologist is warned of the possibility of such a lesion.

Stress fractures

Some fractures occur without any traumatic incident and are caused by repeated, minor stresses on the affected part of the skeleton. The patient experiences pain but often defers seeking medical attention for a few weeks as the pain is not severe. Radiographs show a linear crack in the bone. There is virtually never any displacement. Evidence of healing, with callus formation and well-organized periosteal reaction, is sometimes well established by the time of the initial radiological investigation (*Figure 2.32*).

Common sites to be affected are the necks of the second, third and fourth metatarsals ('march fractures', seen particularly in soldiers after marching or foot stamping on a parade ground); the tibial shaft (in athletes and ballet dancers); the lower ribs ('cough fractures' arising from a bout of coughing); and the pars interarticularis of one of the lower lumbar vertebral arches. Crack fractures of

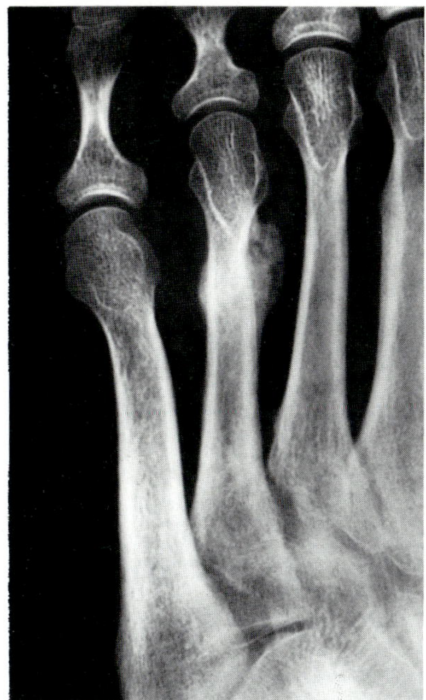

Figure 2.32. March fracture of the fourth metatarsal: highly calcified callus and a small crack. There was no history of injury; pain had been felt in the foot for 3 weeks

Figure 2.33. Spondylolisthesis. Forward slipping of L5 on S1. The defect in the neural arch, which has disrupted the normal hook-like stabilizing action of the arch, is clearly seen (arrow)

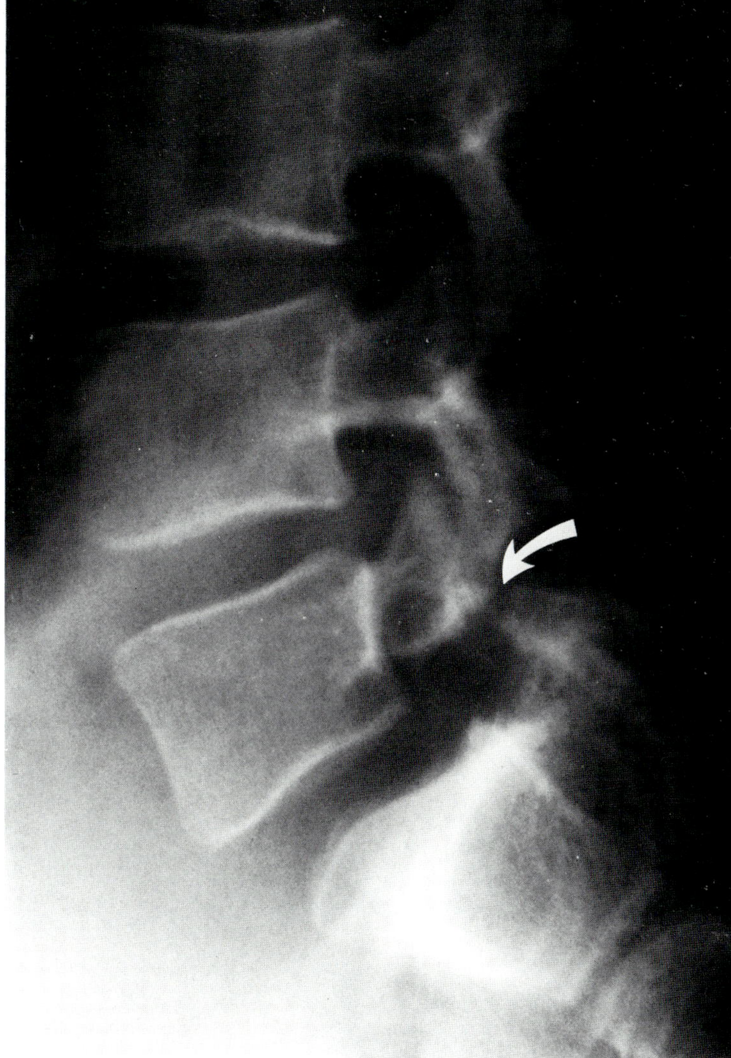

the pars interarticularis give rise to the condition known as spondylolysis, manifest clinically by mild, persisting low-back pain. Unlike stress fractures occurring at other sites there is a tendency for these fractures to remain ununited. Pars interarticularis defects are sometimes visible on standard anteroposterior (AP) and lateral views of the lumbar spine, but at other times oblique views are required for their demonstration.

In the normal individual the hook-like action of the posterior articular joints of the spine withstands the tendency for forward subluxation of one vertebra on the vertebra below. When fractures of the pars interarticularis develop, this stabilizing mechanism is lost, and with repeated stresses on the spine the fractured vertebra may slide forwards on its neighbour immediately below and give rise to the condition of spondylolisthesis (*Figure 2.33*).

Avascular necrosis of bone

Deprivation of blood supply to an area of bone results in bone death—avascular necrosis. The cause of the ischaemia is often obvious: trauma causes laceration and disruption of supplying vessels; radiotherapy kills osteocytes and damages blood vessels; too rapid decompression of deep-sea divers results in bone infarction due to release of bubbles of nitrogen from the bone marrow into the circulation (Caisson disease). In the group of conditions described in this section under 'Osteochondritis' the factor responsible for the ischaemia is at times less certain. In at least some of these conditions trauma is responsible for the disruption of the blood supply leading to bone necrosis. Whether trauma is the causative factor in all cases, it is important to remember that sterile avascular bone necrosis is the feature common to all of these conditions: despite the implication of the word osteochondritis, there is no infective or other inflammatory component.

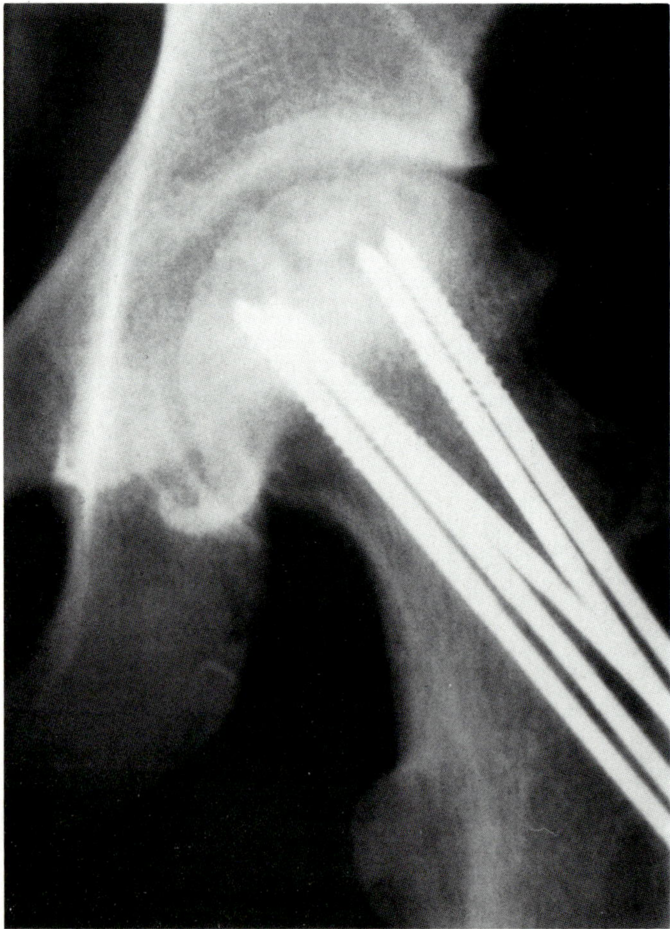

Figure 2.34. Post-traumatic avascular necrosis of head of femur. Dense femoral head with areas of demineralization. Some irregularity of articular surface due to crumbling. Previous screw fixation of femoral neck fracture

Post-traumatic bone necrosis

There are three sites at which post-traumatic avascular necrosis is particularly likely to occur: the head of the femur after a fracture of the neck, the proximal fragment of the scaphoid after a fracture of the body or waist of the bone (*Figure 2.34*), and the body of the talus after a vertical fracture through the middle of this bone. Radiological changes are not immediately apparent, since entirely devascularized bone undergoes neither resorption nor sclerosis. However, if a fracture is treated by immobilization in plaster, some disuse osteoporosis is usually visible in the fractured and surrounding bones after an interval of several weeks. In these circumstances a site of avascular necrosis will be indicated by the relatively greater density of the avascular segment, which does not undergo osteoporosis. This feature is not usually apparent for 1–3 months after the injury. Later, some true increase in density may occur due to crumbling and condensation of the dead fragment.

Some months after the injury, new vessels may grow into the dead bone. This process of revascularization produces patchy areas of demineralization where the dead bone is resorbed, and areas of sclerosis where new bone is laid down on top of the scaffolding of dead trabeculae.

Osteochondritis

Osteochondritis of the femoral head epiphysis (Perthes' disease)

The clinical onset of osteochondritis of the hip is insidious and may occur in a child as young as 3 years but is most common between the ages of 5 and 10. The child feels slight pain in the hip or limps when walking.

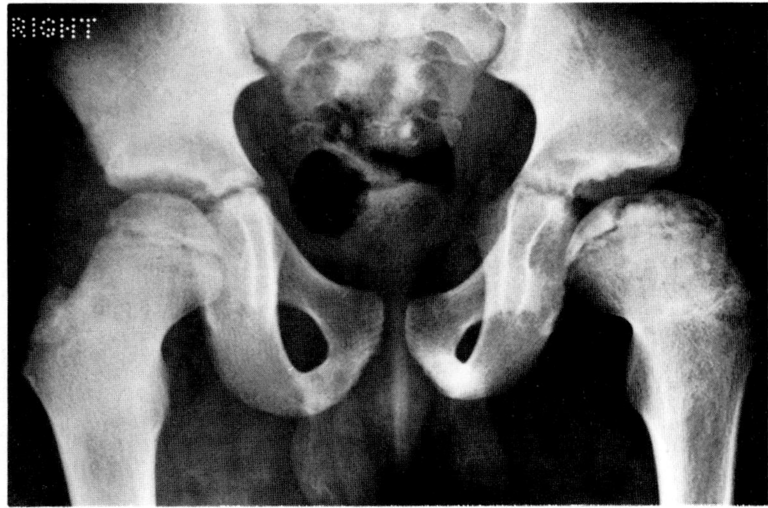

Figure 2.35. Perthes' disease (osteochondritis) of the left hip in a boy aged 7 years: the joint space is wide; the epiphysis of the femoral head is fragmented and shows subarticular lytic areas together with areas of increased density; the head is displaced laterally; the femoral neck is short and wide. There is slight irregularity of the acetabulum secondary to the femoral head changes

The X-ray changes are usually apparent by the time the symptoms develop but they may be delayed for about a month. The joint space is normal or slightly increased, and the epiphysis of the femoral head is flattened, irregular and fragmented. The femoral neck may be short and wide, while the calcium content and trabecular structure of the adjacent bone appears normal (*Figure 2.35*). These changes are in direct contrast to those visible in tuberculosis (*see* page 58). The condition is usually unilateral and, when this is so, the appearances of the normal hip act as a useful control during examination of the affected one.

A radiograph is of value in the initial diagnosis, and serial radiographs are useful in following the progress of the lesion. The first follow-up radiograph should be taken about 3 months after the preliminary one. The fragmentation of the femoral head becomes less marked in due course, and eventually the bone structure returns to normal—although the head usually remains flatter, and the neck wider, than normal. Residual deformity of the femoral head, which predisposes to osteoarthritis, is less likely to occur if the lesion is discovered early and the limb rested from weight bearing until healing is complete.

Osteochondritis of the tibial tuberosity (Osgood–Schlatter's disease)

Fragmentation and separation of the epiphysis of the tibial tuberosity (*Figure 2.36*) in Osgood–Schlatter's disease may be associated with pain. Some overlying soft-tissue swelling is to be expected. The age of onset is later than in Perthes' disease of the hip, being between 12 and 16 years, while the course is more rapid and healing may be complete within a few months. Trauma is usually a causative factor.

Osteochondritis of the navicular (Köhler's disease)

This disease is seen in children between the ages of 3 and 7 years. The child may complain of slight pain in the foot, although

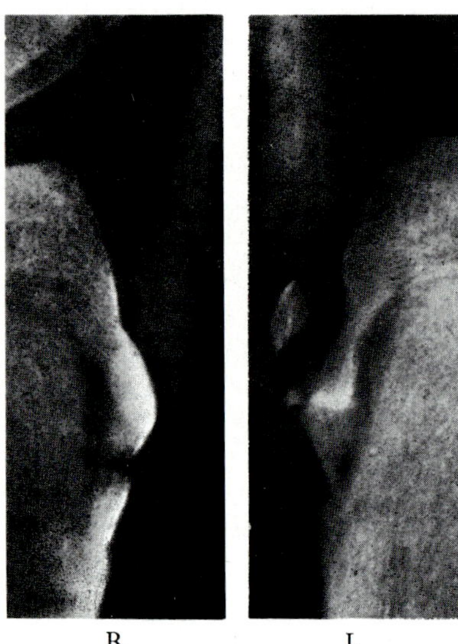

Figure 2.36. Osteochondritis of tibial tuberosity (Osgood–Schlatter's disease) in a female aged 12 years. The left knee epiphysis is displaced forwards and fragmented; the right is normal. There was slight pain on the left; recovery was rapid

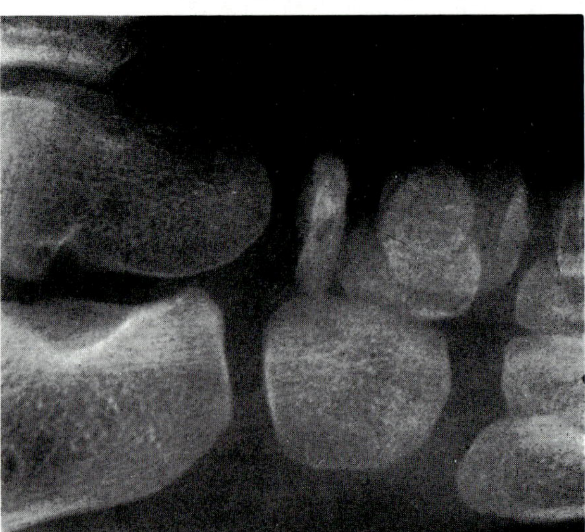

Figure 2.37. Osteochondritis of navicular (Köhler's disease) in a male aged 5 years. There is fragmentation and flattening of the navicular bone with a wide joint space. There was very slight pain in the foot

occasionally the condition is found accidentally when the foot has been radiographed for some other reason. Radiographs show a variable degree of fragmentation and patchy increase in density of the navicular. The joint spaces are not decreased and the surrounding bones show no decalcification (*Figure 2.37*). Healing usually takes place in a few months and when this is complete there is no residual deformity.

Osteochondritis of the head of the second metatarsal

This may cause slight pain in the foot. The metatarsal head is flattened and fragmented and the neck widened, while the joint space is either normal or widened. A small, separated piece of bone is often seen in the affected area. The pain and fragmentation disappear rapidly, but irregularity of the articular surface may persist, predisposing to osteoarthritis. The heads of the third and fourth metatarsals and the base of the first metatarsal are sometimes the sites of similar changes.

Osteochondritis of the lunate (Kienböck's disease)

Pain in the wrist is sometimes due to osteochondritis of the lunate. In a radiograph, the bone appears dense and fragmented and sometimes smaller than normal because of compression; the joint spaces are normal (*Figure 2.38*). The lesion is usually seen in young adults but may occur in older people. There is often, but not always, a history of recent trauma to the wrist.

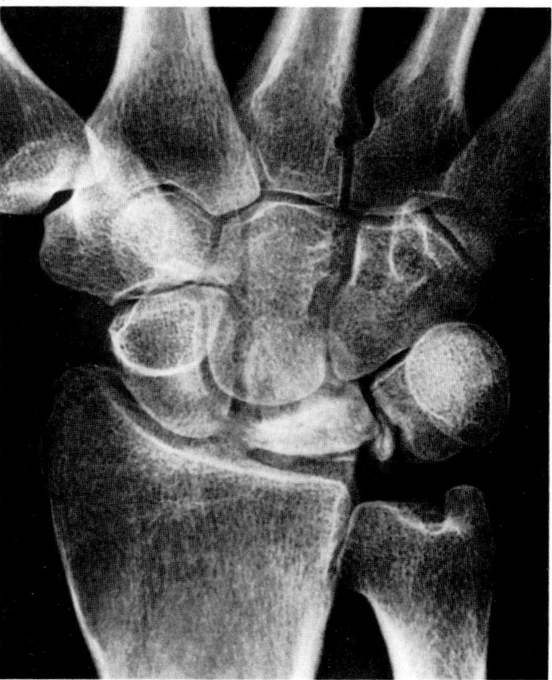

Figure 2.38. Osteochondritis of the lunate: the lunate is dense and fragmented, and the joint spaces are normal. There was no history of injury; slight pain was felt in the wrist for 6 weeks

Osteochondritis of the thoracic spine (juvenile osteochondritis)

This disease occurs in young people between the ages of 10 and 20. There may be some pain in the back, or scoliosis and kyphosis. The exact pathology of the lesion is uncertain. The abnormality may be confined to one disc or vertebra or it may be seen in several, the affected ones often being separated by apparently normal discs and vertebrae. The dorsal spine and the upper lumbar region are most commonly affected.

Four types of X-ray changes are seen, either singly or in combination, the severity of each varying from case to case.

1. Local defects and some irregularity of the superior or inferior angle of the vertebral body (*Figure 2.39*).

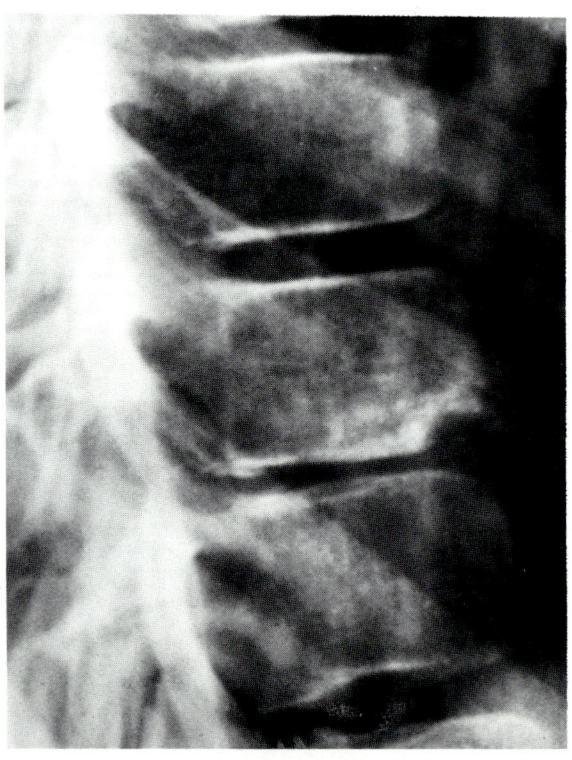

Figure 2.39. Osteochondritis of the thoracic spine in a girl aged 11. Narrow disc space; erosion of the anteroinferior aspect of the body of the affected vertebra; no shadow to suggest an abscess. Slight pain but no physical signs. Lesion healed after many months

2. A diminished disc space. Sometimes the X-ray appearances indicate herniation of the disc into the vertebral body. This is seen as a well-defined defect with a sclerotic margin within the substance of the vertebral body. At other times the cause of the diminished disc space is not apparent.
3. Fragmentation of the epiphyseal ring.
4. A slight degree of wedge-shaped collapse of the vertebral body. This is a relatively late change.

Minor manifestations of these lesions are commonly seen in radiographs of the lower dorsal spine in patients with no symptoms. The more severe changes, such as those shown in *Figure 2.39*, are usually associated with symptoms and thus represent a true patholo-gical entity. After a long period during which the X-ray appearances remain unchanged, healing gradually takes place, usually leaving some residual wedge-shaped deformity of the vertebral body.

The combined appearance of a narrow disc space and erosion of the vertebral end-plate (*Figure 2.39*) is difficult to distinguish from the changes of tuberculosis in the early stages. The non-progressive nature of the lesion, the paucity of signs or symptoms, and the absence of a paravertebral abscess usually ensure the correct diagnosis after a period of observation.

Osteochondritis dissecans

In this condition a small fracture forms on the convex articular surface of one of the joints, and the small fragment so produced may become separated to lie within the joint. The sites most commonly affected are the medial femoral condyle, the proximal articular surface of the talus, the capitellum of the lower end of the humerus, and the head of the first metatarsal. The condition occurs particular-ly in young adults, is commoner in males than in females, and a history of trauma can often be elicited.

By the time symptoms of pain are present bone changes are usually visible on X-ray examination. A well-defined semilunar area of erosion, about 5–10 mm in size, is seen on the articular surface of the bone (*Figure 2.40*). The fragment so separated may still be in position (*Figure 2.40*), or it may be seen lying loose within the joint. This condition is the commonest cause of an intra-articular loose body, which may produce intermittent locking of the joint and predispose to the development of secondary osteoarthritic changes.

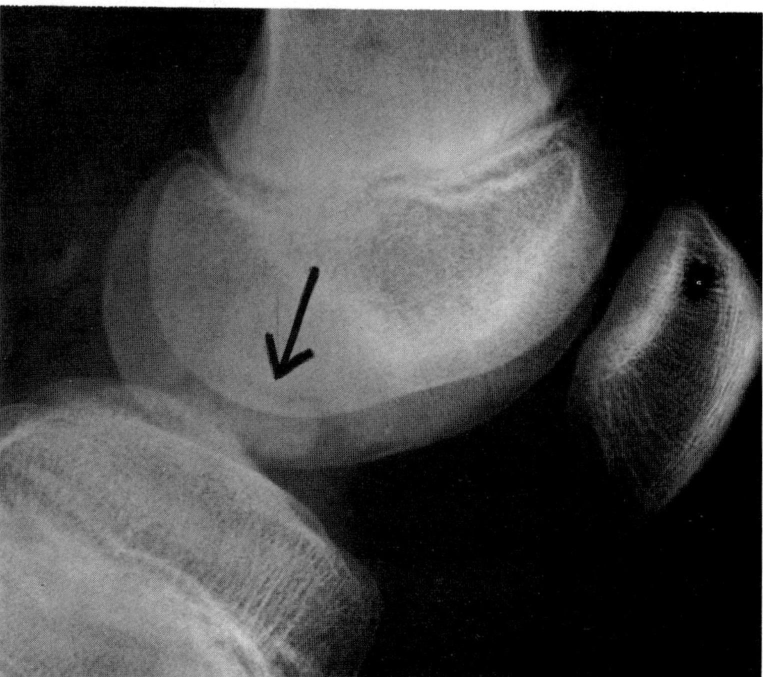

Figure 2.40. Osteochondritis dissecans of the lower end of the femur in a boy aged 12: the arrow points to a curved fracture line, separating off a fragment of the ar-ticular portion of the femoral condyle. There was a history of pain in the knee for 12 weeks

Slipped upper femoral epiphysis (adolescent coxa vara)

In young people between the ages of 12 and 17 years, separation of the head from the neck of the femur may occur during normal use of the limb. Clinically the onset is insidious, with slight pain in the hip or knee and a slight limp. On examination some limitation of movement may be found, especially of internal rotation. The condition is commoner in males, and there is a tendency for overweight boys to be affected.

On X-ray examination, the head of the femur is seen to be displaced medially and posteriorly in relation to the neck. In the early stages the displacement is slight, and may be visible only in a lateral view. (It should be remembered that in the lateral view the trochanters lie partly posterior to the neck and proximal shaft of the femur, and displacement of the femoral head therefore occurs to the side of the trochanters (*Figure 2.42*)).

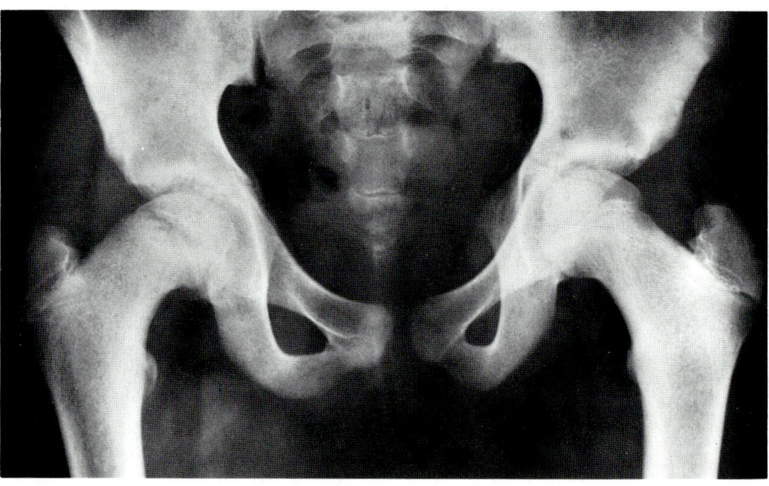

Figure 2.41. Slipped right femoral epiphysis in a girl aged 13. The head is rotated medially in relation to the neck. The epiphyseal plate is widened (translucency between head and neck) due to separation. There was no history of trauma, but 3 weeks' fairly severe pain and limping

On the anteroposterior view, medial displacement of the femoral head is sometimes evident when comparison is made with the opposite side. In about one third of cases, however, the condition is bilateral. Displacement of the head may be apparent if a line is drawn on the radiograph continuing the lateral border of the femoral neck proximally. This line should normally intersect the lateral part of the head, but if the epiphysis is displaced it may fail to do so. This is obvious in the case illustrated in *Figure 2.41*.

Radiographs are not only useful in diagnosis; by showing the amount of displacement of the head on the neck, they are also useful when a decision is being made on whether manipulative reduction is necessary. Reduction seems to increase the risk of avascular necrosis of the head and is therefore better avoided if the displacement is slight. Where operative fixation with threaded wires or screws is undertaken, serial radiographs are indicated from time to time to

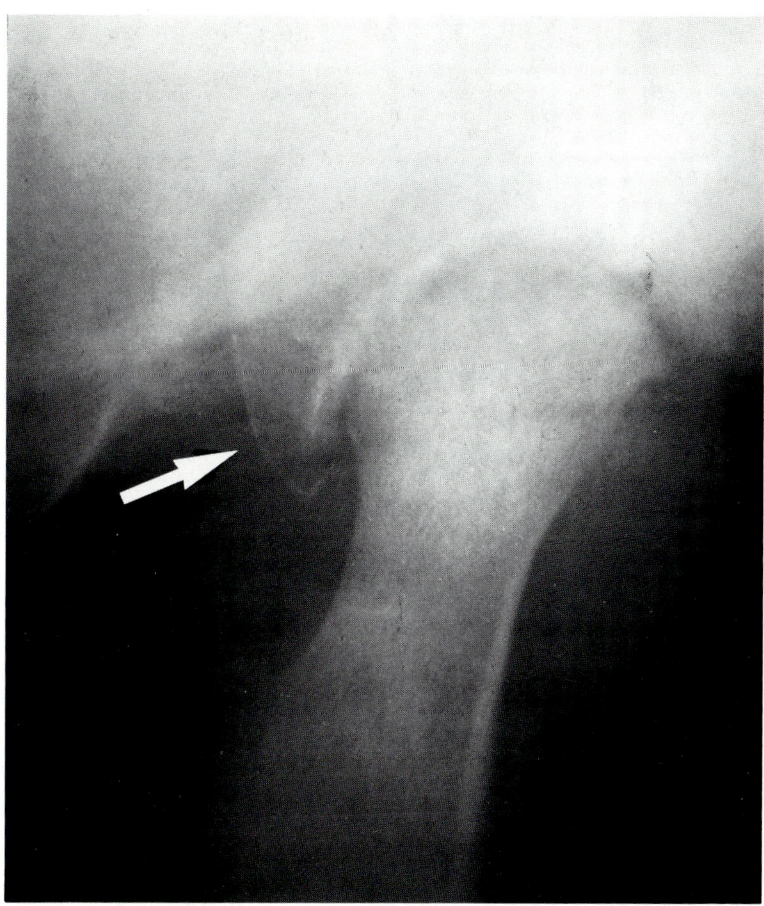

Figure 2.42. The same hip as in *Figure 2.41*, lateral view. The head is rotated posteriorly in relation to the neck. The arrow points to the posteroinferior part of the epiphysis

show whether the position has been maintained. This is important, since persisting deformity predisposes to osteoarthritis in later life.

Infection of a bone or joint

Acute osteomyelitis

Indications for radiology

Acute osteomyelitis usually presents with pain, fever, leucocytosis, and local swelling and tenderness.

A bone may become infected through the blood-stream, or directly as a result of missile wounds, compound fractures, or local spread from nearby inflammation. The metaphysis is the usual site of involvement in haematogenous infection. In children the epiphyseal cartilage plate acts as a barrier to the spread of infection (*see Figure 2.46*), so that it is unusual for septic arthritis to complicate osteomyelitis except in those regions in which the metaphysis lies

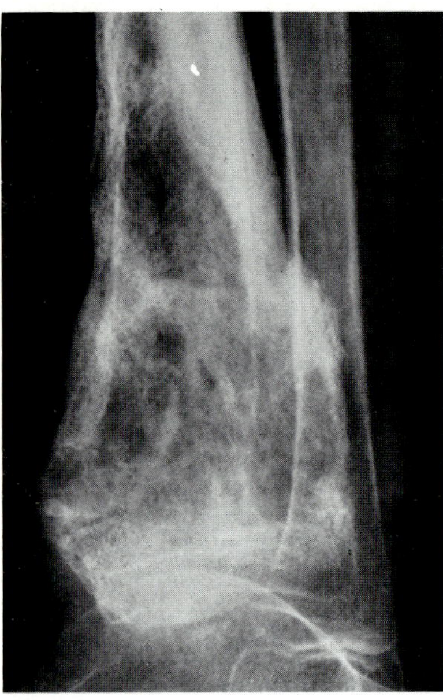

Figure 2.43. Plain radiograph of the tibia in a case of osteomyelitis of 5 weeks' duration. The bone destruction and periosteal new bone formation are clearly seen. The presence of a sequestrum is suggested but difficult to prove

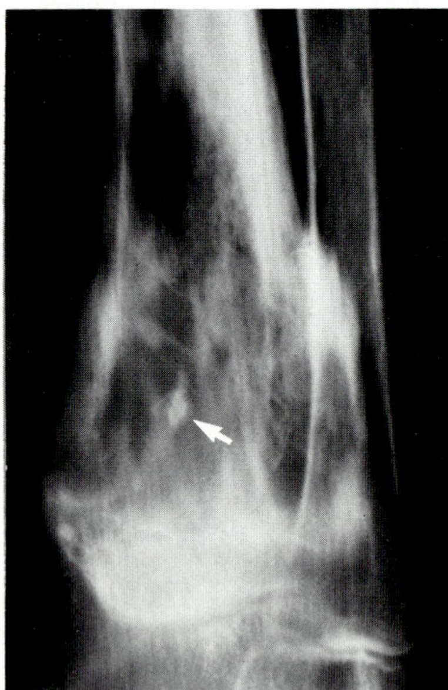

Figure 2.44. Tomogram of the same bone, showing a small dense (white) shadow centrally, confirming the presence of a sequestrum (arrow)

wholly or partly within the joint. These include the proximal humerus, the elbow, and both ends of the femur. With direct infection, the site of osteomyelitis does of course correspond with the site of injury or local soft-tissue inflammation.

In either blood-borne or direct infection, there is a latent period between the onset of the bone infection and the appearance of X-ray changes. During this period—which is never shorter than 10 days and may be much longer, especially in compound fractures—the bone may be heavily infected, and on surgical exploration pus may be seen between the trabeculae or between the cortex and periosteum. It is therefore essential not to delay treatment until changes are seen in the radiographs; it is also unnecessary to radiograph a bone before the tenth day of the infection, except in certain sites—for instance the hip region—where swelling of the soft parts inaccessible to palpation may be detected in the radiograph.

After 14–21 days have elapsed, it is usually necessary to make an X-ray examination in order to see the amount of bone change that has taken place. Usually the infection is adequately controlled by chemotherapy and only minimal changes are seen radiologically. At other times considerable change may occur although the infection may appear clinically to be well controlled. Further radiographs, taken a week or so after the initial ones, will show whether the bone changes are spreading or resolving and will usually show whether sequestra are present.

A sequestrum tends to prevent healing, even with adequate chemotherapy, and will as a rule require surgical removal. Occasionally sequestra cannot be easily seen in a plain radiograph (*Figure 2.43*) although they may be clearly demonstrated in a tomogram (*Figure 2.44*), so that tomography is indicated in cases of delayed healing when no sequestrum is visible in the plain radiograph.

An occasional late result of osteomyelitis is a sinus opening onto the skin. When this is present it is often useful to examine the extent of the sinus and to see whether it reaches to the surface of the bone or to a cavity or sequestrum within the bone. Contrast medium can be injected into the sinus for this purpose and two radiographs taken at right angles to each other to show the extent of the opacified sinus track.

X-ray appearances

The earliest X-ray change in acute osteomyelitis may be either a small area of bone erosion or calcification beneath the raised periosteum, or both changes may coexist (*Figure 2.45*). Unless the infection is successfully suppressed, bone destruction and new bone formation will proceed on a considerable scale. Pieces of bone, isolated from their blood supply and surrounded by areas of osteoblastic bone absorption, will die. These sequestra may become well demarcated at any time after the third week of infection. They are often relatively dense, and stand out in the radiograph as white bone masses against the surrounding living bone, which may be decalcified by osteoblastic absorption, and therefore transradiant (*Figure 2.46*).

Figure 2.45. Osteomyelitis of the tibia 17 days after onset (no treatment): there is an area of deep bone erosion towards the lateral side and some periosteal new bone. On the medial side, where the periosteum has been raised by pus, the new bone formation is still separated from the cortex by a transradiant area; on the lateral side the new bone formation has already reached the cortex

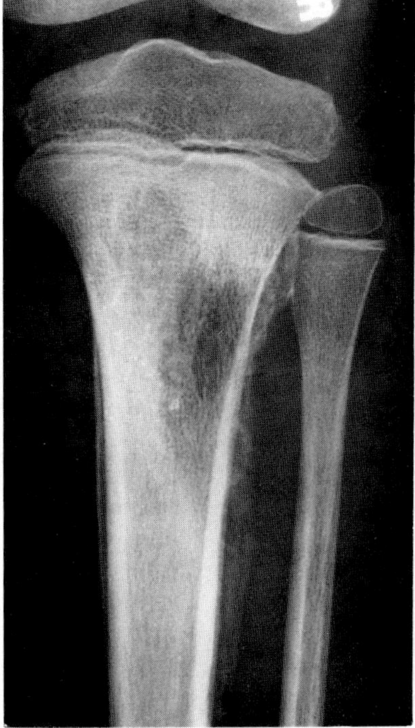

Figure 2.46. (right). Osteomyelitis of the tibia 28 days after onset (no penicillin). There is extensive erosion and periosteal new bone, and a large sequestrum centrally (arrow). The spherical transradiancy adjacent to the sequestrum is the result of an antecedent surgical drill hole for drainage. Note that the lesions do not extend across the epiphyseal plate

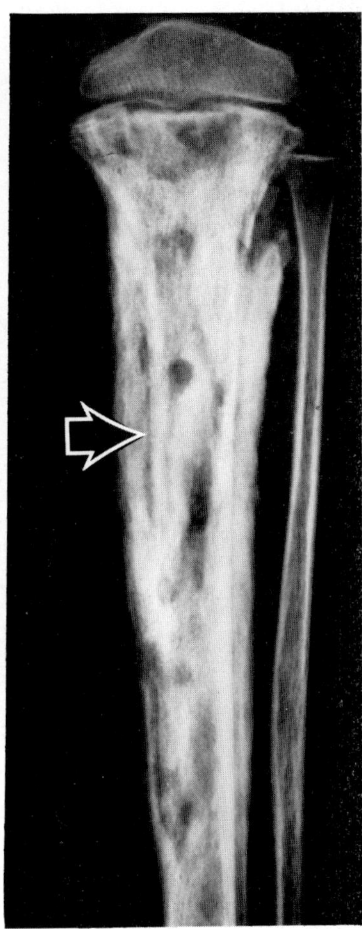

Value of radiology

Generally speaking, the X-ray changes are extensive in blood-borne bone infection, although they will be much modified in cases treated early with antibiotics. In other types of infection, such as that associated with a compound fracture, the radiographs often underrate the amount of bone disease and quite small X-ray changes—such as a small area of erosion or periostitis—may be highly significant; sometimes delay in callus formation is the only X-ray evidence of infection in the fracture area.

X-ray changes of osteomyelitis are more evident in some regions than in others. In the bones of the vault of the skull there are often no X-ray changes to be seen despite a known infection. On the other hand, apparently extensive erosion in a radiograph of a terminal phalanx may represent only a small amount of actual bone damage, since the excessive absorption of the calcium elements (which causes the X-ray appearances) is not necessarily associated with serious matrix disease; if the matrix damage is slight, rapid regeneration of the bone will be visible in the radiograph after successful treatment.

Chronic blood-borne bone infection

Sometimes a blood-borne infection, instead of having an acute dramatic onset, starts insidiously—with relatively inconspicuous symptoms and physical signs. An example of this is a Brodie's abscess (chronic bone abscess). By the time the patient seeks medical advice the latent period after the onset of infection may already have elapsed and the characteristic X-ray changes may already be visible. These comprise a circular or oval area of bone destruction with some sclerosis of the margin. A small area of periosteal new bone is usually seen when the lesion is near the bone surface (*Figure 2.47*). Sequestra are either not present or are small

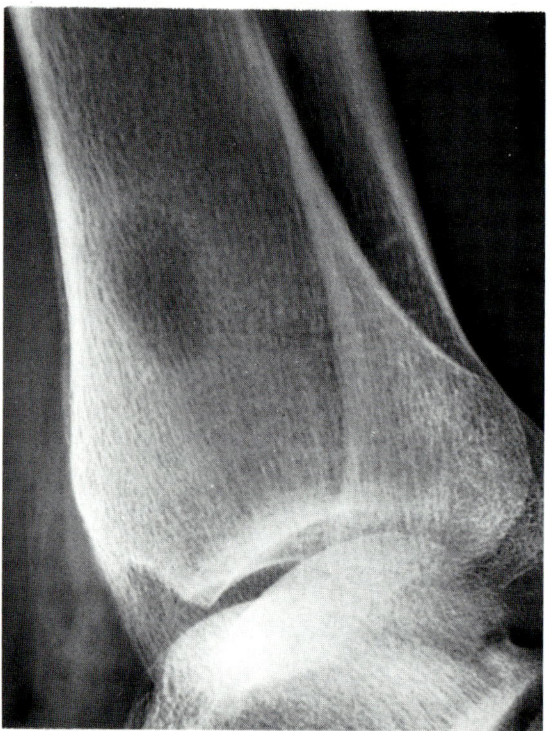

Figure 2.47. Brodie's abscess of the tibia: oval area of erosion and thin white line of periosteal new bone anteriorly; history of pain in the ankle region for the past 4 weeks

and inconspicuous. Brodie's abscesses usually arise in the metaphyseal region.

Other forms of chronic osteomyelitis may produce extensive erosion and periosteal new bone formation. In such cases differentiation from a malignant bone tumour may be difficult both clinically and radiologically (*see* page 81).

Syphilitic infection of bone

Congenital syphilitic osteitis

The skeletal changes in an infant with congenital syphilis are characteristic. Extensive bone destruction occurs in the metaphyseal

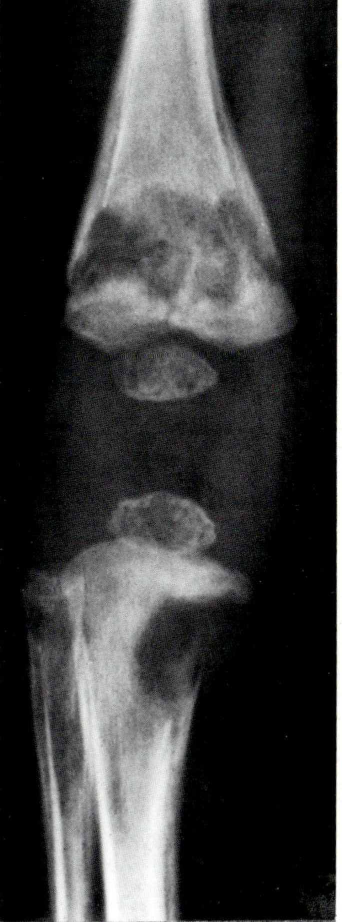

Figure 2.48. Congenital syphilis in a 9-month-old baby: erosions across the diaphysis of the femur and on the medial side of the tibia; periosteal new bone around the shafts. No local signs or symptoms. Possibility of syphilis confirmed by X-ray appearances and positive Wassermann reaction

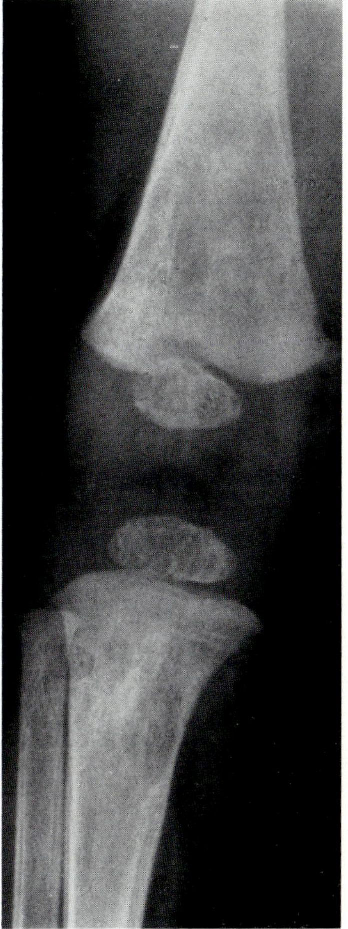

Figure 2.49. The same patient as in *Figure 2.48,* 12 weeks after the beginning of penicillin treatment. The lesions resolved rapidly, and the Wassermann reaction became negative

region and is often accompanied by well-marked periosteal new bone formation (*Figure 2.48*). Any of the long bones or the skull may be affected, but the changes of congenital syphilitic osteitis are most commonly seen on a radiograph of the leg. When the skull is affected, multiple diffuse areas of erosion, about 1 cm in size, may be present.

Radiographs are also of great value in showing the response to treatment. If penicillin therapy is successful, radiographs taken a month after its commencement will show considerable resolution of the bone lesions; after 2 or 3 months the bone changes may be seen to have resolved completely (compare *Figure 2.48*, taken before treatment, with *Figure 2.49*, taken 12 weeks after the beginning of treatment).

Neuropathic joints

The commoner causes of neuropathic joints are diabetes, pain suppression due to prolonged steroid or analgesic intake, neurosyphilis and syringomyelia. Although each of these conditions has its own typical distribution, the changes in affected joints are similar and are illustrated in *Figure 2.50* in a patient suffering from syringomyelia.

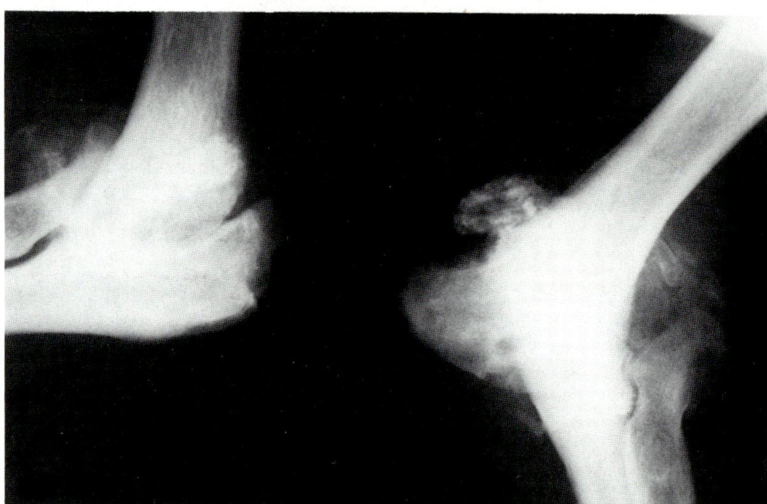

Figure 2.50. Neuropathic left elbow joint; syringomyelia. There is gross joint disorganization with dislocation and fractures and periarticular bone fragments but no osteoporosis

Diminished or absent pain sensation results in failure of rapid reflex correction of abnormal stresses imposed on affected joints. Repeated or isolated injuries in this situation can lead to fractures (which are usually subarticular) or to joint subluxation or dislocation. Progressive disorganization of the joint takes place as a result of further injuries. The fractures do not heal. Sometimes much bone is present within and around the joint: this mainly represents fractured bone, often grossly fragmented, but can also arise from post-traumatic soft-tissue ossification. Eventual resorption of these fragments is common. Since the fractures are painless the patient continues to use the affected limbs, which leads to one of the most distinctive radiological features of neuropathic joints—absence of osteoporosis. Normally in the presence of an unhealed fracture osteoporosis develops due to disuse from chronic pain.

Injuries to the soft tissues are commonly found in association with joint injuries when pain is suppressed. These soft-tissue lesions may become infected, and the infection may spread to the adjacent bone. Radiographic changes of osteomyelitis may therefore be present in limbs showing neuropathic joint changes.

In tabes dorsalis, the most common joints to show neuropathic changes are those of the hips, knees, and lumbar spine. Joints affected by neurosyphilis are sometimes called Charcot joints, named after the French neurologist who first described them in the nineteenth century. Neuropathic joints in the feet are usually due to diabetes, while syringomyelia produces the above features in the joints of the upper limbs including the shoulders. Analgesics and steroids are often taken for joint pain. The relief of suffering that they engender leads to increased use of a joint already diseased by rheumatoid arthritis or other processes, and the greater stresses thereby imposed on the abnormal joint can lead eventually to the development of neuropathic joint changes.

Pyogenic infection of joints (septic arthritis)

The sources of joint infection are similar to those of bone infection. In the early stages the joint space may be increased due to an effusion into it but it very soon tends to diminish as the joint cartilage is destroyed. If the infection is not adequately controlled bone erosion will occur at the articular surface, and there will often be some subperiosteal new bone formation around the shaft nearby, which is a useful diagnostic feature (*Figure 2.51*). There is much

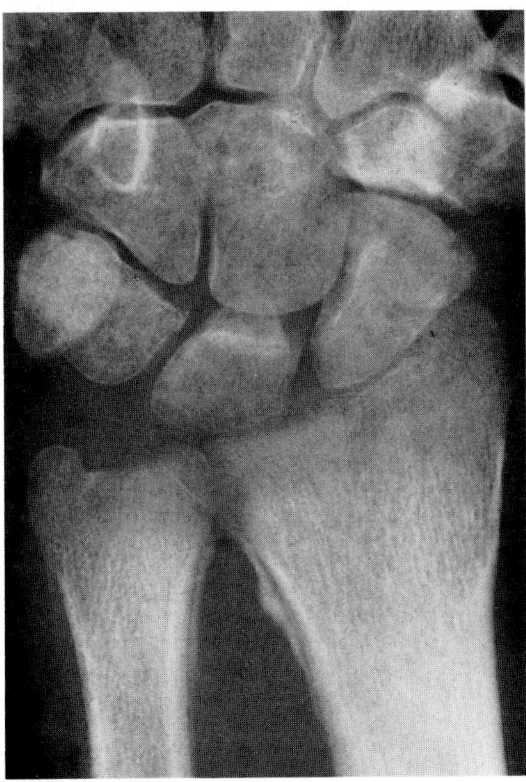

Figure 2.51. Septic arthritis of the wrist joint (staphylococcal): diminished radiocarpal joint space; early erosion of the articular surface; and periosteal new bone around the shaft of the ulna on both sides, and of the radius on the medial side. The general loss of density is rather patchy in distribution

general loss of density of the bones in the joint area, and this may be rather unevenly distributed, giving the bones a mottled appearance. This is not in itself an indication that the infection has spread from the joint to the bones.

Radiographs are useful in confirming the diagnosis in doubtful cases or for observing the course of the infection and the response to treatment in cases where the diagnosis is not in doubt. As healing

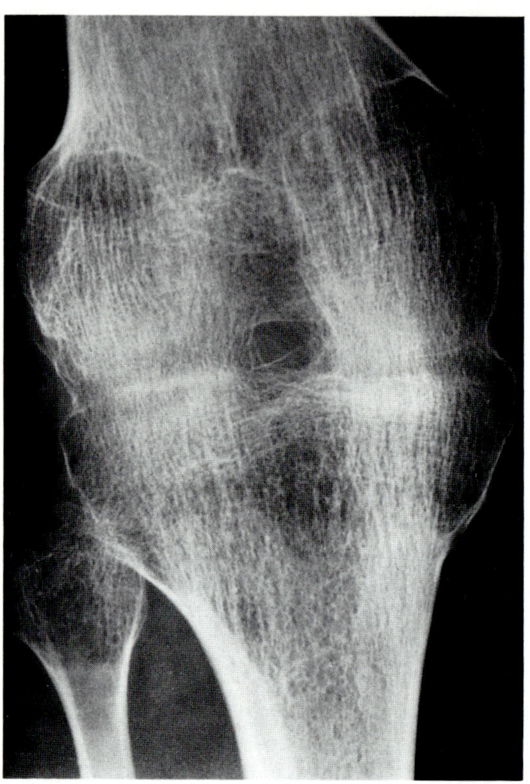

Figure 2.52. Bony ankylosis of the knee following septic arthritis: note the trabecular continuity between the two bones

proceeds, the calcium content will be seen to improve; and if the joint space is not greatly diminished the final functional result may be good. If the joint space is destroyed bony ankylosis can be expected (*Figure 2.52*).

Chronic pyogenic joint infection

Some cases of septic arthritis may take such a chronic and insidious course that it is not easy to distinguish them from a tuberculous joint infection. Since it is important for treatment to know the organism responsible, aspiration or a diagnostic biopsy is often indicated rather than prolonged serial X-ray observation.

Ankylosis of a joint

This may occur as the result of disease or it may be produced by surgical procedures. In the latter instance, radiographs are of value in showing the presence or absence of bone union.

When bony ankylosis is present the radiograph will show continuity of the trabeculae between the two bones (*Figure 2.52*). If this continuity is not seen but the joint is immobile on clinical examination it will not be possible to tell from the radiographs whether the immobility is due to intra-articular adhesions and periarticular contractions or to strong fibrous ankylosis. If adhesions and contractions are the cause, and some preservation of the joint interval is visible in the radiographs, it may be possible to mobilize the joint and restore some degree of movement should this be desirable.

Occasionally the diminished joint space is obscured by periarticular lipping and it is not easy to determine whether trabecular continuity—and therefore bony ankylosis—is present. In this situation tomography will usually provide the information required.

Tuberculous infection of bones and joints

Tuberculous osteomyelitis

Indications for radiography

Chronic or subacute pain and swelling over a bone will indicate the need for an X-ray examination of the affected area. In a tuberculous lesion the onset is rather insidious, and the patient may have little constitutional upset, though in some cases there may be some fever.

Long bones

A tuberculous abscess occasionally develops in a long bone, most commonly in the metaphysis, and its X-ray appearance is very like that of a Brodie's abscess (*see* page 52). However, a tuberculous bone abscess usually shows more erosion and less sclerosis than a Brodie's abscess of the same size. Furthermore, adjacent soft-tissue abscesses tend to be larger in tuberculosis and may partially calcify (*see Figure 2.55*). As in other regions of the body, the possibility of tuberculosis should be considered when calcification is seen within a soft-tissue lesion.

Phalanges

Spindle-shaped swelling of one or more of the fingers of a baby or young child will suggest tuberculous dactylitis. Characteristically,

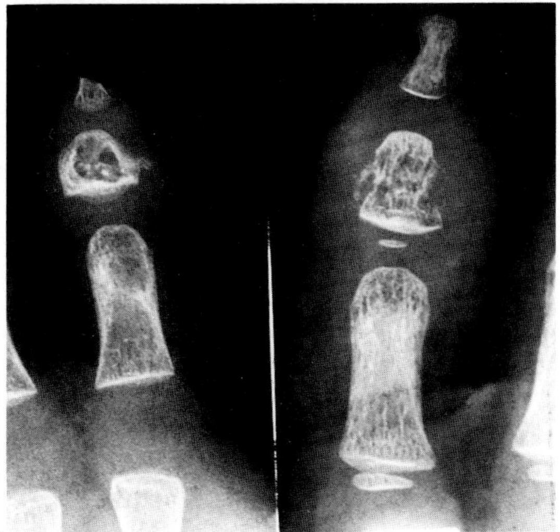

Figure 2.53. Two cases of tuberculous dactylitis (left, in a baby aged 18 months; right, in a baby aged 30 months): central destruction of the middle phalanx with small sequestra; expansion of the affected bone; and considerable soft-tissue swelling, best seen in the second case

there is a combination of destruction and expansion of the affected bone (*Figure 2.53*). The descriptive term spina ventosa (a short bone inflated with air) is applied when the changes are gross. Some periosteal reaction is usually present.

Tuberculous infection of a limb joint

The onset of a tuberculous lesion in one of the joints of a limb is often insidious. Some pain is felt, usually in the neighbourhood of the affected joint; but in the case of the hip joint it may be referred to the knee area. There is limitation of most movements of the joint, some being more restricted than others.

Joint effusions and soft-tissue swellings may be seen at an early stage. Apart from these there is often, but not always, a long latent period between the onset of pain (or other clinical manifestations of arthritis) and the appearance of changes in the radiograph; this latent period may be a matter of months.

X-ray appearances

One of the earliest radiographic changes is a diffuse general loss of density of the bone in the neighbourhood of the infected joint. Another early change is a slight diminution of the joint space. Both can best be detected by comparing the X-ray appearances of the

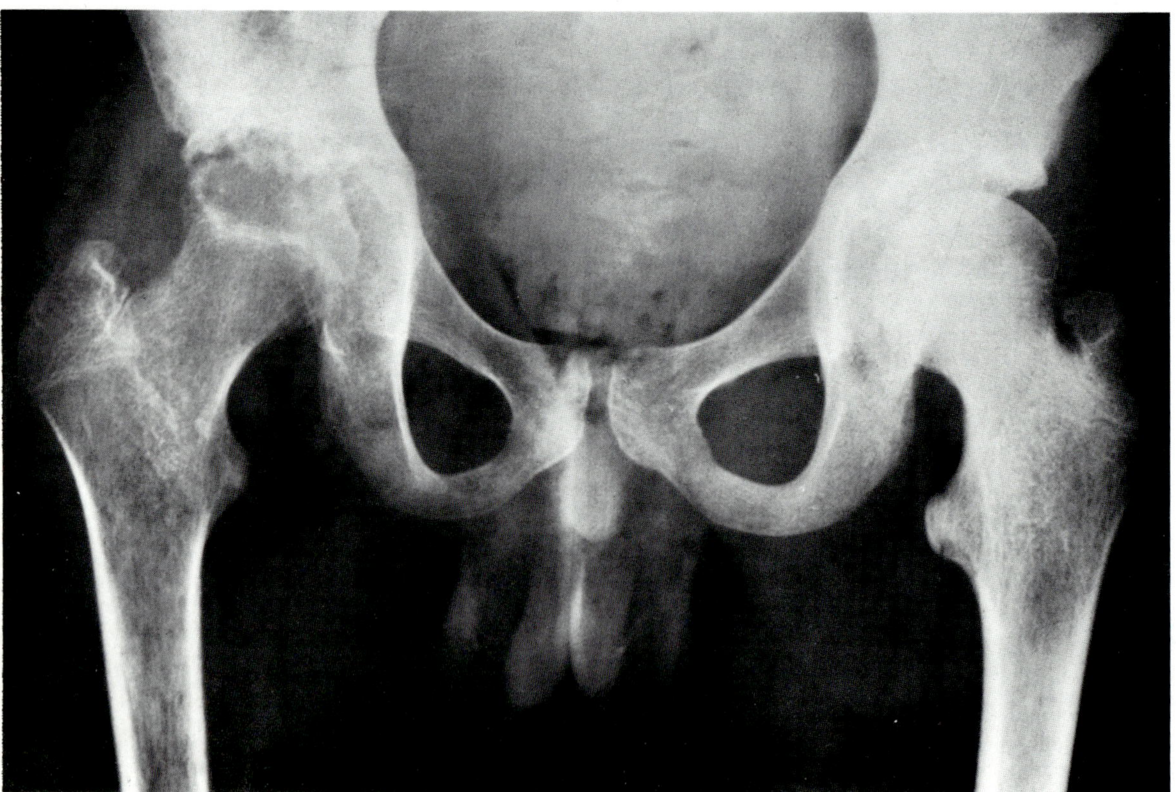

Figure 2.54. Tuberculous lesion of the right hip joint: diminished joint space; erosion of the articular surfaces; and diffuse general loss of density (the thinned cortex appears as a white line round the demineralized shaft)

infected limb with those of the normal joint on the opposite side. For this purpose the two limbs are positioned symmetrically and, when possible, radiographed together on the same film with the same exposure.

As the lesion progresses there may be a more obvious diminution of the joint space and well-marked diffuse loss of density; the trabeculae become indistinct and the remaining cortical layer is thinned out, giving a white 'pencilled' outline to the bone (*Figure 2.54*). Local bone destruction at the articular surfaces, or in the subarticular bone, is the final change. Periosteal new bone formation is usually absent or is an inconspicuous feature, and there is no massive sequestrum formation, although some bone debris a few millimetres in size may occasionally be seen.

Differential diagnosis

The combination of the clinical and X-ray findings will often be sufficient for diagnosis, but sometimes differentiation will have to be made from a chronic pyogenic joint infection or rheumatoid arthritis.

Serial X-ray control during treatment

The patient is treated with chemotherapy and rest of the affected limb in a splint or plaster. As healing advances, the calcium content

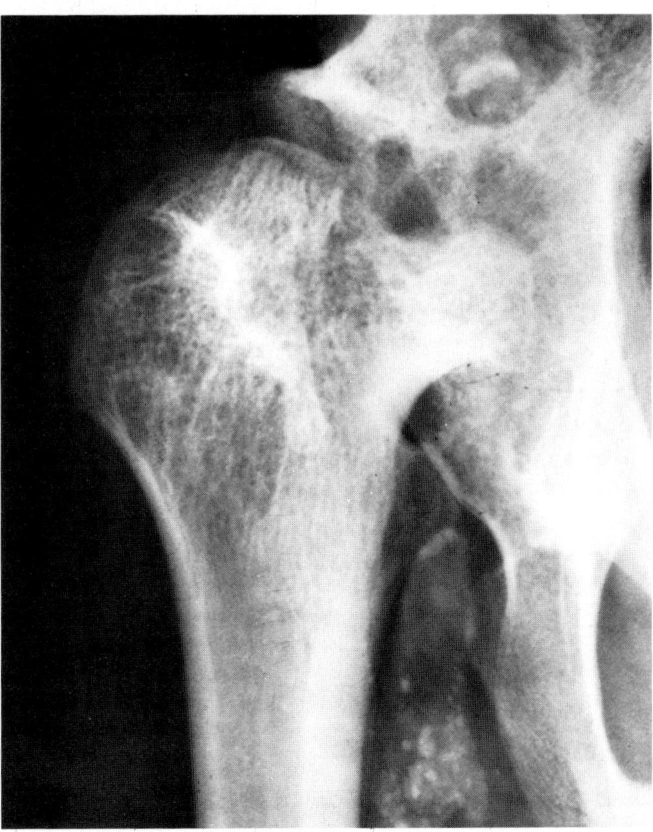

Figure 2.55. Healing tuberculous lesion of the hip joint, 2 years after onset: the trabecular pattern is reforming. There is a cavity with a small sequestrum in the ilium and the shadow of a partly calcified abscess below the lesser trochanter. Destruction of the femoral head has resulted in permanent deformity

of the surrounding bone may be seen to improve but it will not be good until function has been resumed. When healing is complete the trabeculae will reform, although the pattern will usually be abnormal, and punctate areas of calcification may be visible in a healed tuberculous abscess near the joint (*Figure 2.55*). If the joint is appreciably damaged before treatment is instituted, persisting deformity of the articular surfaces is to be expected (*Figure 2.55*) and this will predispose to the development of secondary osteoarthritis.

Infection of the spine

Tuberculosis of the spine

Backache of insidious onset, usually persisting after a trial of bed rest, may indicate a tuberculous lesion.

X-ray appearances

By the time the symptoms of a tuberculous lesion of the spine are present, X-ray changes will usually be apparent. The usual site of

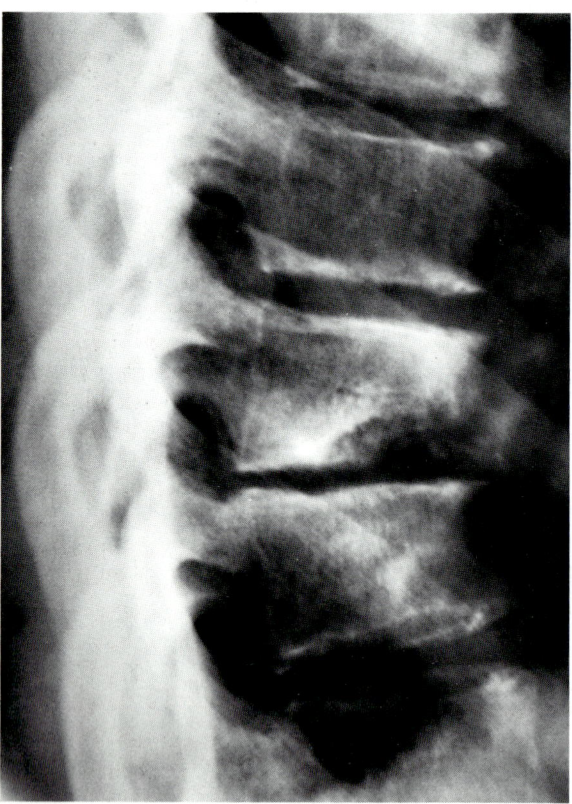

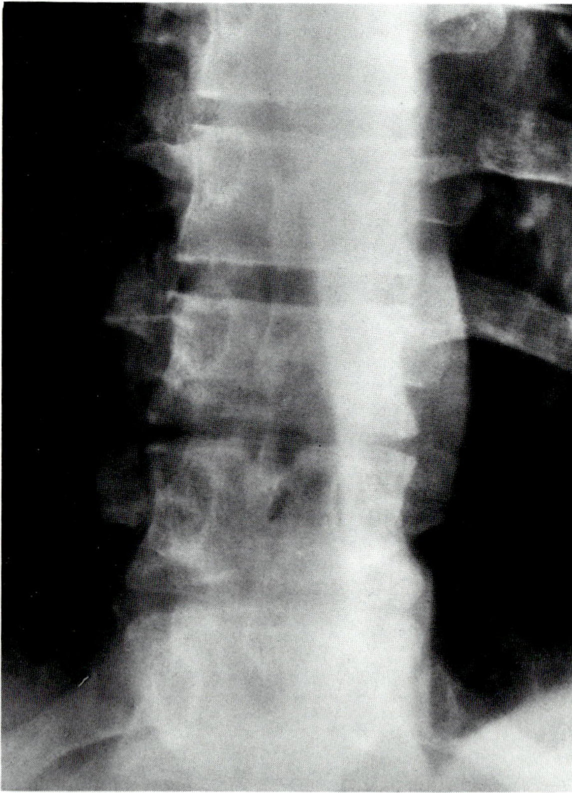

Figure 2.56. Tuberculous lesion of the spine in a male aged 20 (lateral view): erosion of the anteroinferior aspect of the body of T10, and diminished joint space between T10 and T11

Figure 2.57. The same patient as in *Figure 2.56* (posterior view). The shadow with a well-defined convex lateral margin to the left of T9 and 10 indicates a paravertebral abscess. Pain was felt in this part of the back for 5 months

infection is in the vertebral body, most commonly in the anterior part adjacent to the upper or lower articular surface. Tuberculous lesions of the spine are primarily destructive, and it is very rare to see any reactive sclerosis. The infection spreads to the adjacent disc, which is destroyed with consequent radiographic evidence of diminution of the disc space (*Figure 2.56*). Paravertebral abscesses, which can reach very considerable size and which may contain calcification in the healing phase, may accompany the bone changes. In the cervical region the abscess shadow may displace the pharyngeal transradiancy anteriorly, while in the lumbar region it will cause an outward bulging of the shadow of the psoas muscle. In the thoracic region it often has a well-defined lateral convex margin (*Figure 2.57*). This must not be confused with the shadow of the descending thoracic aorta, which should always be separately identified, or with the straight shadows of the normal mediastinal pleural reflections over the sides of the dorsal vertebral bodies.

As the anterior part of a vertebral body bears the brunt of the bone erosion, wedge-shaped collapse is a common occurrence, producing angular kyphosis. After destruction of the disc the infection spreads across the diminished disc space to involve the next vertebra, and finally, if untreated, the two affected vertebrae fuse into a single wedge-shaped bone mass.

In the early stages differentiation from osteochondritis of the spine (*see Figure 2.39*) may be difficult. A positive Mantoux reaction, a raised erythrocyte sedimentation rate (ESR), and local tenderness will favour tuberculosis, but if there is any doubt a therapeutic trial with antituberculous drugs or aspiration may be needed for diagnosis.

The tendency for infections of the spine to spread from bone to destroy the adjoining disc spaces, with radiographic evidence of disc space reduction, provides a useful feature distinguishing infection from metastases of the spine. It is rare for tumour to destroy the disc, so that the disc space is usually preserved in the presence of vertebral body metastases (*see Figure 2.85*). Furthermore, metastases commonly destroy the pedicles (*see Figure 2.84*) while the vertebral arch is rarely involved in infection. Paravertebral masses can accompany both conditions, but tumour masses are generally small while tuberculous paraspinal abscesses can become very large.

Uncommonly, tuberculous infection spreads primarily along the paraspinal ligaments, and paraspinal abscesses can be observed radiologically with absent or only minimal erosions of the vertebral bodies.

Pyogenic infection of the spine

The radiographic changes of pyogenic infection of the spine are very similar to those of tuberculosis, except that in pyogenic infection:

1. Bone destruction is seen on serial films to progress more rapidly, reflecting the more virulent nature of the infection.
2. There is commonly some reactive sclerosis around the margins of destroyed bone, while tuberculous lesions are usually purely destructive.

3. Paravertebral pyogenic abscesses do not reach the large size sometimes found in tuberculous abscesses.

Despite these differences, radiological distinction is often impossible. Pyogenic spondylitis will be suggested clinically by a rapid onset and evidence of sepsis elsewhere and can be confirmed by bacteriological investigation of aspirated pus or bone biopsy.

Miscellaneous joint diseases

Rheumatoid arthritis

Rheumatoid arthritis is characterized by low-grade inflammation of connective tissue, the synovium being particularly affected. This synovial inflammation causes the characteristic bone erosions at the synovial attachments. A pannus of proliferated inflamed synovial tissue grows over and destroys the articular cartilages, leading to a loss of the joint space. In a large percentage of cases rheumatoid factor can be detected in the serum by the latex or Rose–Waaler

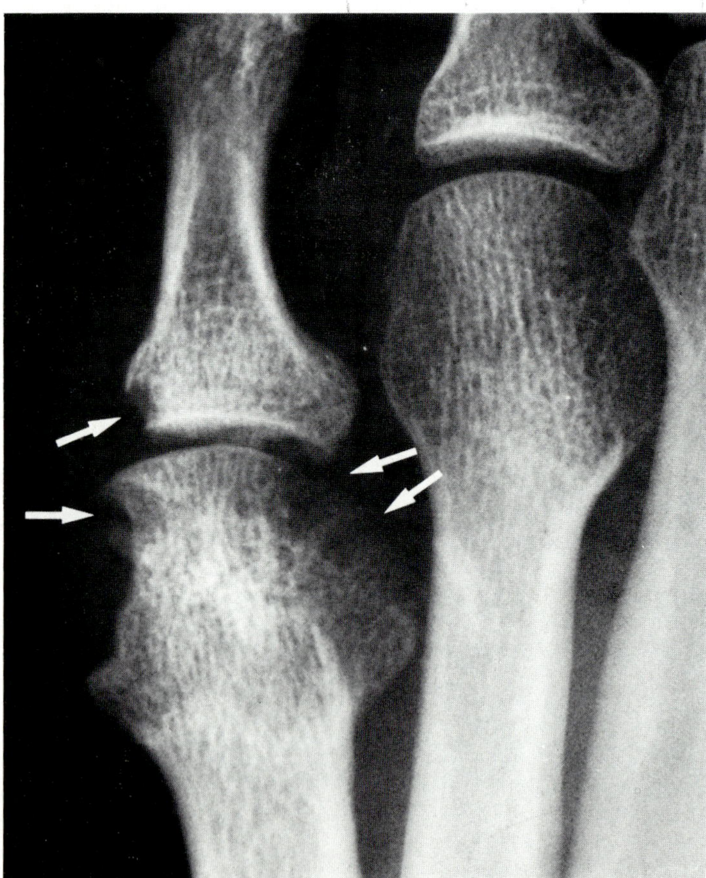

Figure 2.58. Rheumatoid arthritis: erosions at synovial attachments and on articular surfaces of first metatarsal head and base of the proximal phalanx (arrows); slight joint-space narrowing; symptoms of arthritis for 15 months; hands radiographically normal

tests. The ESR tends to be high in the active phase. Some cases have related lupus erythematosus or other collagen diseases. A few patients develop pulmonary fibrosis resembling fibrosing alveolitis (*see* page 221), and a rheumatoid pleural effusion occurs for a time in approximately 10 per cent of cases. The common age of onset of the disease is in the thirties, but the disorder may begin in childhood (Still's disease) or in old age. Symptoms may be confined for a time to one joint, or many joints may be affected from the start.

The small joints of the hands and feet are most commonly affected, the metacarpophalangeal, metatarsophalangeal, and proximal interphalangeal joints being particularly involved. It is rare for the disease to affect the terminal interphalangeal joints (cf. psoriasis, below). The carpus and tarsus and the ulnar styloid are also often sites of disease. In a patient suspected of the condition, therefore, X-rays of the hands and feet should be requested. The large joints of the limbs are often involved later, but it is comparatively rare for the disease to start in one of these joints.

The early radiological changes consist of symmetrical, spindle-shaped soft-tissue swellings over affected joints, demineralization

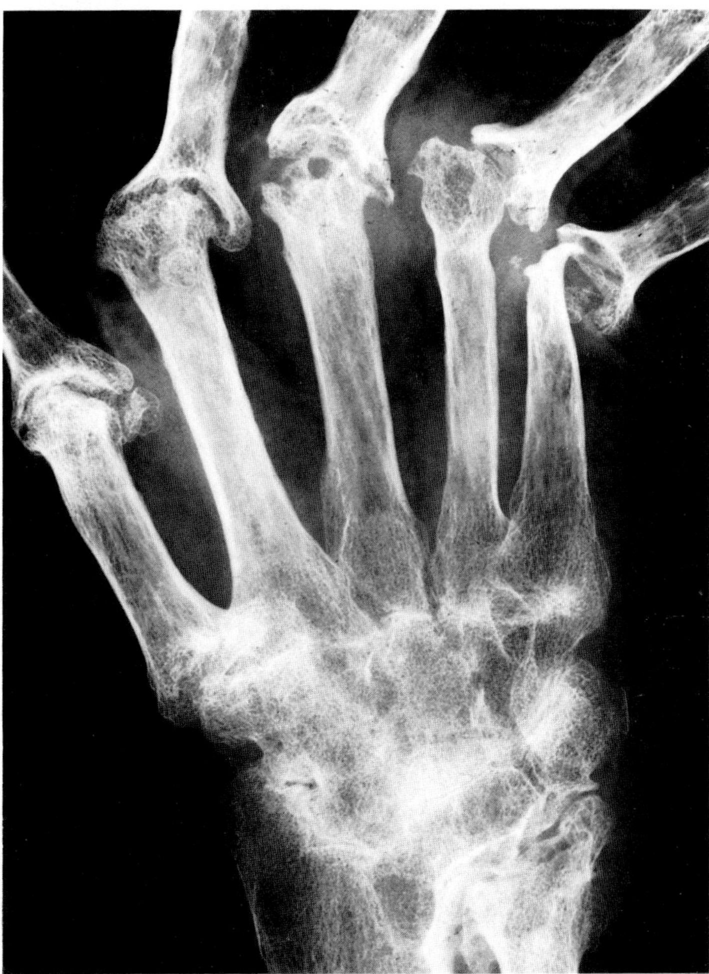

Figure 2.59. Rheumatoid arthritis; arthritis mutilans. Subluxation with ulnar deviation at metacarpophalangeal joints, cup-and-pencil deformity at fifth metacarpophalangeal joint, erosions with sclerotic margins on third metacarpal head, ankylosis of carpal bones, and generalized reduction of bone density. Arthritis had been present for many years

(from hyperaemia) of the subarticular regions, and erosions. The erosions occur at the articular margins (at the sites of synovial attachments) and along the articular surfaces (*Figure 2.58*). In the active phase, the erosions are purely destructive (*Figure 2.58*) but in long standing quiescent or burnt out disease they commonly have sclerotic margins (*Figure 2.59*). A periosteal reaction is often seen on the shafts adjacent to affected joints. Later, there is overt joint space narrowing resulting from destruction of the articular cartilages.

The severe late deformities that may occur in this condition are well illustrated in *Figure 2.59*. The bone ends themselves may become destroyed, causing gross bony deformity (arthritis mutilans). Erosion of a metacarpal head may be complete and this, together with thinning of the shaft and scooping out of the adjacent phalanx, gives a cup-and-pencil type of deformity which may be seen in a very severe case. Multiple subluxations occur, those in the hand classically giving rise to ulnar deviation at the metacarpophalangeal joints. Bony ankylosis, particularly of the carpus and tarsus, may develop.

Value of radiology in rheumatoid arthritis

In a clinically doubtful case the presence of typical bone erosions will confirm the diagnosis; they will be seen in 90 per cent of cases, in

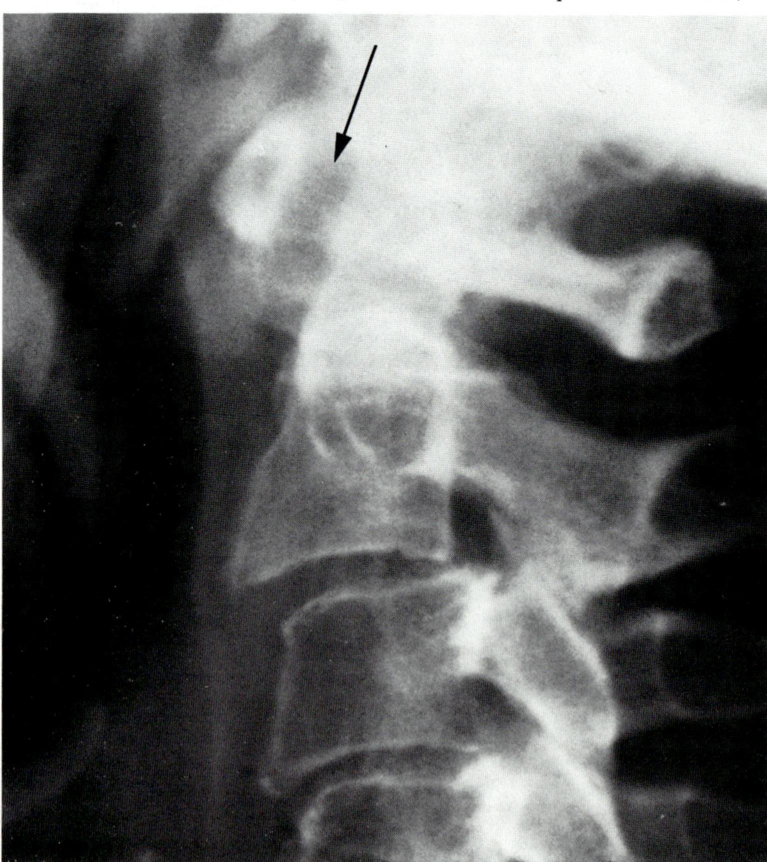

Figure 2.60. Rheumatoid arthritis. Atlantoaxial subluxation. Space between anterior arch of atlas and odontoid peg (arrow) increased from narrow slit to 5 mm. Minor C2/3 subluxation is also present

either the hands or the feet, by the time medical advice is sought. In some 15 per cent the hands are involved clinically but not the feet, yet the radiographs show obvious metatarsal head erosions (*see Figure 2.58*) but no lesions in the hands. In cases radiologically normal at the onset, erosions generally appear within the next 3 years. Radiographs are of value in recording progress and demonstrating the extent of damage to a joint, particularly when surgical procedures are contemplated.

In many cases the hands and feet are most affected, but in others the major disability may arise from involvement of a large joint such as the hip or knee. Rheumatoid arthritis sometimes involves the cervical spine, causing reduction of the disc spaces and fusion of the arches, and (of particular importance) subluxation at the atlanto-axial joint. This can be seen on a lateral radiograph taken with the neck flexed: the odontoid peg of C2 may move away from the anterior arch of the atlas so that the space between them may increase from 2 to 3 mm in the neutral position to 5 mm on flexion (*Figure 2.60*). Occasionally the sacroiliac joints are affected, and distinction between rheumatoid arthritis and ankylosing spondylitis with peripheral joint involvement may depend on the latex test, which is negative in the latter condition.

Erosions similar to those of rheumatoid arthritis occur in ankylosing spondylitis, Reiter's syndrome, psoriatic arthropathy, and the arthritis occasionally found in association with ulcerative colitis and Crohn's disease. In all of these, tests for rheumatoid factor are negative.

Ankylosing spondylitis

The symptoms of ankylosing spondylitis are backache and stiffness. The patient is usually a young adult, and the condition is far commoner in males than in females. The ESR is much raised.

The histological features are similar to those of rheumatoid arthritis: there is chronic inflammation of the synovium and a pannus spreads across an affected joint, destroying the articular cartilages. The distribution, however, differs from that of rheumatoid arthritis. The axial skeleton is mainly affected, and it is comparatively rare for joints of the appendicular skeleton, other than those of the shoulders and hips, to be involved.

In the early stages the sacroiliac joints show widening of the joint space and pitted erosions of the articular cortex (*Figure 2.61*). Later the joint space narrows and may finally ankylose (*Figure 2.62*), and there is considerable sclerosis in the adjacent bone of both the sacrum and the ilium. The joints are usually equally affected.

The posterior joints of the dorsolumbar region of the spine and the costovertebral and costotransverse joints are also affected early in the disease. These changes, however, are difficult to see on standard view radiographs. A more obvious early change in the spine is the development of a squared appearance of the lumbar vertebral bodies. This is brought about by new bone deposition on the

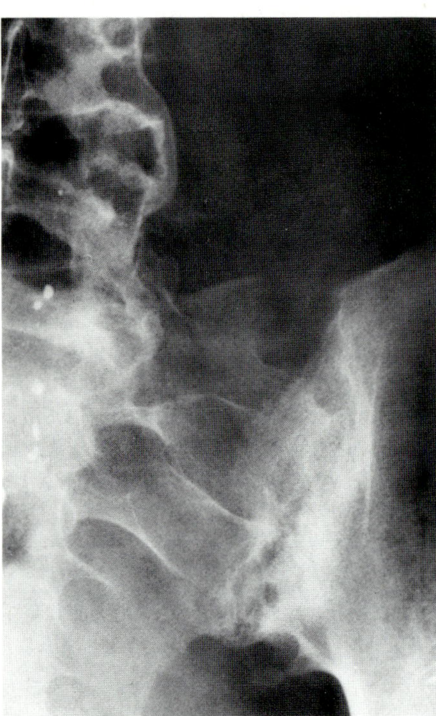

Figure 2.62. Ankylosing spondylitis, late stage. Obliteration of both sacroiliac joints by bony ankylosis; bamboo spine, with ossification between the vertebral bodies (white arrows) and the interspinous ligament (black arrows). History of pain and stiffness in the back for the past 8 years

Figure 2.61. Ankylosing spondylitis. Erosions and sclerosis of subarticular bone of sacroiliac joint, more marked on iliac side; ossification in soft tissues between L4 and L5; similar changes on right side. Low-back pain had been present for 6 years

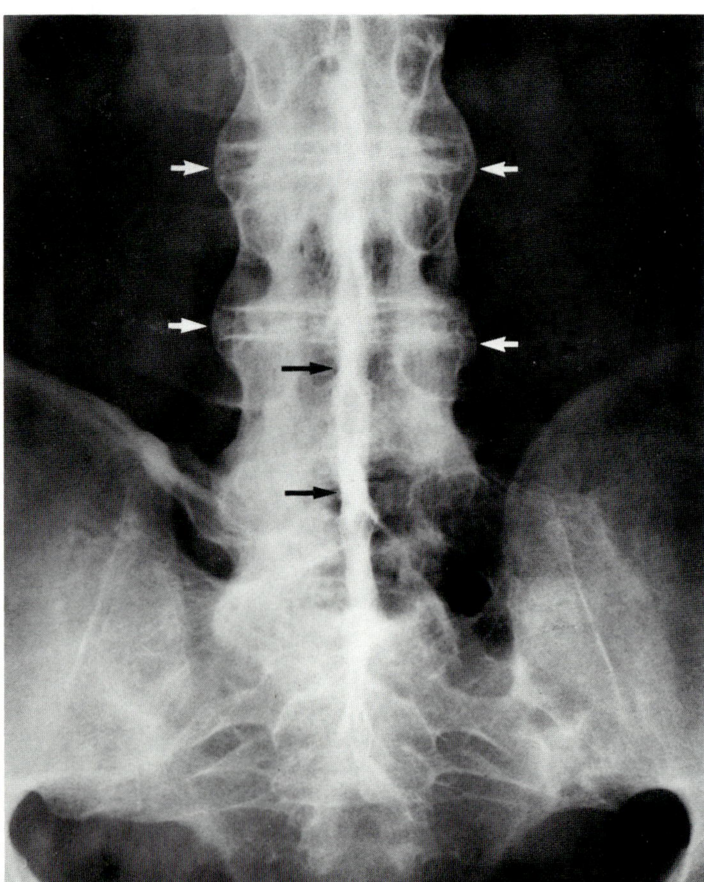

anterior surfaces of the vertebral bodies, and is seen on the lateral view radiographs. Later on, calcification and ossification occur in the paraspinal ligaments and surrounding soft tissues, which, when well developed, cause the condition aptly named 'bamboo spine' (*Figure 2.62*). Ankylosing spondylitis is often confined to the spinal column, but as already mentioned the hip and other large joints may also be involved, in which case the X-ray appearances of these joints will closely simulate those of rheumatoid arthritis.

Reiter's syndrome

The syndrome comprises non-specific urethritis, conjunctivitis and arthritis. The arthritic changes resemble those of rheumatoid arthritis clinically and radiologically, although the gross deformities of rheumatoid arthritis do not develop. Involvement of the sacroiliac joints and development of a bony spur on the plantar aspect of the calcaneum can occur in both diseases but are more common in Reiter's syndrome.

Psoriatic arthropathy

Erosions of articular surfaces and joint space narrowing, similar to the changes of rheumatoid arthritis, occur in psoriatic arthropathy. However, there is an important difference in the distribution of lesions in the two conditions. The interphalangeal joints of the hands, particularly the distal joints, are particularly severely affected in psoriatic arthropathy, while in rheumatoid arthritis the metacarpophalangeal and proximal interphalangeal joints are the main areas of damage, and the terminal interphalangeal joints spared. 'Cup-and-pencil' deformities of the terminal interphalangeal joints are sometimes found in psoriatic arthropathy; these are produced by the extreme destruction of the bone ends, the pointed necks of the middle phalanges lying within the eroded bases of the terminal interphalangeal joints (this appearance has been illustrated in *Figure 2.59*, involving a metacarpophalangeal joint in a patient with rheumatoid arthritis). In the feet the metatarsophalangeal as well as the interphalangeal joints can be involved in psoriatic arthropathy.

Gout

Gout may be suspected if terminal or proximal interphalangeal joints of the hand or the metatarsophalangeal joint of the great toe are swollen, if there is a history of acute episodes of severe pain with swelling and redness over a joint, or if there is chronic swelling and occasional discharge of chalk-like material through the skin.

Radiographs of the hands or feet of a patient with gout may show what appear to be small, well-defined punched-out areas, without a white rim of sclerotic bone, near the articular ends of the bone, or occasionally further away (*Figure 2.63*). These transradiant areas are caused by urate deposits. They can often be distinguished from the erosions of rheumatoid arthritis by their distribution. In gout the

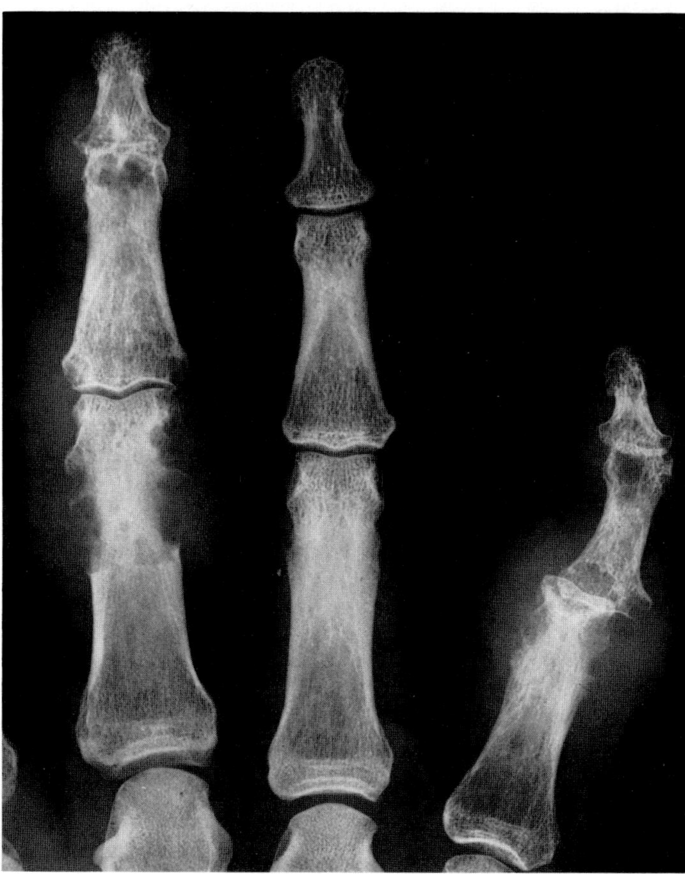

Figure 2.63. Gout. Translucent areas caused by urate deposits in some of the phalanges, near but often not in the joints; these are circular, as if punched out, and are not demarcated by a rim of dense bone. Some joint spaces are diminished. There is no osteoporosis. Gross soft-tissue swelling around affected joints. Occasional attacks of acute pain and swelling around the joints, and a high level of blood uric acid. The metacarpal joints are not involved

proximal and distal interphalangeal joints and the great toe metatarsophalangeal joints are chiefly affected, while in rheumatoid arthritis the predominant distribution is in the metacarpophalangeal, metatarsophalangeal, and proximal interphalangeal joints, with sparing of the terminal interphalangeal joints. Further features that aid radiological differentiation between gout and rheumatoid arthritis are:

1. The periarticular soft-tissue swellings of gout are eccentric and may contain amorphous calcification, while the swellings of rheumatoid arthritis are spindle shaped and uncalcified.
2. Para-articular demineralization is almost always absent in gout.

In gout the serum uric acid will be elevated and the latex test negative. In long standing disease, secondary osteoarthritic changes are commonly seen in affected joints.

Degenerative joint disease

Osteoarthritis

Osteoarthritis is termed secondary when there is a known predisposing cause (most commonly previous trauma to the joint) and primary when there is no obvious preceding joint lesion. In the latter situation repeated stresses on the joint, as may be experienced in heavy manual labour, probably play a significant contributory role. The onset is often insidious. In many cases there may be little or no pain; while in others, particularly when the condition involves a hip or knee, pain may be troublesome and severe. The disease tends to affect either one or two large joints—such as a hip, knee or shoulder—or several small joints, particularly the distal joints of the fingers. The trapezium metacarpal joint and metatarsophalangeal joints of the great toe are commonly affected in the elderly.

Four radiographic changes are seen in osteoarthritis (*Figure 2.64*):
1. Narrowing of the joint space due to loss of the articular cartilages.
2. Reactive sclerosis of the articular surfaces of the bone ends.
3. Formation of osteophytes (small bony projections) at the articular margins.

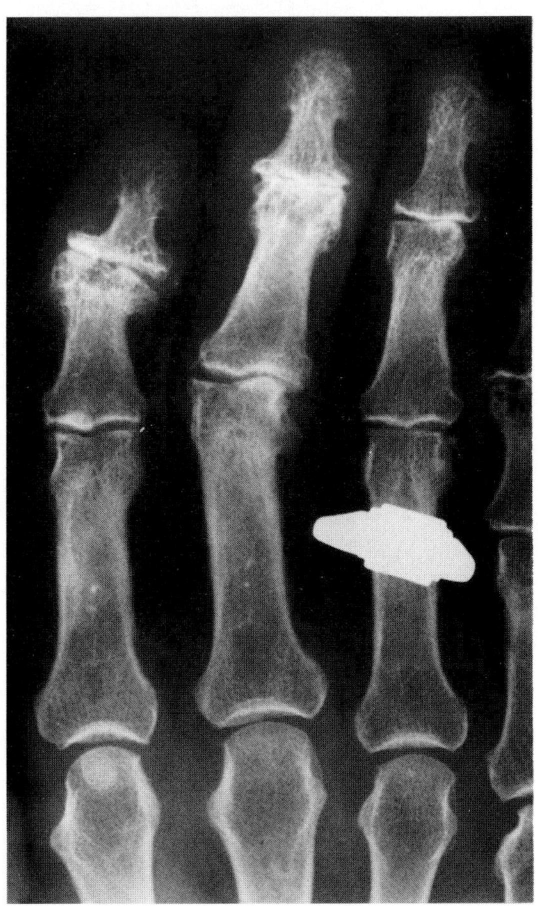

Figure 2.64. Osteoarthritis: joint space narrowing, subarticular bone sclerosis and some marginal osteophyte bone overgrowth affecting interphalangeal joints, particularly proximal interphalangeal joint of middle finger and all distal interphalangeal joints. Compare appearances with those of normal metacarpophalangeal joints

4. Development of cysts in the subarticular regions. These cysts are formed by the repeated pumping of synovial fluid into the bone through minute defects in the damaged articular cartilage. Cysts 3–5 mm in diameter are commonly seen in the first metatarsal head in osteoarthritis of the metatarsophalangeal joint; and larger cysts, 1–2 cm in diameter, may be present in the ilium when the hip joint is affected.

Spondylosis

Degeneration of the intervertebral discs produces radiographic changes of disc-space narrowing, subarticular sclerosis and marginal osteophyte formation, similar to the first three features described in the section on osteoarthritis (*Figure 2.65*). Degenerative disc

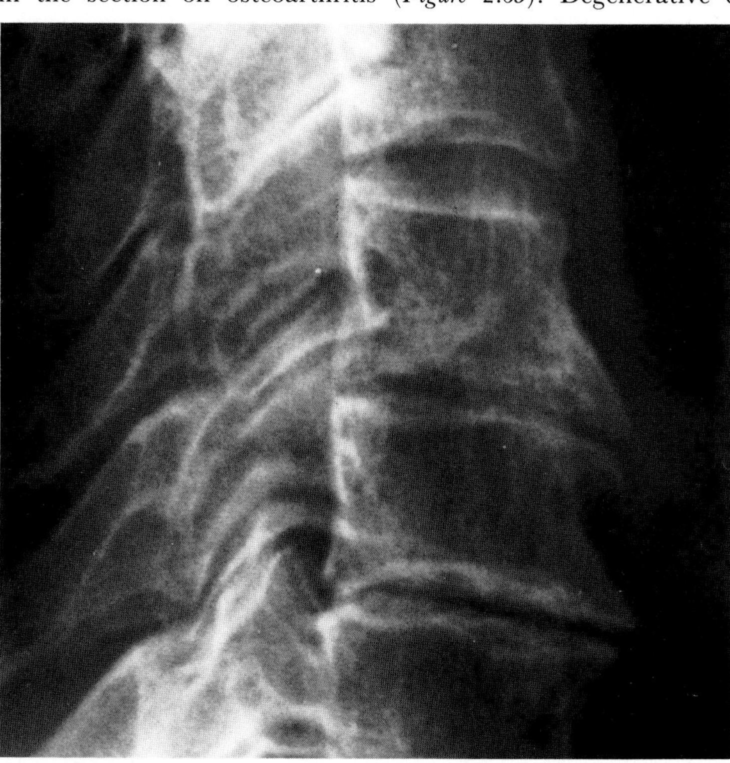

Figure 2.65. Spondylosis: joint space narrowing, subarticular sclerosis and marginal osteophyte formation affecting lower two disc spaces. Compare with normal disc space above

disease (spondylosis) is seen most commonly in the lower cervical spine and at the lumbosacral junction. In the cervical region osteophytes may press on the spinal nerves as they pass through the intervertebral foramina, giving rise to severe nerve root pain. Encroachment on the intervertebral foramina by osteophytes is best seen on oblique views of the cervical area.

Striking osteophyte buttressing around synovial joints and the intervertebral discs is often seen as an incidental finding in an asymptomatic patient X-rayed for some unrelated purpose. Osteophytes can be regarded as providing a protective mechanism, adding stability to a joint subjected to abnormal stresses.

Generalized reduction of bone density

A widespread reduction in bone density may be seen in radiographs in the following situations:
1. When there is deficient formation of the bone matrix of osteoid tissue—osteoporosis.
2. When there is defective calcification of the matrix of osteoid—osteomalacia in the adult, rickets in children.
3. In hyperparathyroidism.

A widespread reduction in bone density may represent the sole radiographic abnormality in the early stages of any of these conditions. Difficulties in diagnosis at this stage are intensified by the facts that radiological determination of reduction in bone density is usually made by subjective assessment, and progressive loss of skeletal mass occurs as a normal physiological event after middle age, so that the findings have to be considered in the context of the patient's age. It must also be borne in mind that the radiographic appearances may result from the coexistence of more than one disease, e.g. both osteoporosis and osteomalacia. In the more advanced stages, radiological signs indicating a specific diagnosis may develop—e.g. Looser's zones indicating osteomalacia, sub-periosteal bone erosion and expanding bone cysts (brown tumours) indicating hyperparathyroidism.

Osteoporosis

The causes of a generalized deficiency in the formation of the osteoid matrix are:
1. Endocrine disorders: Cushing's syndrome, thyrotoxicosis (this, however, rarely causes radiologically recognizable osteoporosis) and hypogonadism.
2. Drug-induced osteoporosis: from steroids and heparin.
3. Dietary deficiencies: starvation (e.g. famine, anorexia nervosa) and vitamin C deficiency (scurvy). Osteoporosis is the only skeletal abnormality produced by scurvy in adults: the striking radiological features of scurvy in childhood are described below.
4. Post-menopausal and senile osteoporosis: post-menopausal osteoporosis produced by reduced oestrogen secretion; and senile osteoporosis occurring in elderly men, probably due in part to reduced androgen formation. Decreased mobility may also be a contributory factor in the development of post-menopausal and senile osteoporosis, which are the commonest forms of the condition.
5. Congenital osteogenesis imperfecta probably results from a congenital defect of osteoid deposition.
6. Idiopathic osteoporosis: osteoporosis occurring in young adults for which no cause can be found.

Leukaemia in childhood and myelomatosis can sometimes present with a generalized reduction in bone density without evidence of well-defined lytic areas (*see Figure 2.90*).

As has already been mentioned, the early radiological changes of osteoporosis consist of a widespread reduction of bone density. The bone cortices are thinned. It should be remembered that the primary defect in this condition is a deficient formation of bone matrix: the matrix that does form is normally mineralized. The thinned cortex is therefore seen as a well-mineralized rim (*Figure 2.66*).

There is a tendency for the trabeculae that bear the brunt of major stresses on the skeleton to remain well developed and consequently to stand out conspicuously relative to the rest of the skeleton.

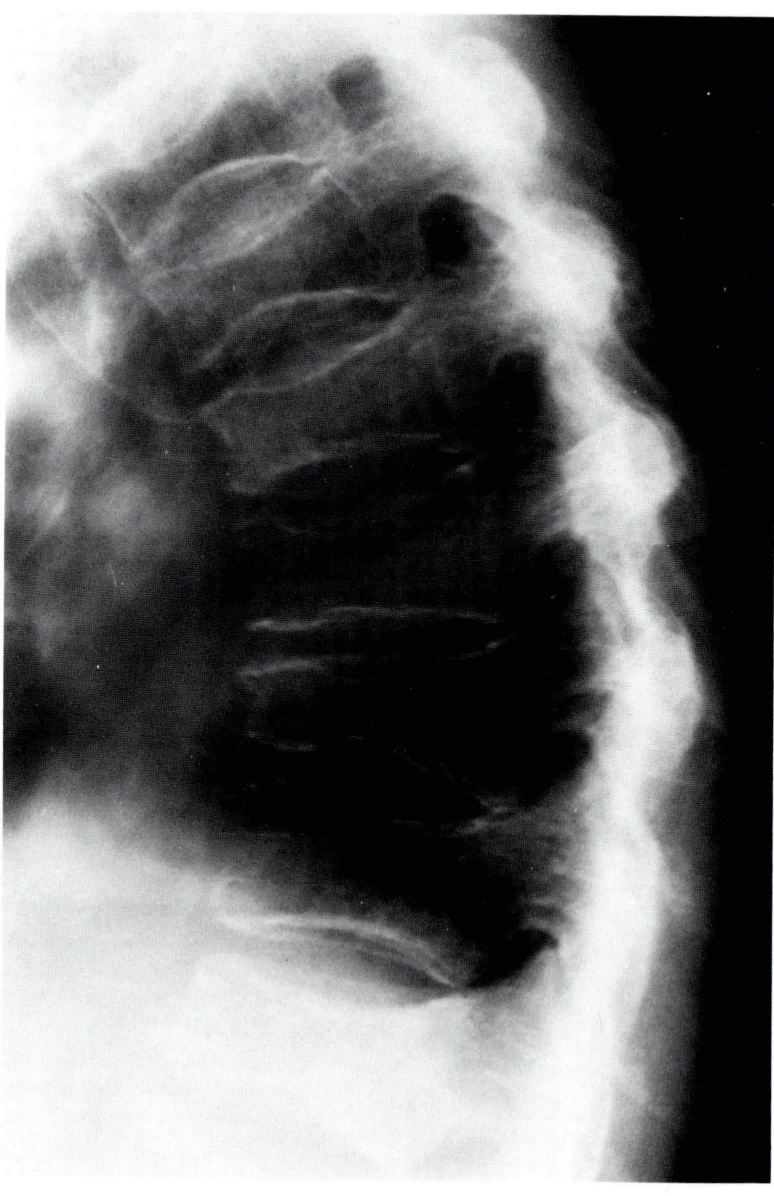

Figure 2.66. Osteoporosis: generalized skeletal demineralization, multiple vertebral compression fractures, thin but nevertheless intact white cortical line around each vertebral body, and no callus formation

Later, numerous fractures arise in the weakened skeleton from normal stresses or trivial trauma, and the presence of these is the most distinctive radiological feature of osteoporosis. Such fractures are particularly common in the bodies of the dorsal and lumbar spine, the femoral necks and the ribs. The dorsal and lumbar vertebral fractures are commonly patchily distributed, fractured vertebral bodies being separated from each other by bodies that are intact (*Figure 2.66*). Generally, callus formation indicating healing is impaired. There is, however, one important exception to this: when osteoporosis results from disorders causing Cushing's syndrome or from iatrogenic steroid therapy, extensive calcification may be seen in excessively abundant new matrix formed around the fracture sites. Despite the florid radiographic appearances, the calcification takes place in incompletely formed osteoid that lacks the strength of normal matrix. Steroid excess can sometimes be recognized radiologically as the cause of the osteoporosis by this singular appearance of exuberant pseudocallus formation.

Osteoporosis that is localized in distribution occurs with disuse (as when a fractured limb is immobilized in plaster) and in situations of focal hyperaemia (as in tuberculous and rheumatoid arthritis). Osteoporosis limited to one region is easier to recognize in the early stages than generalized osteoporosis since comparison can be made in doubtful cases with unaffected regions of the skeleton, particularly with the identical region on the opposite side.

Scurvy

As mentioned above, scurvy developing in adults from deficient vitamin C intake produces widespread osteoporosis, similar in appearances to osteoporosis from other causes. In children, however, the radiological features are characteristic and diagnostic of the condition. The disease is not found before the age of 6 or 9 months, as the child is protected during this period with vitamin C derived from the mother.

The characteristic radiological features of scurvy are illustrated in *Figure 2.67*. There is delayed skeletal development, due to deficient osteoid formation in the metaphyses and epiphyses. The skeleton is generally osteoporotic, with thin, sparse trabeculae and thin cortices. In contrast to this, the osteoid that is present in the metaphysis and epiphysis is well mineralized: this results in a characteristic, dense, transverse, metaphyseal band and a ring-like epiphyseal halo. Osteoid formation is particularly defective in the region immediately beneath the white metaphyseal band, which produces a narrow, submetaphyseal, transradiant band. This area of deficient bone formation is particularly fragile and is responsible for another characteristic radiological change of scurvy—bony spurs or beaks at the metaphyseal margin resulting from metaphyseal corner fractures. Since vitamin C deficiency causes abnormal capillary fragility, there is a tendency for large subperiosteal haematomas to form at the time of these fractures. These haematomas subsequently calcify, causing a striking radiological appearance.

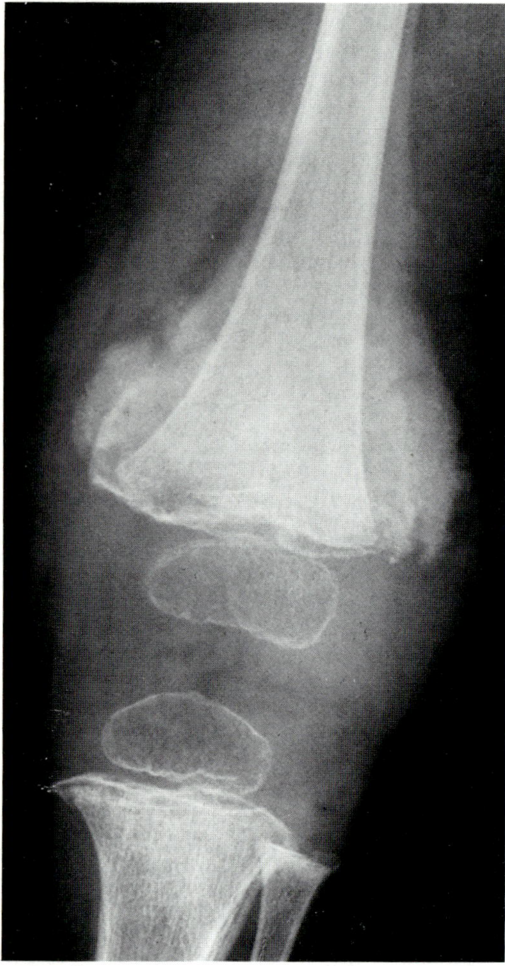

Figure 2.67. Scurvy in a child aged 3: 'halo' appearance of epiphyses, dense metaphyseal band with translucent band immediately beneath it (best seen on medial side of tibia), metaphyseal corner fractures (medial side of femur and tibia), and calcifying lower femoral subperiosteal haematomas

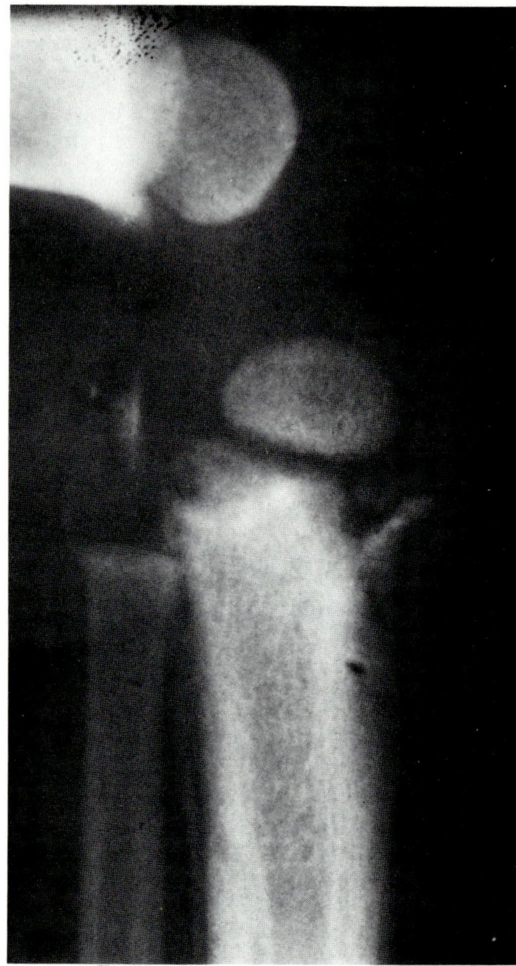

Figure 2.68. Battered baby syndrome. Metaphyseal corner fractures and subperiosteal new bone formation; in addition, there is displacement by trauma of the upper tibial epiphysis; the bone texture is normal

The radiological features of scurvy need to be distinguished from those of the battered baby syndrome. In this latter condition metaphyseal corner fractures and subperiosteal haematomas also develop. However, epiphyseal fracture separations may be present as further evidence of violent trauma, and the bone texture is normal (*Figure 2.68*).

Osteomalacia and rickets

Both of these conditions are due to a deficient mineralization of the normally formed osteoid matrix. The disorder is termed osteomalacia when it is present in the adult skeleton and rickets when it develops in childhood.

Causes

The following are the causes of osteomalacia and rickets:
1. Dietary deficiencies of vitamin D, or vitamin D and calcium, occurring in association with inadequate exposure to sunlight.
2. Disorders of malabsorption causing impaired absorption of vitamin D, or vitamin D and calcium, from the gut.
3. Certain renal disorders, including renal tubular acidosis (e.g. Fanconi's syndrome), chronic renal failure from any cause, vitamin-D resistant rickets, and hypophosphataemia.
4. Hypophosphatasia (a hereditary deficiency of the enzyme alkaline phosphatase, which is necessary for the formation of calcium phosphate).
5. Prolonged anticonvulsant therapy. These drugs induce changes in liver microsomal enzymes, leading to conversion of vitamin D to inactive metabolites.

Radiological features of osteomalacia

The distinctive radiological feature of osteomalacia is the presence of Looser's zones. These are linear translucencies, 2–3 mm wide, extending either perpendicularly or obliquely into the bone from the cortical margin. They are commonly 1–2 cm long (*Figure 2.69*). A characteristic feature of Looser's zones is that they tend to occur symmetrically on the two sides of the body. The sites most commonly affected are the necks and proximal shafts of the femora on the

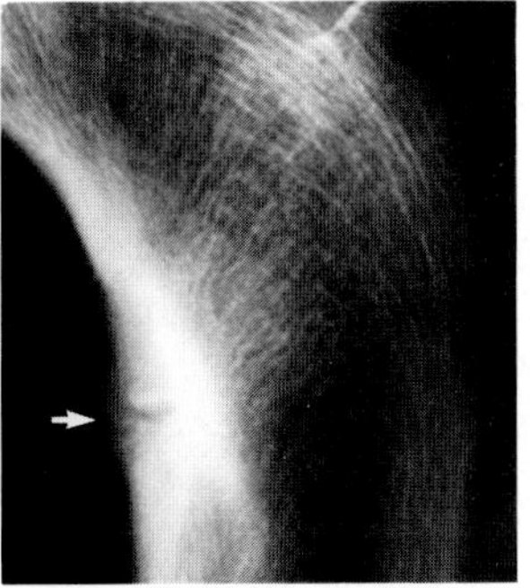

Figure 2.69. Osteomalacia with Looser's zone; horizontal transradiant zone 1 cm long across the cortex in the region of the lesser trochanter

Figure 2.70. Osteomalacia of the spine in a woman of 38, caused by dietary insufficiencies: biconcave vertebral bodies resulting from pressure on the softened bones by the discs

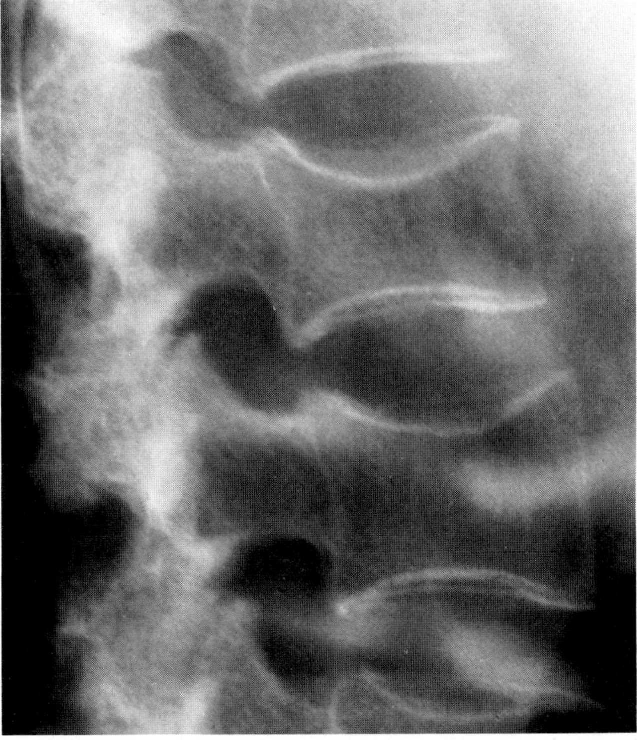

medial sides (*Figure 2.69*), the pubic rami, the lateral borders of the scapulae, and the lower ribs. It is generally accepted that Looser's zones arise from stress fractures (fractures occurring during normal activities) and that they represent seams of osteoid that have formed in the process of healing but have failed to undergo normal mineralization. In the early stages the margins of Looser's zones are ill-defined, but after several weeks or months the margins become well-defined and slightly sclerotic.

As the term osteomalacia implies, the bones are soft as a result of deficient mineralization, and bowing and other alterations of shape arising from normal forces on the skeleton constitute the second distinctive radiological feature of the condition. Thus the pelvis may acquire a triradiate rather than an oval shape, and bilateral coxa vara deformities and bowing of the lower limbs may develop from the weight of the erect body upon them. The thoracic cage becomes bell shaped due to indrawing of the lower ribs. A dorsal kyphosis develops, and the dorsal and lumbar vertebral bodies become characteristically biconcave (*Figure 2.70*). This change tends to be quite generalized in contrast to the scattered infractions of the spine seen in osteoporosis.

Accompanying these changes, the skeleton is seen to be generally poorly mineralized.

Radiological features of rickets

As in osteomalacia, radiological features indicating failure of mineralization of osteoid, and evidence of bone softening and widespread reduction in bone density, are shown in patients with rickets. Changes due to failure of mineralization of osteoid are, however, particularly marked in the growing metaphyses and epiphyses, and the distribution of deformities due to bone softening is in some respects different from that seen in the adult.

Deficient mineralization of normally formed osteoid at the bone ends results in a wide transradiant band at the metaphysis. The line of calcification adjacent to this broad band is irregular (*Figures 2.71 and 2.73*). In the wrist, crawling results in splaying and cupping of the soft distal radial and ulnar metaphyses (*Figure 2.71*). When the child starts to walk, similar metaphyseal splaying develops in the long bones of the lower limbs and is accompanied by bowing which at times is extremely pronounced. The epiphyses are small or invisible altogether as a result of defective mineralization. Other characteristic bone changes to be seen in rickets are swellings of the anterior rib ends at the costochondral junctions and bossing of the parietal region of the skull. In severe cases there is general decalcification of the bones.

Radiography is valuable not only in diagnosis. The extent of the bone changes seen in the radiographs will give evidence of the severity of the condition and will act as a record from which the response to treatment can be judged. For these purposes, a radiograph of one wrist is adequate. In rickets due to vitamin D deficiency response to treatment is rapid, and some evidence of healing may be observed in the radiograph at the end of a fortnight.

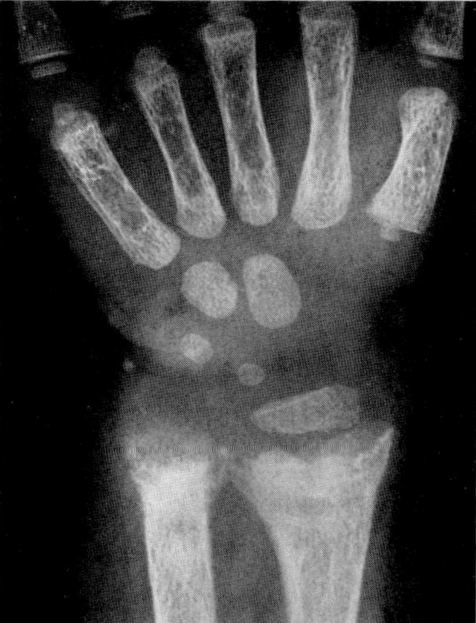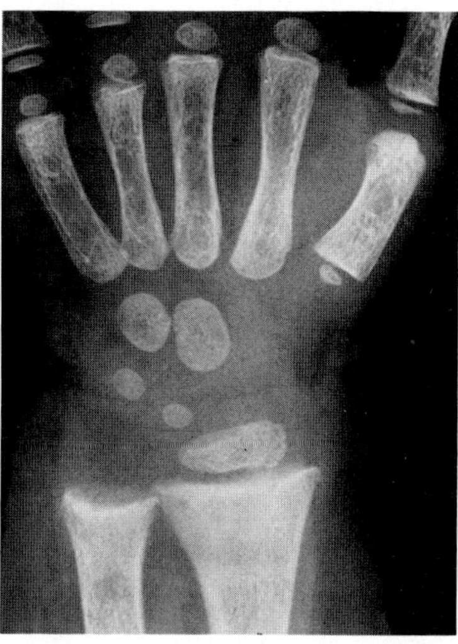

Figure 2.71. Active rickets in the wrist of a child aged 2: the metaphyses of the radius and ulna are splayed out and concave distally; the line of the provisional zone of calcification is ill-defined and irregular

Figure 2.72. The same wrist as in *Figure 2.71*, 6 weeks later, after vitamin D therapy. The metaphyses are no longer splayed out and are almost straight. The zone of calcification has reformed in a well-defined white line

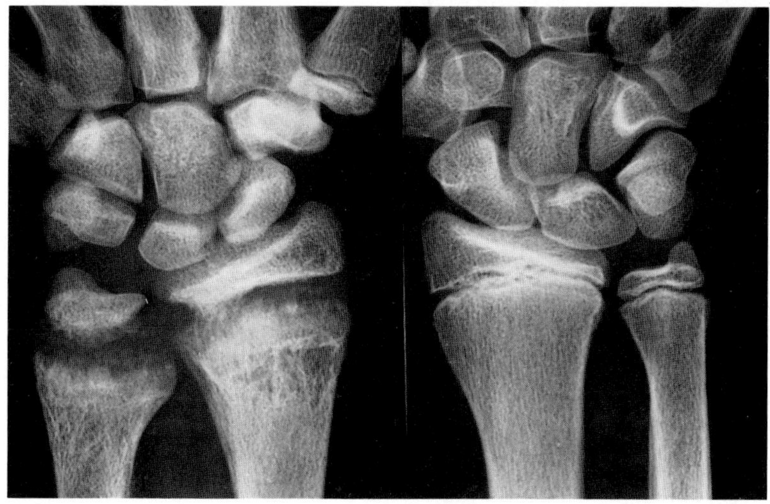

Figure 2.73. Renal rickets in a boy aged 12 (the patient's wrist on the left, that of a normal child of the same age on the right); broad transradiant band of uncalcified osteoid at metaphysis, irregular line of calcification adjacent to this

In 6 weeks healing should be almost complete and, unless there are residual bone deformities, the X-ray appearances should be normal—that is, the lower end of the radius no longer splayed out, and the metaphysis almost straight and showing normal mineralization (*Figure 2.72*).

Hyperparathyroidism

Primary hyperparathyroidism

The patient with primary hyperparathyroidism may complain of little apart from weakness and nausea until a spontaneous fracture takes place, or there may be symptoms from renal calculi, or a bone abnormality may be found in an incidental radiograph (such as a cyst-like area in a rib on routine radiography of the chest).

Hyperparathyroidism exists when there is a sustained inappropriately high secretion of parathyroid hormone. In the primary form this is usually due to a single adenoma of one of the parathyroid glands. Increased parathormone secretion results in:

1. Increased absorption of calcium by the gut.
2. Diminished renal tubular reabsorption of phosphate and increased tubular reabsorption of calcium.
3. Resorption of bone (there is in fact increased bone formation as well as bone resorption, but the net effect is one of bone resorption).

There are therefore several factors contributing to the hypercalcaemia found in hyperparathyroidism.

Radiological appearances

Only 25–35 per cent of patients with hyperparathyroidism have radiologically detectable bone disease. Typical changes include phalangeal subperiosteal cortical resorption, cyst-like transradiant areas, a coarsened trabecular pattern, and sometimes an obvious reduction in bone density.

Cortical resorption   Subperiosteal phalangeal erosions, seen particularly on the radial sides of the middle phalanges of the three middle fingers, are diagnostic of hyperparathyroidism (*Figure 2.74*). Furthermore, this is the commonest bone change to be found in primary hyperparathyroidism and is virtually always present if there are other bony manifestations of the disease, such as cyst-like areas or a coarsened trabecular pattern; the exception to this is that the subperiosteal erosions may disappear before these other changes in the healing stage.

Other common sites of cortical erosion are the outer end of the clavicle, the femoral neck on the medial side, and the medial surface of the proximal tibia (*Figure 2.75*). In the hands, erosions of the tufts of the terminal phalanges may also be present (*Figure 2.74*).

Bone cysts   Bone cysts, or 'brown tumours' of hyperparathyroidism, may be quite small or they may be large and produce considerable expansion of the bone (*Figures 2.75 and 2.76*). The margins of the cysts are well-defined but there is no surrounding white rim of sclerosis. A pathological fracture may occur through a weakened cystic area of bone. Brown tumours need to be differentiated from other conditions producing cyst-like bone lesions, e.g. fibrous dysplasia. When a bone cyst is discovered incidentally, the hands should be X-rayed: if subperiosteal erosions of the phalanges are absent, hyperparathyroidism as the cause of the cyst can virtually always be excluded.

Coarsened trabecular pattern   A coarsened trabecular pattern (*Figure 2.76*) is produced when some of the trabeculae become demineralized and thus invisible in the radiograph, while the remainder are

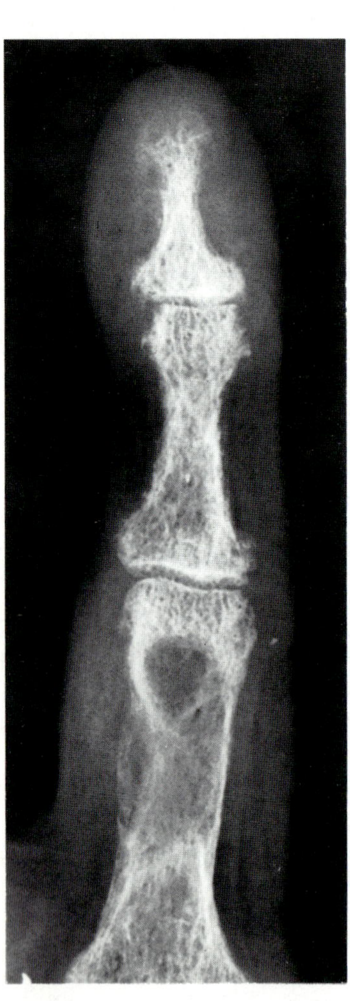

Figure 2.74. Primary hyperparathyroidism: subperiosteal erosions along shaft of middle phalanx, and erosions of tuft of terminal phalanx; brown tumour in proximal phalanx

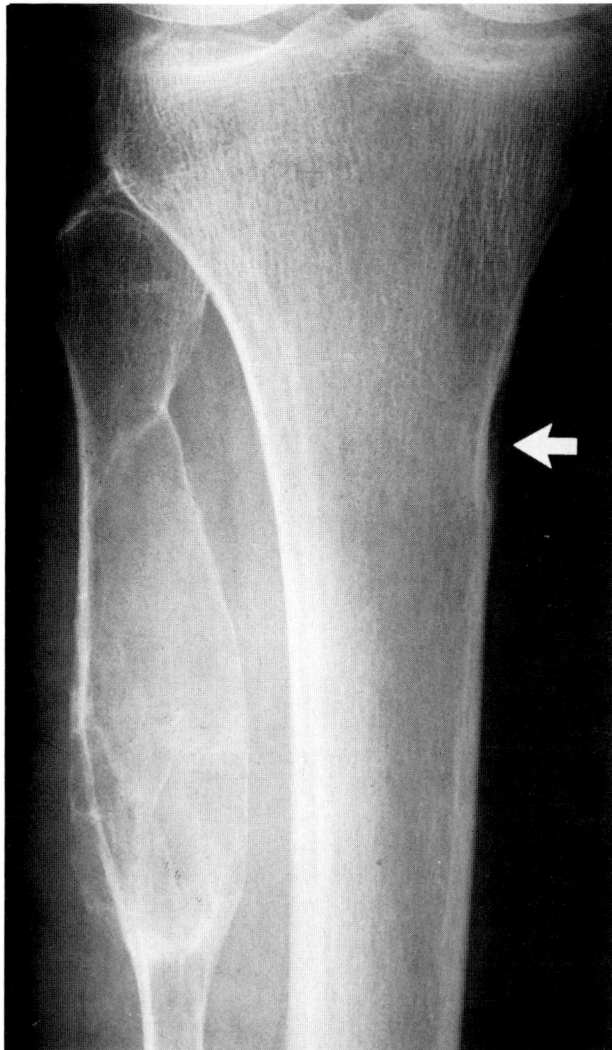

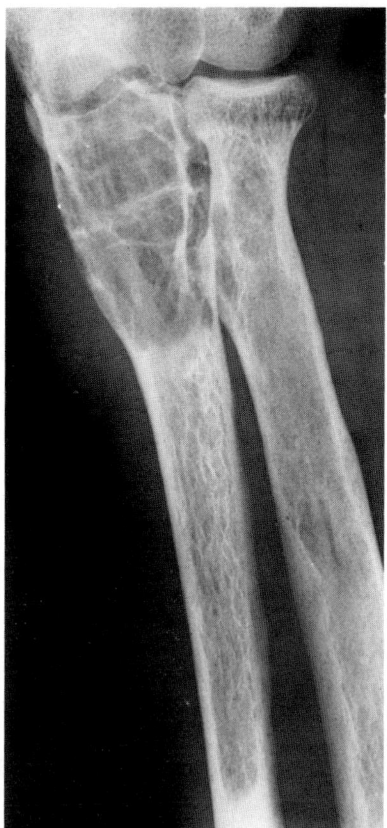

Figure 2.76. Primary hyperparathyroidism: coarse trabecular pattern shown in ulna below a brown tumour; male aged 25 years; parathyroid adenoma removed with recovery

Figure 2.75. Primary hyperparathyroidism: cyst-like lesion of fibula with expanded cortex over it; cortical erosion on medial side of proximal tibia (arrow)

widely spaced and stand out more clearly against the relatively transradiant background. In the skull, demineralization may give rise to a mottled appearance of the vault (pepperpot skull). Hyperparathyroidism may cause nephrocalcinosis and renal calculus formation. Calcification within and around joints occurs only very occasionally in the primary form of the disease.

Secondary hyperparathyroidism

Secondary hyperparathyroidism may develop in renal failure, in dietary rickets, and in conditions causing malabsorption. Parathyroid hormone secretion is increased in response to the hypocalcaemia present in these conditions, the hormone causing increased intestinal calcium absorption and resorption of calcium from bone. The increased secretion of parathyroid hormone also reduces tubular

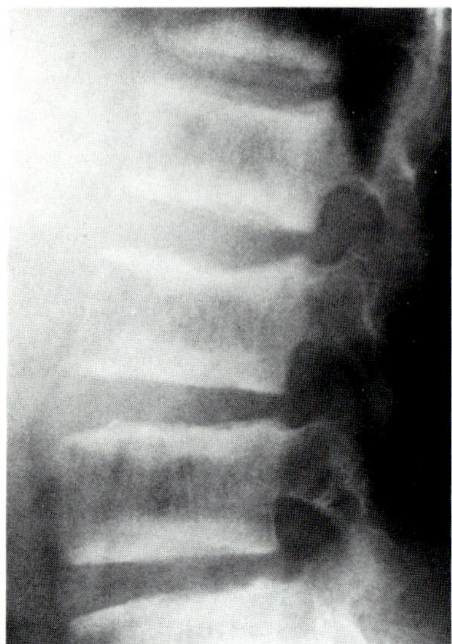

Figure 2.77. Chronic renal failure and secondary hyperparathyroidism: 'rugger-jersey' spine (sclerosis of upper and lower thirds of vertebral bodies, some demineralization of middle thirds)

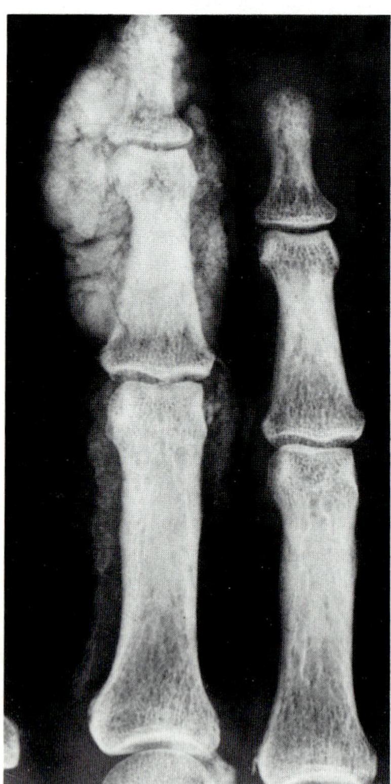

Figure 2.78. Secondary hyperparathyroidism; extensive calcification in the soft tissues

resorption of phosphate and the serum phosphate level falls, except in chronic renal failure when retention of phosphate may occur due to the reduced glomerular filtration rate. Phosphate retention, by lowering the serum calcium level still further, is an additional important factor in the development of secondary hyperparathyroidism in chronic renal disease. Usually the degree of secondary hyperparathyroidism is greater in chronic renal failure than in nutritional deficiency or malabsorption of vitamin D, and the radiological changes are correspondingly more marked.

Radiological appearances

As in the primary form of the disease, the commonest skeletal manifestation of secondary hyperparathyroidism is the presence of subperiosteal erosions, seen particularly in the middle phalanges of the fingers but also affecting the sites mentioned in the description of the primary disease. Brown tumours are less common in secondary than in primary hyperparathyroidism. In the secondary form a distinctive change may be seen in the spine, consisting of sclerosed vertebral bone ends separated by a demineralized central band (*Figure 2.77*). The descriptive term 'rugger-jersey spine' is given to this appearance. Skeletal manifestations of rickets or osteomalacia may accompany those of secondary hyperparathyroidism.

Nephrocalcinosis and renal calculi are rarer in the secondary than in the primary form of the disease. In contrast to the primary disease, soft-tissue calcification affecting particularly the subcutaneous tissues and blood vessels is a common and sometimes striking radiological feature of secondary hyperparathyroidism (*Figure 2.78*).

Bone cysts and neoplasms

Radiographs of a bone are usually indicated when there is chronic local pain, a swelling in connection with the bone, or a spontaneous fracture, suggesting the possibility of a cyst or bone tumour. On the other hand, an unsuspected cyst or tumour may be found when radiographs are taken for some other purpose.

Diagnosis from the X-ray appearances, or even from tissue obtained at biopsy, is not always easy. Accurate diagnosis of bone cysts and tumours is particularly dependent on close consultation between the clinician, radiologist and pathologist. When the differential diagnosis of a suspected bone neoplasm is being considered, the following should be taken into account:

1. Age of the patient. Many bone tumours present within well-defined age ranges, and primary malignant bone tumours and lymphomas affect in general a younger age group than do bone metastases and myeloma.
2. Sex of the patient. Sometimes useful: for example, breast carcinoma with bone metastases is exceedingly common in females, rare in males.

3. Whether the lesions are single or multiple. This information is useful in diagnosis (e.g. primary bone tumours are usually single, metastases almost invariably multiple) and in treatment.
4. Site of the lesion. Certain tumours may involve particular areas of the skeleton (e.g. metastases are confined largely to the red-marrow areas and are exceptionally rare in the extremities) or a particular site within a bone (e.g. giant-cell tumours of long bones always involve the subarticular region).

Most bone cysts and tumours produce lytic defects, but some tumours are either bone or cartilage forming or induce a sclerotic bone reaction, giving rise to areas of increased radiographic density

Table 2.1 Radiographic features of bone cysts and neoplasms

Feature	*Benign*	*Malignant*
Margin of lytic defect	Smooth and very well defined with sharp transition between abnormal and normal bone: sometimes rim of sclerosis	Hazy, 2–3 mm wide transition band between the defect and normal bone
Localized expansion of bone	Common	Rare, except sometimes in plasmacytoma and in metastases from kidney and thyroid
Overlying cortex	Thinned (discontinuous when a fracture has occurred through the weakened area of bone)	Destroyed
Periosteal new bone formation	Not a feature, except in osteoid osteoma and after a pathological fracture	Seen in some sarcomas, e.g. Ewing's sarcoma. Very uncommon in metastases
Associated soft-tissue mass	Absent	May be present, indicating extension of tumour into the adjacent soft tissues

(*see Figure 2.86*). The radiographic features shown in Table 2.1 are useful in distinguishing benign bone cysts and tumours from malignant tumours, typical examples of which are illustrated in *Figures 2.75* and *2.82* respectively.

Table 2.1 shows that the radiographic features of lytic malignant bone tumours (such as metastases, lymphomas, sarcomas and plasmacytomas) may closely resemble those of osteomyelitis. The soft-tissue mass accompanying malignant bone tumours is localized, while the swelling associated with bone infection tends to be diffuse. Differentiation between the two conditions is usually obvious on clinical grounds, but confusion may arise.

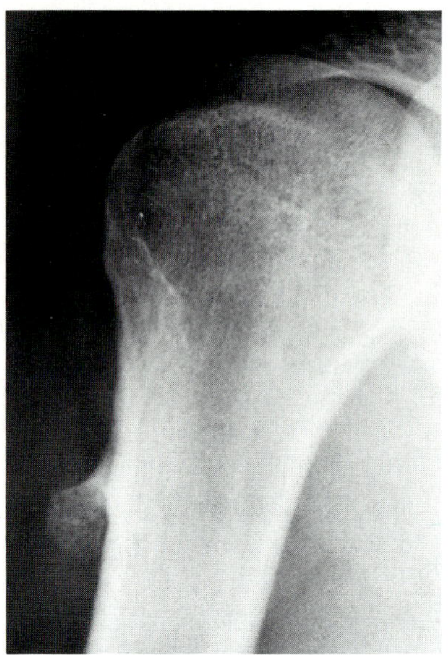

Figure 2.79. Osteochondroma: bony lump showing normal trabecular structure arising from proximal shaft of humerus; cartilage cap not calcified in this case; patient complained of painless, hard lump

Cysts and benign tumours of bone

Osteochondroma (cartilage-capped exostosis)

An osteochondroma is a common cause of a hard lump near the end of a long bone. This consists of a localized excrescence of bone covered with a cartilaginous cap. The tumour may be sessile or pedunculated, usually arises in the metaphyseal region (most commonly of the proximal humerus or around the knee), and characteristically points away from the nearby joint (*Figure 2.79*). Single or multiple lesions may be present: the latter situation is usually hereditary and termed diaphyseal aclasia. The importance of the condition is that occasionally a chondrosarcoma arises in the cartilaginous cap: the incidence of this complication is less than 1 per cent when the tumour is solitary but approximately 10 per cent in diaphyseal aclasia. Malignant change is suggested by onset of pain and a rapid increase in size.

Cystic and cyst-like bone lesions

A bone lesion containing solid material (e.g. chondroma, fibrous dysplasia, and brown tumour of hyperparathyroidism) may resemble a bone cyst in radiographic appearance. Such a lesion may be described as cyst-like. The X-ray features have already been described: sharply defined, smooth, and sometimes sclerotic margin; cortical thinning and sometimes expansion; no periosteal reaction unless a pathological fracture has occurred; no associated soft-tissue swelling (*see Figures 2.75 and 2.76*). When such a lesion is seen the following should be considered in the differential diagnosis:

1. Simple bone cyst. Usually discovered during childhood or adolescence. Commonly in the proximal metaphysis of the humerus, femur or tibia.
2. Fibrous dysplasia. In this condition fibrous tissue is laid down instead of bone. The affected area may be oval and cyst-like, or the whole region of bone may be abnormal in shape and somewhat expanded, with strands of opaque bone running across areas of transradiancy. There may be only a single lesion, or several bones may be affected. Usually there are no other clinical manifestations, but a rare form in girls is associated with precocious puberty and skin pigmentation (Albright syndrome). Common sites are the upper end of the femur or tibia, the skull and the ilium. The lesions may first be detected during childhood or adolescence; they progress to a certain size and do not increase in size when general growth ceases. Sometimes they regress in middle age. The condition is benign. A non-osteogenic fibroma may give rise to a rather similar isolated transradiant zone, demarcated by a rim of dense sclerotic bone. This benign tumour of fibrous tissue most commonly involves the metaphyses of long bones, particularly around the knee.
3. Hyperparathyroidism—*see* page 78 and *Figures 2.75 and 2.76*.
4. Brodie's and tuberculous abscesses—*see* pages 52 and 57 and *Figure 2.47*.

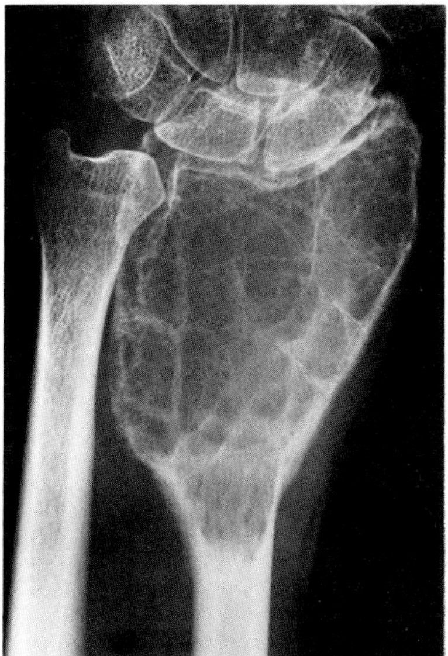

Figure 2.80. Giant-cell tumour: markedly expanding, cystic lesion of lower end of radius, crossed by coarse, bony strands giving a foam-like appearance; thinned cortex

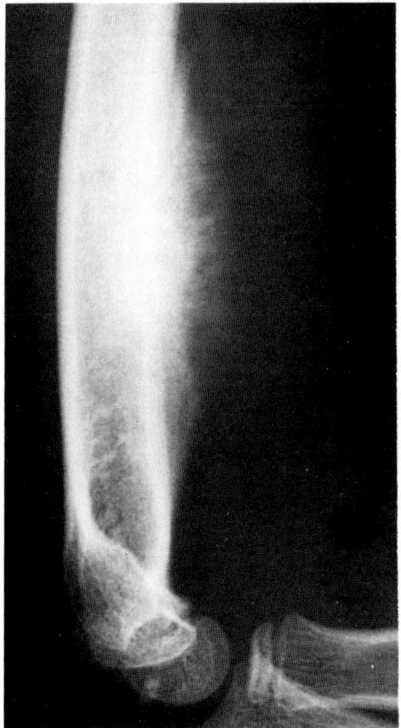

Figure 2.81. Osteosarcoma: new bone formation perpendicular to the shaft of the humerus, giving a 'sun-ray' appearance; subperiosteal new bone at proximal and distal ends of tumour

5. Chondroma. As with other tumours of cartilaginous origin a chondroma may contain flecks of calcification.
6. Benign osteoblastoma. Flecks of calcification or bone may be present within the tumour.
7. Haemangioma.

To this list should be added the following four tumours which characteristically involve the ends of long bones and which may produce considerable bone expansion.

8. Giant-cell tumour. Occurs at ages 20–40, i.e. found only after epiphyseal fusion. Characteristic subarticular location, usually in long bones. Bone expansion (*Figure 2.80*). Locally malignant, so hazy margin and adjacent soft-tissue mass may be present.
9. Aneurysmal bone cyst. Occurs at ages 10–30, i.e. before or after epiphyseal fusion. Arises in shafts of long bones and may extend to subarticular region after epiphyseal fusion. Also found in axial skeleton. Entirely benign. Well-defined margins. Degree of bone expansion sometimes very considerable.
10. Chondroblastoma. Occurs at ages 10–20. Most arise in epiphyseal plate, and involve both sides of plate. As with other cartilaginous tumours, chondroblastomas may contain flecks of calcification.
11. Chondromyxoid fibroma. Occurs at ages 20–30. Occurs in metaphyseal regions and may extend to epiphyses. Resembles aneurysmal bone cysts.

Cystic expansion, but often with the obvious radiographic hallmarks of malignancy (*see* above) may also be found in plasmacytoma and in some secondary tumours, e.g. metastases from kidney and thyroid.

Malignant bone tumours

The general radiographic features of malignant bone tumours have been described on page 81. Metastases account for the great majority of these tumours.

Primary bone sarcomas

These tumours in general involve a younger age group than do secondary deposits: osteosarcomas and Ewing's tumours usually present during childhood or young adulthood, and fibrosarcomas most commonly occur in adults in their thirties. The exceptions are chondrosarcomas, which develop during middle age, and sarcomas complicating Paget's disease.

Fibrosarcomas are usually purely destructive and radiologically resemble lytic metastases. Chondrosarcomas, in addition to the typical destructive changes, may contain areas of calcification, and osteosarcomas areas of calcification and ossification (*Figure 2.81*). In the latter condition, numerous spicules of new bone may be laid down in the soft tissues at right angles to the bone surface, which gives a 'sunray' appearance, or periosteal new bone formation may occur along the shaft adjacent to the tumour.

Ewing's sarcomas may present in long or flat bones. In long bones, the midshafts are typically involved, mottled or more confluent poorly defined areas of destruction are seen and a periosteal reaction which may be laminated giving the appearance of an onion skin may be present. The appearances can be radiologically indistinguishable from those of osteomyelitis. Ewing's sarcoma generally presents between the ages of 10 and 25: entirely similar appearances are seen in metastatic neuroblastoma in children under 3 years of age, and in reticulum-cell sarcoma in patients aged 20–40.

Secondary deposits in bone

When a patient is known to be suffering from a malignant neoplasm in some part of the body, the occurrence of pain in a bone area, or a spontaneous fracture, is an indication for radiology and sometimes for an isotope bone scan. While primary carcinomas of most tissues may metastasize to bone, secondary bone deposits from tumours of

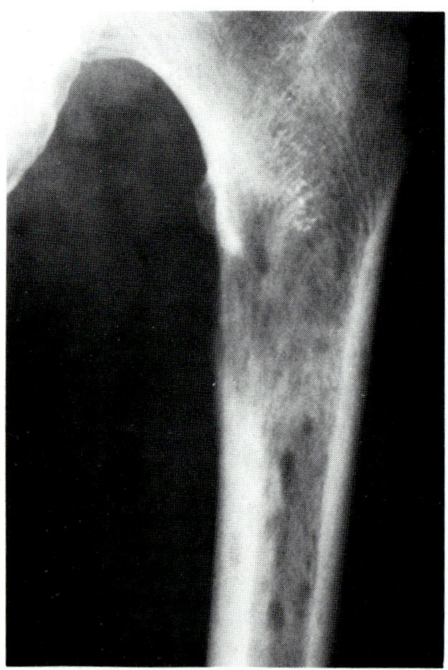

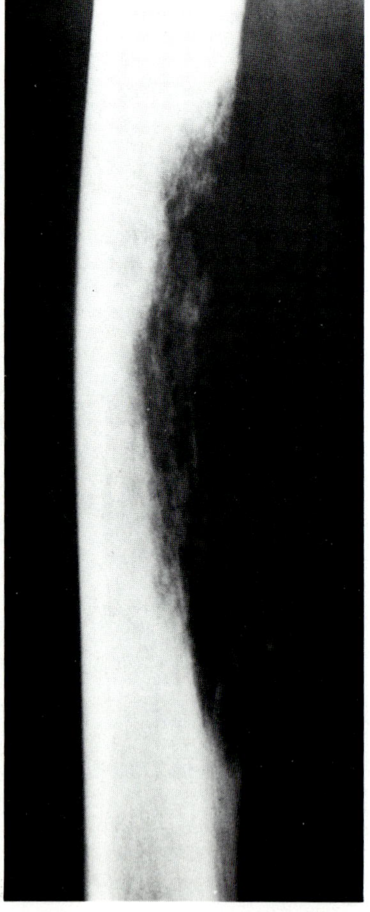

Figure 2.82. Lytic metastasis in left femur: bone destruction in proximal shaft with ill-defined margin and without any sclerotic rim; cortex destroyed on medial side; primary bronchial carcinoma

Figure 2.83. Lytic metastasis in right femur: very large, purely destructive lesion with ill-defined margin; no reactive sclerosis or periosteal reaction; primary bronchial carcinoma

the bronchus, breast, prostate, kidney and thyroid are particularly common.

Sometimes secondary deposits are found in a bone when radiographs are being taken for some other purpose and no primary tumour can be discovered on routine clinical investigation. In such cases a radiograph of the chest should be obtained, since the primary tumour may be an asymptomatic bronchial carcinoma. An intravenous urogram may also be helpful, since an occult renal-cell carcinoma is sometimes the source of such deposits. In the absence of gastrointestinal symptoms or positive faecal occult bloods, barium investigation of the gastrointestinal tract for a possible primary tumour of the gut is almost invariably unrewarding and should not be undertaken. Ultrasound or computed tomography examination of the pancreas occasionally discloses an asymptomatic tumour of the body or tail.

The characteristic X-ray appearances of a lytic metastasis have already been described: an area of bone destruction with ill-defined margins and a 2–3 mm wide zone of transition between the erosion and the normal bone; no surrounding rim of sclerosis; cortical destruction without periosteal reaction; and sometimes a soft-tissue mass (*Figures 2.82 and 2.83*). A secondary deposit is at times indistinguishable radiologically from a primary malignant bone neoplasm.

Metastases in the spine most commonly involve the pedicles and vertebral bodies. The pedicles are clearly seen on the anteroposterior view as paired oval shadows lying on either side of the midline, superimposed on the shadows of the vertebral bodies. Each pair of pedicles should be carefully examined in turn for any evidence of destruction or sclerosis (*Figure 2.84*). In the presence of a scoliosis, the pedicles on the inner aspect of the spinal curvature are often invisible on the anteroposterior view: this should not be misinterpreted as an indication of bone destruction.

A metastasis in a vertebral body typically causes destruction of the trabeculae and cortex, and a compression fracture of the weakened bone (*Figure 2.85*). The tumour very rarely spreads to the discs, so that the adjoining disc spaces are preserved. This is a useful point in differentiating a metastasis from infection of the spine: infection spreads readily from the initial focus in a vertebral body to destroy the adjacent disc, resulting in disc-space narrowing (*see Figure 2.56*). It is sometimes less easy to distinguish between a vertebral body metastasis and osteoporotic vertebral collapse. In a metastasis, however, frank bone destruction with loss of continuity of the cortical white line may be seen (*Figure 2.85*), one or both of the pedicles of the affected vertebra may be destroyed, and the texture of the skeleton may elsewhere be normal. In osteoporotic vertebral collapse, on the other hand, the cortical margin—although locally fractured—is complete, the pedicles are preserved, and the skeleton shows a generalized reduction in density (*see Figure 2.66*).

Certain bone metastases engender an osteoblastic bone reaction, resulting in areas of increased density in the radiograph, or a combination of lytic and sclerotic deposits may be present (*Figure 2.86*). By far the commonest causes of these appearances are prostatic carcinoma in male patients and breast carcinoma in female

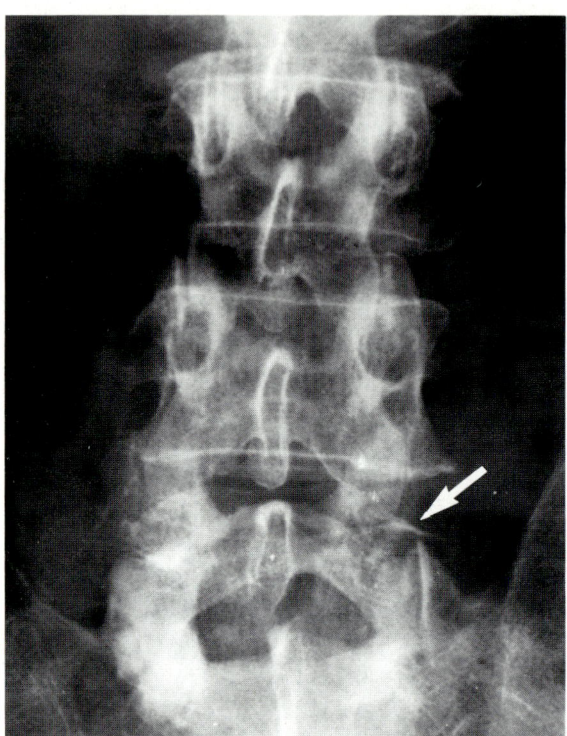

Figure 2.84. Metastasis in left pedicle of fifth lumbar vertebra. This pedicle is destroyed (arrow), while the right pedicle of L5 and the paired pedicles of L3 and L4 are clearly visible

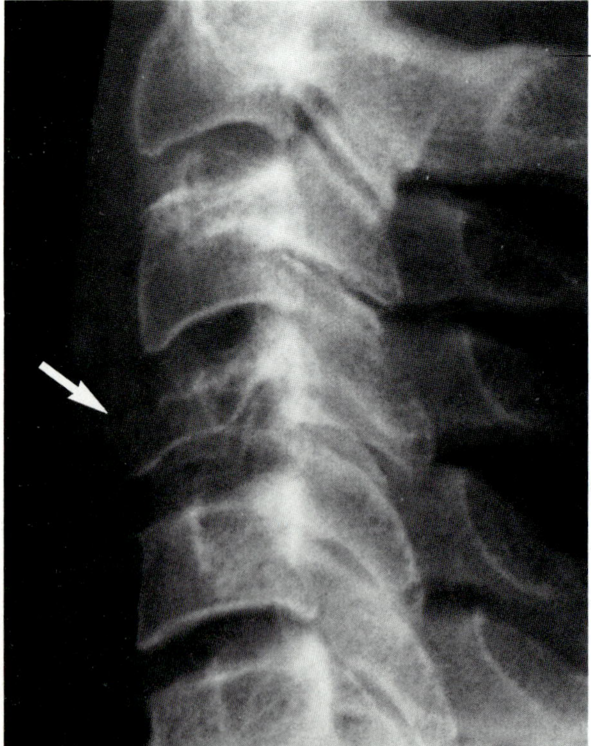

Figure 2.85. Metastasis of body of fourth cervical vertebra: pathological compression fracture with obvious bone destruction (loss of the cortical white line anteriorly and anterosuperiorly—arrow); no narrowing of adjacent disc spaces

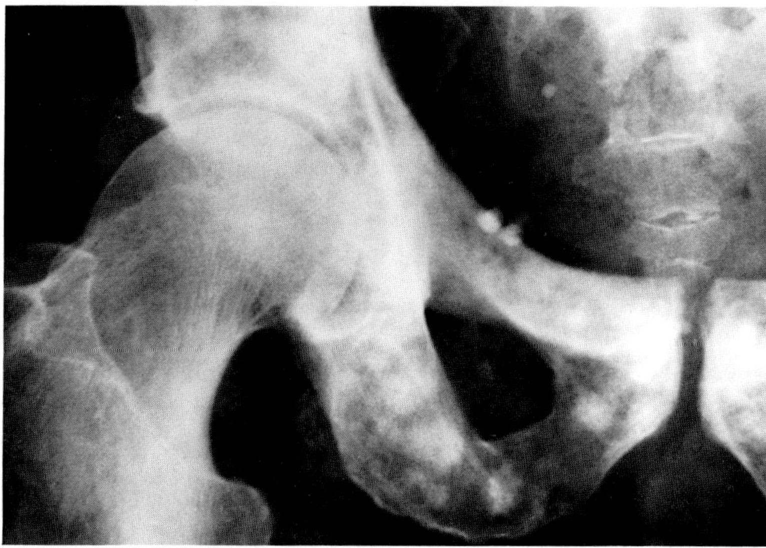

Figure 2.86. Secondary deposits in the pelvis (osteoblastic type): areas of increased density; no cortical thickening; primary prostatic carcinoma (The two opacities overlying the inner pelvic rim are phleboliths in the soft tissues.)

patients. Uncommonly, secondary deposits from other primary carcinomas (including bronchus, bladder, pancreas, stomach and colon) and carcinoid tumours of the alimentary tract may give rise to osteoblastic metastases.

Bone lesions in lymphoma may be lytic, sclerotic or a mixture of the two. While the radiographic appearances can be indistinguishable from those of metastases, the patient with lymphoma is often in a considerably younger age group. Myelosclerosis also engenders an osteoblastic bone reaction: a plain film of the abdomen will show gross enlargement of the spleen in this condition.

The radiographic features of sclerotic metastases must be distinguished from those of Paget's disease. The latter can usually be readily recognized by the distinctive cortical thickening, bone enlargement, bone softening, and alteration of trabecular structure (*see Figure 2.91*). Since Paget's disease and prostatic carcinoma are conditions of old age, both may coexist in the same patient.

In destructive types of deposit, some recalcification may occur subsequent to radiotherapy or endocrine therapy. This usually commences 2 or 3 months after treatment has been started. After stilboestrol therapy for osteoblastic secondary deposits from prostatic carcinoma, there is usually little change in the radiological appearances of the bones.

Bone metastases are more accurately detected by isotope bone scan than by radiographs, and sometimes the scan provides the only evidence of bone disease (*Figure 2.87*). Since the isotope scan is non-specific (*see* page 11) radiographs must be taken of regions of scan abnormality. These radiographs may show the typical appearances of bone metastases, confirming the diagnosis, or they may show 'hot' areas attributable to other causes such as degenerative joint disease. When the radiographs are entirely normal, it can reasonably be assumed that multiple 'hot spots' on the scan in a patient with a known primary carcinoma indicate the presence of bone metastases.

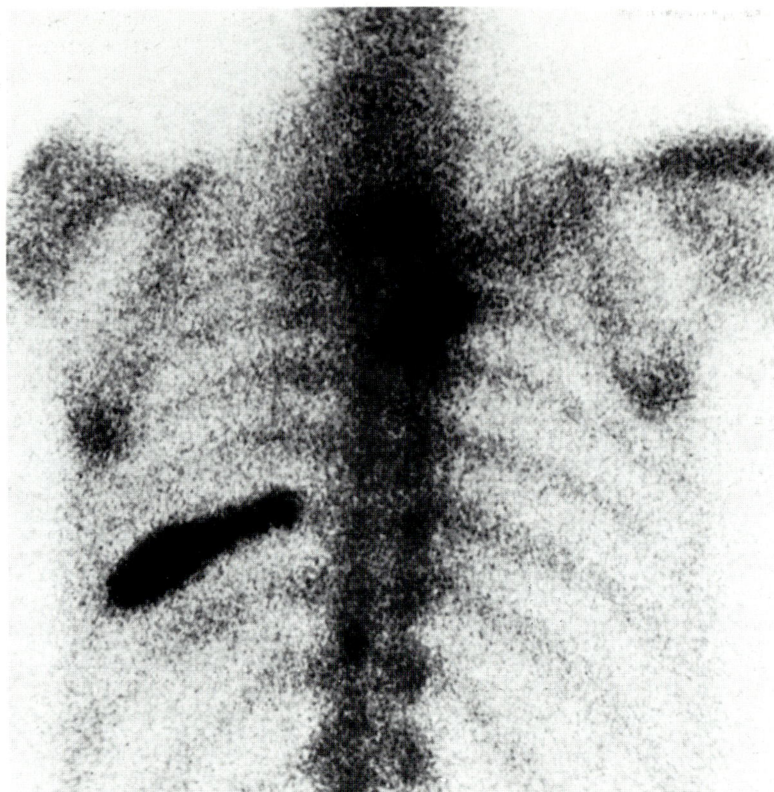

Figure 2.87. Radioisotope bone scan (posterior scan, gamma-camera recording): 'hot spots' due to metastases shown in upper dorsal vertebrae, eleventh dorsal vertebra, and left ninth rib; no X-ray abnormality at time of examination, but bone destruction shown on radiographs 2 months later; primary bronchial carcinoma

Myeloma

Multiple myeloma can simulate carcinomatosis radiologically but is distinguishable from it by the absence of a known primary lesion and the presence of Bence Jones proteins in the urine, an abnormal serum electrophoretic pattern with excess of gamma globulin, and myeloma cells in a marrow biopsy sample. The eroded areas are usually small, 2–5 mm in size (*Figures 2.88* and *2.89*), but occasionally a few isolated larger areas of erosion are seen.

A common presenting symptom in a person aged over 55 is persistent lower dorsal backache. Lateral view radiographs may show diffuse trabecular loss with or without compression of one or several vertebrae (*Figure 2.90*), an appearance similar to that of spinal osteoporosis from any cause. In such cases, typical well-defined 5 mm erosions may be visible in the skull or pelvis, suggesting the condition.

Occasionally a large isolated erosion with cortical expansion is seen in a single bone, when the lesion may be referred to as a plasmacytoma. In most of these cases generalized myelomatosis develops at a later date, sometimes only after an interval of several years. Very occasionally the bone lesions of myeloma are sclerotic.

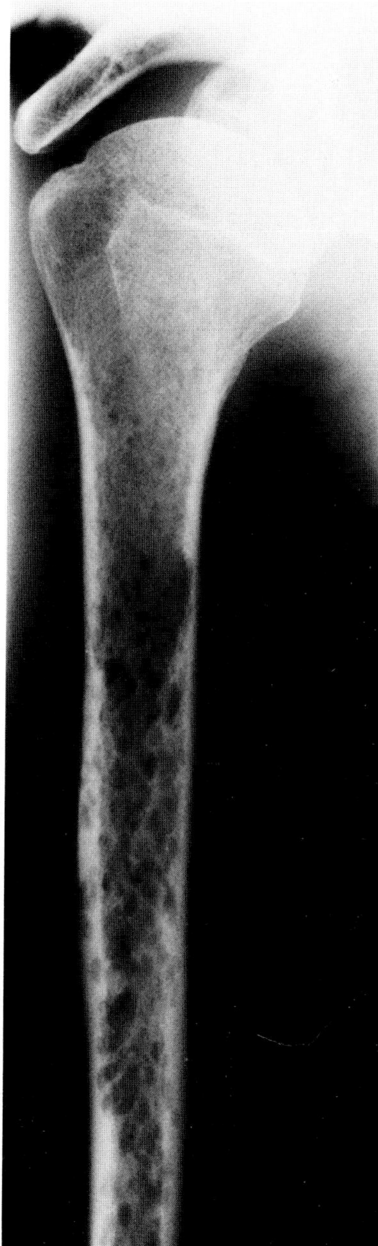

Figure 2.88. Myeloma: multiple 2–5 mm diameter well-defined lytic lesions in shaft of humerus; no rim of sclerosis

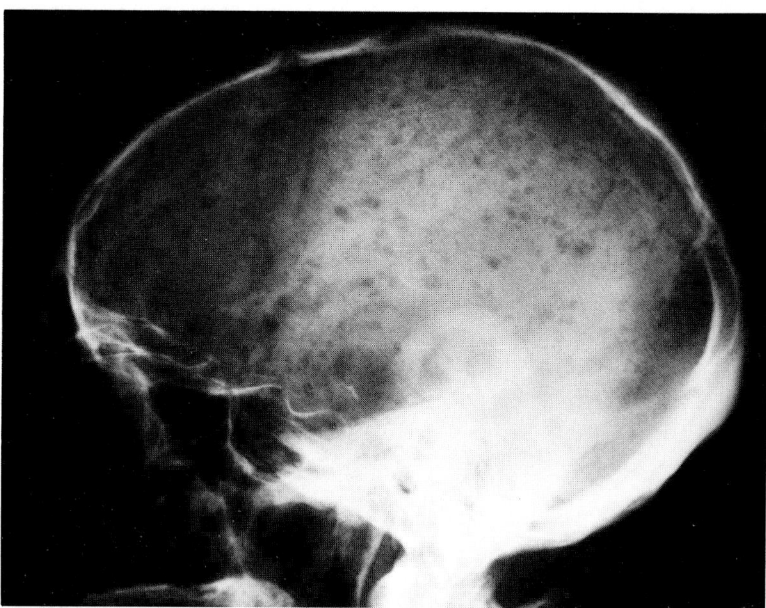

Figure 2.89. Myeloma: lesions in skull are well defined, as if 'punched out'; same patient as in *Figure 2.88*

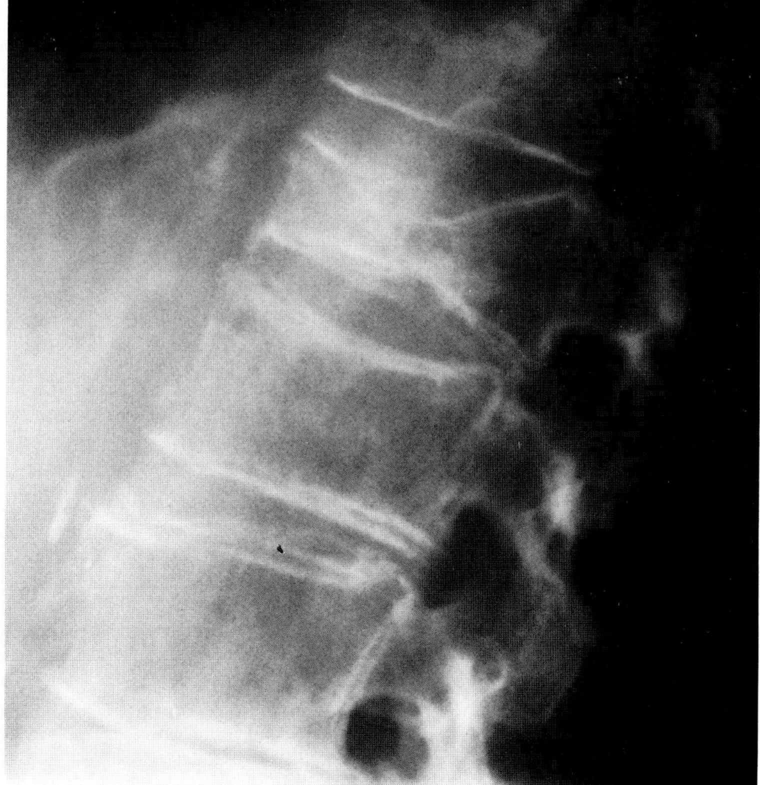

Figure 2.90. Myeloma affecting spine: generalized demineralization with collapse of the twelfth dorsal and first lumbar vertebral bodies

Paget's disease

An elderly patient suffering from Paget's disease may complain of a slight pain in the bones, bowing of the legs with increasing kyphosis, and sometimes enlargement of the head. More commonly, there are no symptoms and the condition is discovered incidentally from radiographs taken for some other purpose.

There are four characteristic X-ray features of Paget's disease:
1. Thickening of the cortex, producing enlargement of the affected bone (*Figures 2.91 and 2.92*). This feature, which is usually very obvious, is of the utmost value in differentiating Paget's disease

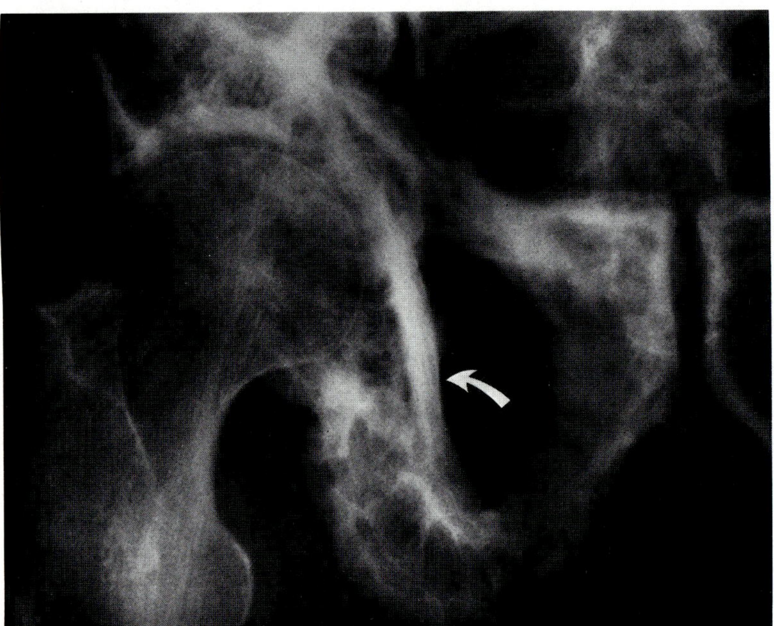

Figure 2.91. Paget's disease of the pelvis: the cortex is thickened (arrow), causing enlargement of the bone; the pattern of the trabeculae is coarse and irregular

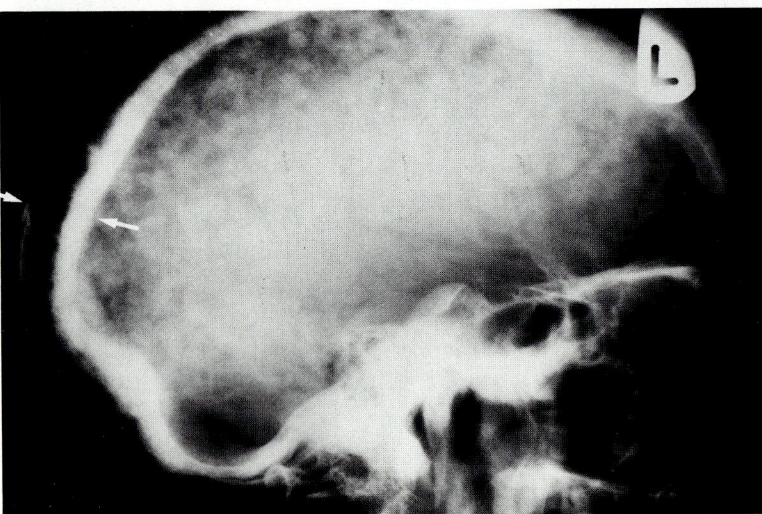

Figure 2.92. Paget's disease of the skull: there is characteristic thickening of the vault (arrows); mixed lytic and sclerotic areas are present

from other common causes of mixed lytic and sclerotic bone lesions, e.g. metastases from prostatic carcinoma (*see Figure 2.86*).

2. Bone softening, causing bowing of the femur and tibia, protrusio acetabuli, kyphosis and basilar impression.
3. Mixed lytic and sclerotic areas (*Figure 2.92*).
4. Development of a very coarse trabecular pattern (*Figure 2.91*). This is also a useful feature in differentiating Paget's disease from sclerotic metastases.

Not all of the above changes may be present: deformity due to bone softening, for example, may not be evident, or the lesions may be entirely lytic with no radiographic evidence of sclerosis in the early stages.

Several bones are usually affected but the condition may be confined to a single bone such as the clavicle. The pelvis is the most common site of Paget's disease. The distribution of the lesions within a bone is variable. The whole of the long bone, or only the distal or proximal parts, may be affected. Virtually without exception, Paget's disease involves, and extends in continuity from, the subarticular region of a long bone: the diagnosis should be seriously questioned if changes are seen in the midshaft only. Sometimes only one vertebra is affected. This will appear denser than normal, and will be flattened, but it will also show an increase in width that will serve to distinguish the appearances from a sclerosing secondary deposit.

Associated bony lipping of the joint margins is often seen, especially around flattened vertebrae, or in the hips when the femora are bowed.

A primary osteosarcoma is found more often in a bone affected by Paget's disease than in a normal bone, and may show in a radiograph as an area of ill-defined erosion with occasional faint sun-ray linear calcifications projecting out at right angles to the cortex into a soft-tissue mass.

The bones tend to be rather brittle, and transverse rather than oblique fractures may occur. Union is usually satisfactory. Sometimes pseudo-fractures are seen, identical histologically and in radiological appearance to Looser's zones of osteomalacia (*see Figure 2.69*). The common sites for these in Paget's disease are along the convex outer surfaces of bowed weight-bearing bones.

The soft tissues

Foreign bodies

Radio-opacity of foreign bodies

Foreign bodies containing atoms of relatively high atomic weight are usually clearly visible on X-ray examination. Fragments of iron, even if no larger than 0.5 mm, can be seen. Foreign bodies will, of course, be more clearly detectable through thin parts, such as the palm, than through denser and thicker parts, such as the abdomen. Particular care is required in examining the tissues overlying bone, as small foreign bodies are least easy to see when superimposed on dense skeletal structures.

Non-opaque foreign bodies, with a density much the same as that of skin and muscle, will not be directly visible even if they are quite large. In this group are included wood splinters and thorns, cartilage such as fishbones (these may calcify, however, and thus be opaque), swabs, aluminium, and plastics (such as buttons, thimbles and dentures). So-called 'lead' pencils are made of wood and graphite and are relatively non-opaque. Glass fragments show much variation in their radio-opacity, depending on whether they contain a small percentage of lead; those that contain none at all are usually invisible. Brick and stone fragments are often only moderately opaque. Most rubber tubes and bands are non-opaque unless they are specially impregnated with substances containing atoms of high atomic weight.

If an object similar to the suspected foreign body is available—such as the other half of a broken denture, a similar button, or another piece of the broken glass—it should be examined for radio-opacity through the part of the patient in which the foreign body is suspected of being lodged. It is no use taking a radiograph of the test object without intervening tissue of suitable density, for even a rose petal can be demonstrated radiologically if there are no substances except air between the film and the X-ray tube. If the object is found to be opaque, and yet no opaque foreign body can be seen in the suspected area, the diagnosis of a foreign body can be confidently excluded.

In some locations and in favourable circumstances, non-opaque foreign bodies may be demonstrated radiologically by indirect methods (*see* below, pages 93 and 95).

Localization of radio-opaque foreign bodies

An opaque foreign body may need to be localized radiologically in relation to nearby anatomical structures or to a marked point on the skin surface. Localization relative to nearby structures, unless they are bony ones, may be very difficult; in the case of nerves, it is impossible by radiological means. Relationship to the viscera can sometimes be demonstrated by outlining the latter with a contrast medium; possible damage to the viscera caused by the transit of the foreign body through the tissue can also be revealed in this way.

Localizing in relation to a mark on the skin surface is usually easy and accurate. The various methods of achieving this fall within the province of the radiologist and need not be described here. Whatever means are used, the following precautions should be observed: radiographs should be taken with the part positioned in the same way as it will be at operation; care must be taken to see that the mark on the skin is not obliterated by skin sterilization at operation; the interval between localization and removal must be as short as possible, since the foreign body may change its position in the meantime on account of muscle movements, or may erode into a blood vessel or hollow viscus; and a mobile X-ray unit should be available so that localization can be checked rapidly and efficiently during the operation if necessary. Foreign bodies should be removed in the operating theatre under suitable aseptic conditions and not in the X-ray department.

Swallowed foreign bodies in the alimentary tract

A radiological examination is indicated whenever a patient is suspected of having swallowed an object that might have become impacted in the oesophagus or lower in the alimentary tract. The examination should be carried out as soon as possible. The radiologist should be informed of the nature of the object that may have been swallowed, and if there is any doubt as to its radio-opacity he should be given a test object (such as a similar button, or the other half of a broken denture) if one is available.

A radio-opaque swallowed foreign body, lodged in the oesophagus, will be seen in a plain radiograph. A lateral view will be required to confirm that a foreign body in the neck lies within the oesophagus and not in the trachea. If there is doubt as to whether an opaque foreign body is actually within the oesophagus, this can be dispelled by a barium examination; swallowed barium will be seen to surround the object if it lies in the oesophageal lumen.

A non-opaque foreign body in the oesophagus can be demonstrated only by a barium swallow examination. If the opaque barium is diverted round it a constant transradiant zone will mark the position of the body, or the barium may adhere to it, leaving residues of barium after the main column has passed on into the stomach. A small sharp object, which cannot be demonstrated by any other means, may sometimes be revealed by getting the patient to swallow pellets of cotton wool soaked in barium. The passage of these may be seen on fluorscopy to be temporarily arrested at the level of the foreign body.

A swallowed opaque body in the abdomen may be watched radiologically from day to day as it travels through the intestine. If it is detained in the stomach for more than 2 days the interval between each X-ray observation can be increased to 3 or more days. If it should remain in the same area for an unduly long time its exact site may be demonstrated on barium meal and follow-through examination, although the stomach or colon is often sufficiently well outlined by swallowed air in the plain radiograph for the position of the opaque object to be inferred. A final radiograph should always be taken in the theatre just before any operation for removal of a foreign body in the abdomen in case of a recent alteration in its position.

Inhaled foreign bodies in the bronchi

If the patient is suspected of having inhaled a foreign body radiological search is indicated as early as possible, however indefinite the history or small the foreign body, and before any symptoms have appeared.

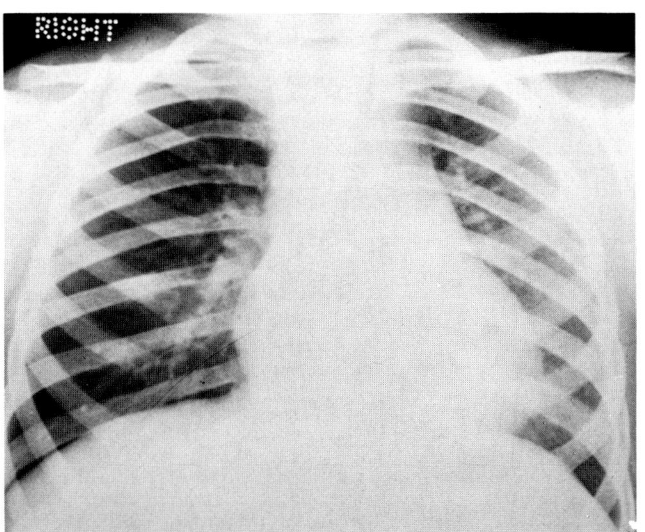

Figure 2.93. Peanut in right main bronchus (inspiration). The right lung is more transradiant than the left, and the vessels are smaller; later bronchoscopic removal, and thereafter equal transradiancy and vessel size

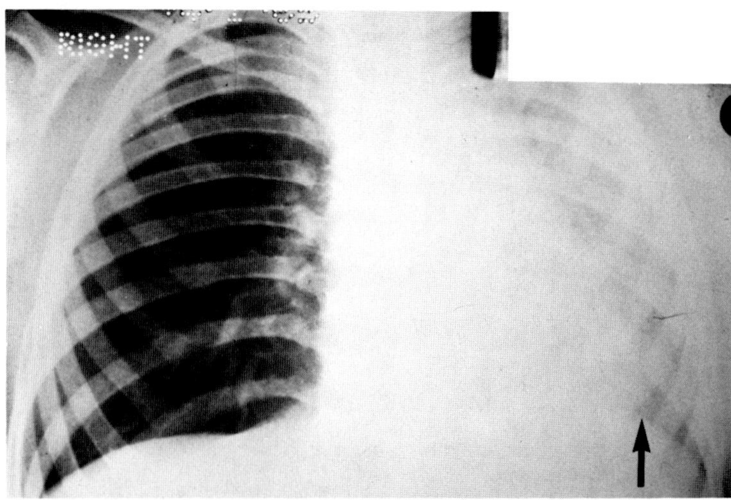

Figure 2.94. The same case as in *Figure 2.93* (expiration). Arrow marks the left dome, which has moved upwards more than the right; normal deflation and opacity of the left lung. The heart is moved to the left by air trapping on the right side, which remains transradiant

A radio-opaque object lodged in the trachea or in a bronchus will be seen in a plain radiograph, and its exact position can usually be shown if both anterior and lateral views are taken. If it is small and of relatively low density (as in the case of a tooth fragment) fluoroscopy as well as plain radiographs may be necessary to demonstrate its presence.

Sometimes tomography is helpful, especially in differentiating an inhaled piece of tooth from a calcified gland near the bronchus. When the foreign body is non-opaque its presence can be suspected if there is a homogeneous shadow with fissure displacement, indicating a lobar or segmental atelectasis, or if there is some ill-defined patchy clouding from distal consolidation.

Occasionally, a peanut or similar non-opaque object will act as a check valve, air passing the foreign body as the bronchus widens on inspiration but becoming trapped early in expiration as the bronchial calibre is reduced. The lung or one lobe will then show vessel narrowing due to diminished blood flow and will be slightly more transradiant than the other side (*Figure 2.93*); this effect is much accentuated in a radiograph taken on expiration, the normal side then becoming less transradiant as it deflates (*Figure 2.94*) but the affected side remaining unchanged. In some cases there are no radiological abnormalities, and bronchoscopy should therefore never be withheld solely on account of a negative radiological examination.

Penetrating foreign bodies in the thorax

An object in the thorax often cannot be localized with sufficient accuracy from anterior and lateral view radiographs, and fluoroscopy is often very helpful for this purpose. If the foreign body is near the periphery it may be particularly important to decide whether it is in the lung or in the chest wall. A foreign body in the lower half of the lungs will tend to move downwards on deep inspiration and upwards on expiration, while one in the intercostal tissues will do the reverse. Also, by rotating the patient it is usually possible at one stage, when the foreign body is seen tangentially, to establish whether it is in the lung.

Non-opaque foreign bodies in wounds

When a sinus track persists after an extensive wound or at operation and it is suspected that there may be a non-opaque foreign body (such as a swab or piece of clothing) at the bottom of the track, it may be possible to confirm the suspicion by an injection of iodized oil into the sinus. If the foreign body absorbs the oil it will show a characteristic opaque pattern on X-ray examination.

Foreign bodies in the eye

When a radio-opaque body is believed to be lodged in the eye a radiological examination may be indicated to confirm its presence and localize it in relation to the cornea. Fragments in the eye needing radiological confirmation are likely to be very small. Steel fragments will be visible in the radiographs even if they are no larger than 0.5 mm, but objects of lower atomic weight—such as certain alloys, brick, cement or radio-opaque glass—will not be visible unless they are larger. Foreign bodies in the eye that are not radio-opaque cannot be demonstrated radiologically.

The combination of anterior and lateral view radiographs may give undoubted evidence of the presence of a foreign body in the eye, or may exclude a radio-opaque foreign body. If a shadow is seen, and there is some doubt whether it represents an object actually in the eye or one just outside it, a further X-ray examination can be made relating the shadow to the eye movements. For this purpose two anterior view radiographs are taken whilst the patient keeps his head absolutely still, the eye (but not the head) being turned to the right for the first exposure and to the left for the second; if a lateral view radiograph is being taken the eye must be turned upwards and downwards for the two exposures. If the foreign body is in the eye it will be seen in two positions in the developed radiograph; whereas if it is in the lid or extraorbital tissue, it will be seen in the same position, having remained stationary during the two exposures. When the patient looks left or down, the shadow cast by a body in the anterior half of the eye will move left or down; but if in the posterior half of the eye, it will move right or up.

For any radiological test relating the image of a foreign body to the movement of the eye it is essential that the patient should be in a co-operative state and able to keep his head and eye still during the exposures and to turn the affected eye in the required direction. Such tests may be impracticable if multiple fragments are present in the eye, since identification of any single fragment in the two exposures may be impossible.

Soft-tissue calcification

Arterial calcification, shown on the radiograph as linear or tubular shadows, is commonly seen in the elderly in the walls of the aorta and other large arteries such as the iliac, femoral, splenic and carotid. In diabetes the extent of arterial calcification may be striking (*see Figure 2.98*), affecting even the small vessels of the extremities. Phleboliths, which represent thrombosed veins, can be seen within the pelvis in most adults. These appear on the radiograph as circular or oval opacities, commonly with a tiny central translucency (*see Figure 2.86*). This last feature is sometimes helpful in distinguishing between phleboliths and lower ureteric calculi.

Post-traumatic soft-tissue calcification and ossification have already been discussed (*see* page 25 and *Figures 2.8* and *2.9*), as has calcification in the supraspinatus tendon (*see* page 27 and *Figure 2.10*). Calcification may develop in gouty tophi around affected joints (*see* page 67) and calcification in the soft tissues is a common feature of secondary hyperparathyroidism (*see* page 80 and *Figure 2.78*). The radiographic appearances of calcification in children or adolescents with dermatomyositis may be quite singular: at times the body appears virtually encased by linear calcium deposits in the soft tissues (*Figure 2.95*).

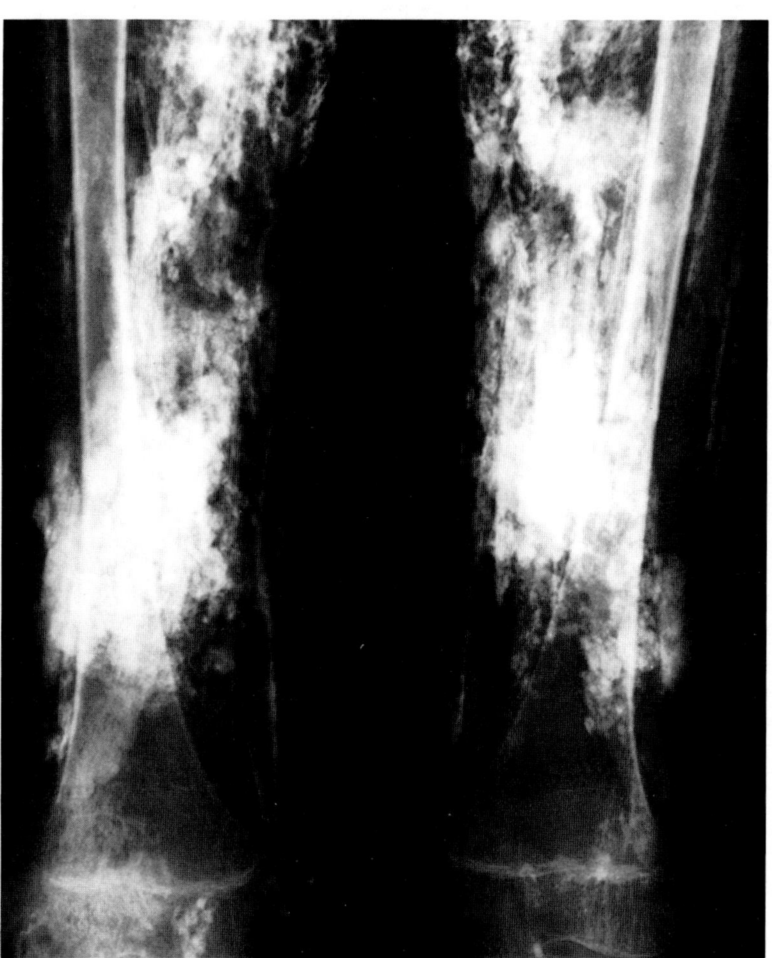

Figure 2.95. Dermatomyositis in an adolescent girl; massive calcification in the soft tissues of the thighs, in places forming linear bands

Tuberculosis is such a common cause of pathological calcification within the organs and tissues of the body that the possibility of this diagnosis should be considered whenever abnormal calcification is seen. While calcification occurs during the healing phase of the disease, adjacent areas of active infection often coexist. In the soft tissues, calcification may be found in tuberculous abscesses (*see Figure 2.55*), or in cervical, axillary or other lymph nodes.

Several parasites may calcify after they die in the soft tissues, and give rise to diagnostic appearances. The dead cysts of cysticercosis

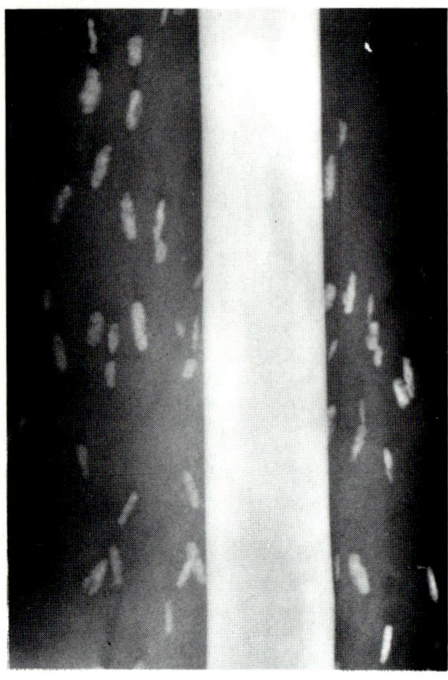

Figure 2.96. Cysticercosis; numerous calcified cysts in the soft tissues of the thigh

produce characteristic multiple oval opacities, approximately 1 cm by 2–3 mm, within the muscles and in general aligned in the directions of the muscle fibres (*Figure 2.96*). The female guinea worm may show as a coiled thread, 2 or 3 mm wide and up to 1 m long, beaded along its length and often seen in the leg. The coiled loa-loa worm is very much smaller, and in patients in endemic areas is sometimes visible on the radiograph in the soft tissues of the hands and feet.

Finally, radiologically demonstrable calcification is occasionally present in tumours, either benign (e.g. thyroid adenomas) or malignant (e.g. fibrosarcomas and liposarcomas).

Gas in the soft tissues

Subcutaneous emphysema

Air may spread from the lung to the soft tissues of the chest wall after injury to the pleura and lung surface. The common causes of this are rib fractures (the sharp fracture margins lacerating the underlying soft tissues) and thoracentesis. On the radiograph pockets and streaks of air are seen in the soft tissues lateral to the rib margin, and the muscle bundles of the pectoral muscle may be outlined by air in the surrounding tissues. The volume of air tracking in the soft tissues may be extreme, creating a striking radiographic appearance (*Figure 2.97*).

Air entering the soft tissues of the chest wall in the above circumstances may track upwards into the neck. Alternatively, air

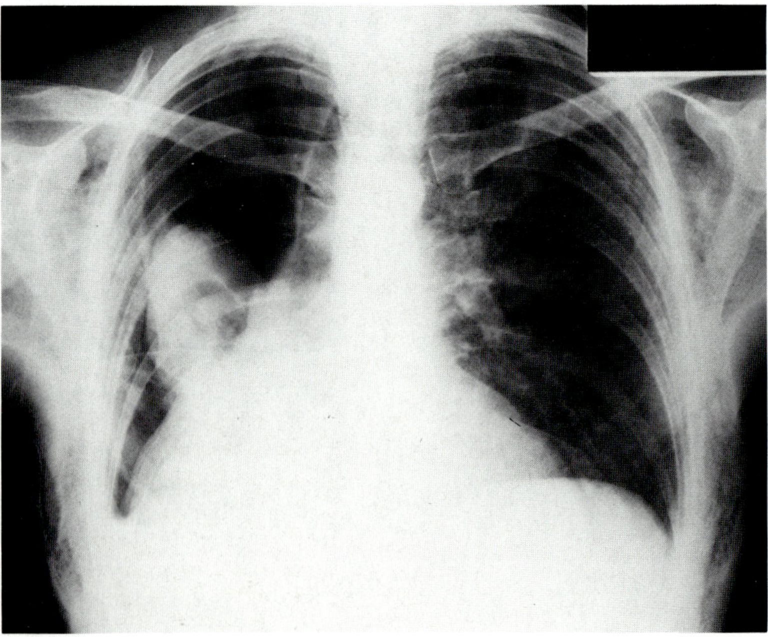

Figure 2.97. Subcutaneous emphysema and right pneumothorax

may spread into the neck when a pneumomediastinum (air within the tissues of the mediastinum) develops. Conditions giving rise to pneumomediastinum include oesophageal perforation, either spontaneous or as a complication of oesophagoscopy.

Gas gangrene

Gas produced by infection with gas-forming organisms is occasionally seen in the soft tissues. The commonest organism to give rise to this is *Clostridium perfringens* (welchii), but occasionally *Clostridium septicum* and even *Escherichia coli* may be responsible for gas formation. Gas gangrene is a relatively uncommon complication of wounds but is sometimes seen in uncontrolled diabetics, the infection spreading in ischaemic tissues. Radiographs show swelling of, and collections of gas pockets within, the infected tissues (*Figure 2.98*). While gas gangrene is essentially a clinical diagnosis, radiographs can be useful in the detection of early cases.

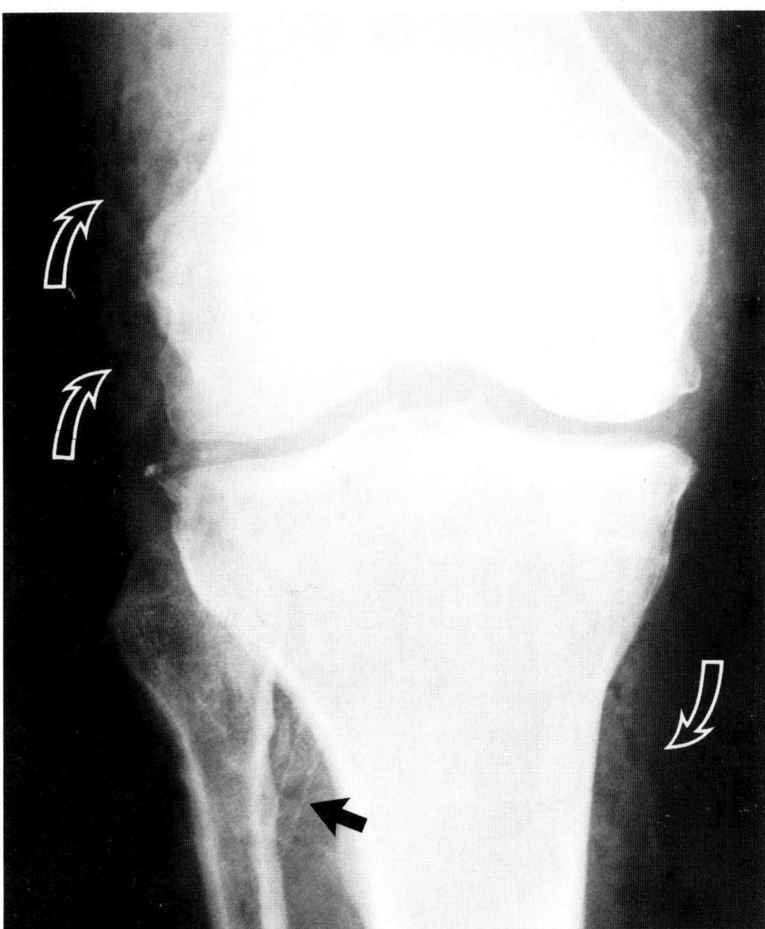

Figure 2.98. Gas gangrene: uncontrolled diabetic with severe ischaemia of lower limb; extensive gas formation in the soft tissues (open arrows); *Clostridium perfringens* isolated; arterial calcification (closed arrow)

3 Radiology of the abdomen

The stomach and duodenum

Hiatus hernia and disorders of the cardia

These are discussed in Chapter 5.

Gastric and duodenal ulcers

Suspicion of a gastric or duodenal ulcer usually arises when a patient complains of epigastric pain (as opposed to discomfort) which occurs between $\frac{1}{2}$ and 3 hours after eating and which is relieved by more food and by alkalis. The pain is usually experienced daily for several weeks and may then be followed by a remission of symptoms for several weeks or months, after which it commonly returns. This regular sequence is not always present, however, and the nature, site, duration and time of onset of the pain can vary considerably from patient to patient. A patient with a duodenal ulcer, for instance, may feel pain to the right of the midline and may be wakened by this during the night, while a penetrating gastric ulcer may cause pain in the back which is sometimes continuous although accentuated after meals. Localized tenderness in the upper abdomen is often present. Vomiting is a common symptom of gastric ulceration.

When a patient is suspected of having a peptic ulcer he should be referred for a barium meal examination. This examination should be performed before medical treatment is started, since the radiographic features of an acute ulcer may disappear quite rapidly with treatment. If treatment has been started a normal result may therefore be obtained, and doubt as to the correctness of the presumptive clinical diagnosis will remain.

However, the X-ray appearances of ulceration, although in close agreement with the operative findings, do not necessarily bear a temporal relationship to the patient's symptoms. In some patients a gastric ulcer can be seen radiologically during the long period of freedom from symptoms, while in others periodic pain of the type associated with peptic ulceration may be felt without any radiological, gastroscopic or operative evidence of disease.

Double-contrast barium meal examination, as described in Chapter 1, is now undertaken routinely in most X-ray departments. A number of films are obtained to show the mucosa of every region of the gas-distended stomach and duodenum coated with a fine layer of barium. In areas where a pool of barium is present much detail will be lost but deformity of the stomach may be obvious (*see Figure 3.11*). It is useful for the medical student and doctor to see barium meals being performed: this allows for a thorough understanding of the reasons for the views commonly obtained and the special features to look for on these views. By witnessing examinations the peristaltic movements of the stomach and duodenum can be appreciated, and these form a very important part of the examination. For instance, localized gastric rigidity and loss of peristalsis occur in the presence of invasion of the gastric wall by malignant tumours.

Radiological features of gastric ulcers

Benign gastric ulcers are usually sited on the lesser curve and adjacent posterior wall aspects of the body or antrum of the stomach. Ulcers produced by the drugs aspirin, indomethacin, and phenylbutazone commonly arise in the antrum. When an ulcer is seen in profile it forms a triangular or square or irregular shaped projection from the line of the stomach (*Figure 3.1*). Spasm of the gastric muscle produced by irritation at the level of the ulcer may produce an incisura (indentation of the gastric wall opposite the ulcer). When the ulcer is seen end-on (*en face*) it is accompanied by a number of gastric folds which converge on and typically run to the edge of the ulcer crater (*Figure 3.2*). These converging lines are important for two reasons. First, they help to draw attention to a tiny ulcer which might otherwise be overlooked. Secondly, they form an important feature in distinguishing benign ulcers from ulceration occurring in gastric carcinomas, since in a carcinoma the mucosal folds do not reach to the edge of the ulcer. These converging lines are more prominent in chronic ulceration and during healing than in acute ulceration. The acute ulcer may be surrounded by a collar of oedema.

An ulcer may penetrate through the gastric wall, in which case its base may be formed by pancreas, liver or omentum. In this situation the barium-filled projection of the ulcer may be very large, and a fluid level may be seen within it in the erect view.

Very considerable fibrosis may occur when chronic ulcers heal. This can give rise to an 'hour-glass' stomach, produced by gross fibrotic scarring with stricture formation at the level of a chronic ulcer of the body of the stomach (*Figure 3.3*). Healing with fibrosis of

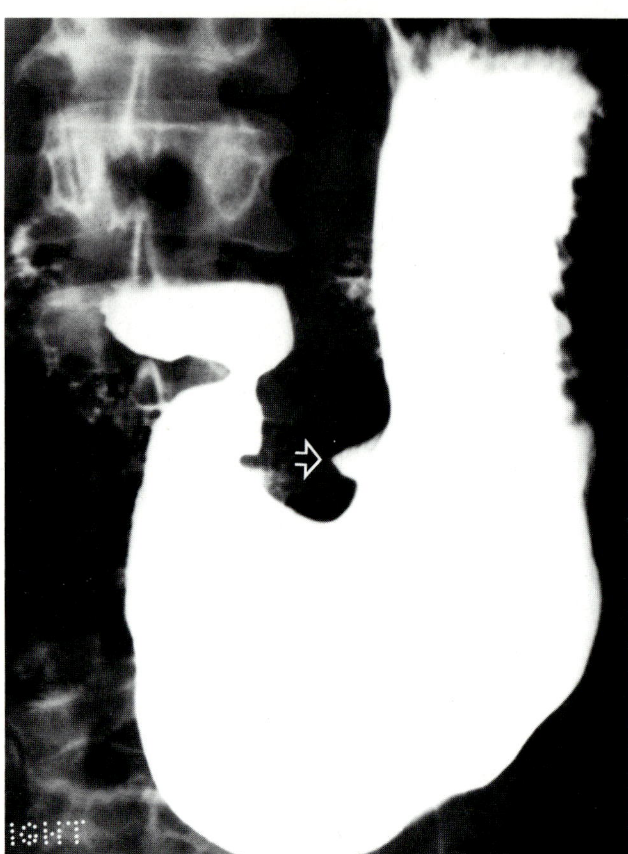

Figure 3.1. Simple lesser curve gastric ulcer, seen in profile (arrow). Ulcer lies outside the line of the lesser curve

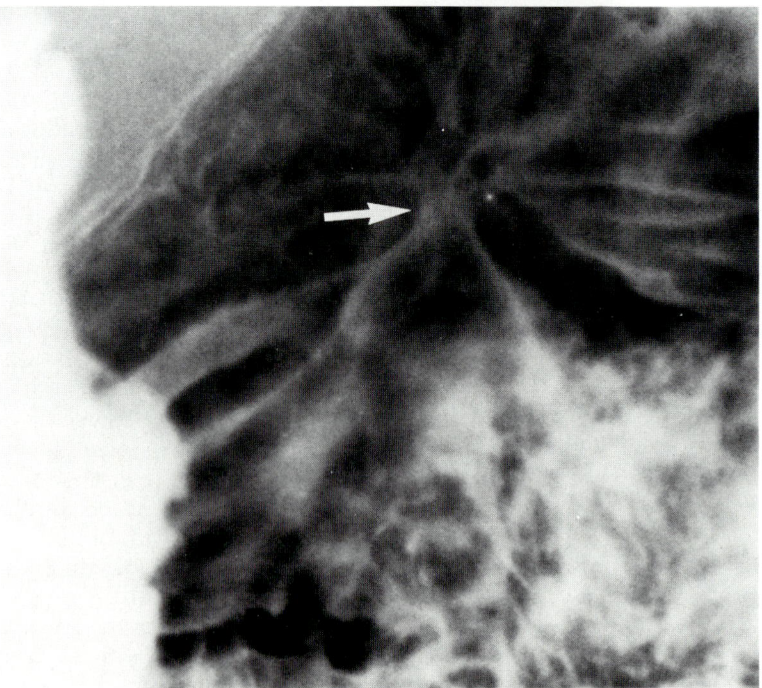

Figure 3.2. Simple gastric ulcer, seen *en face* (arrow). Mucosal folds converge on, and reach to the edge of, the ulcer

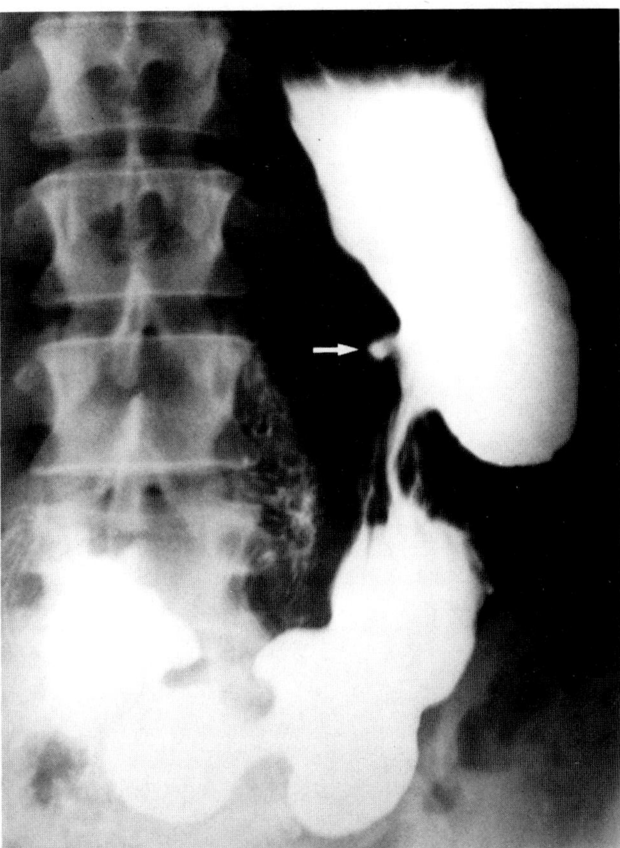

Figure 3.3. Hour-glass stomach. Severe constriction of body of stomach resulting from fibrosis from chronic ulceration. There is also an active ulcer (arrow) on the lesser curve above the level of the constriction

an ulcer in the region of the pyloric canal can result in pyloric obstruction, as described below.

There are two common conditions from which a gastric ulcer should be distinguished:

1. Gastric diverticulum. This usually occurs near the cardia. The features which allow distinction from a gastric ulcer are that a diverticulum is typically flask shaped with a narrow neck, has mucosal folds extending into it, shows some change of shape on examination by fluoroscopy, and has no incisura on the opposite wall.
2. Gastric carcinoma—*see* pages 111 and 112.

Radiological features of duodenal ulcers

Duodenal ulcers are most commonly situated in the cone shaped duodenal cap, but occasionally arise in the second part of the duodenum. The radiological features are similar to those of gastric ulcers. Thus the ulcer crater may be seen filled or lined with barium on the double-contrast view, mucosal folds converge to the edge of the ulcer, and the cap may be deformed by spasm or, in the case of chronic ulceration by fibrosis (*Figure 3.4*). In chronic ulceration the

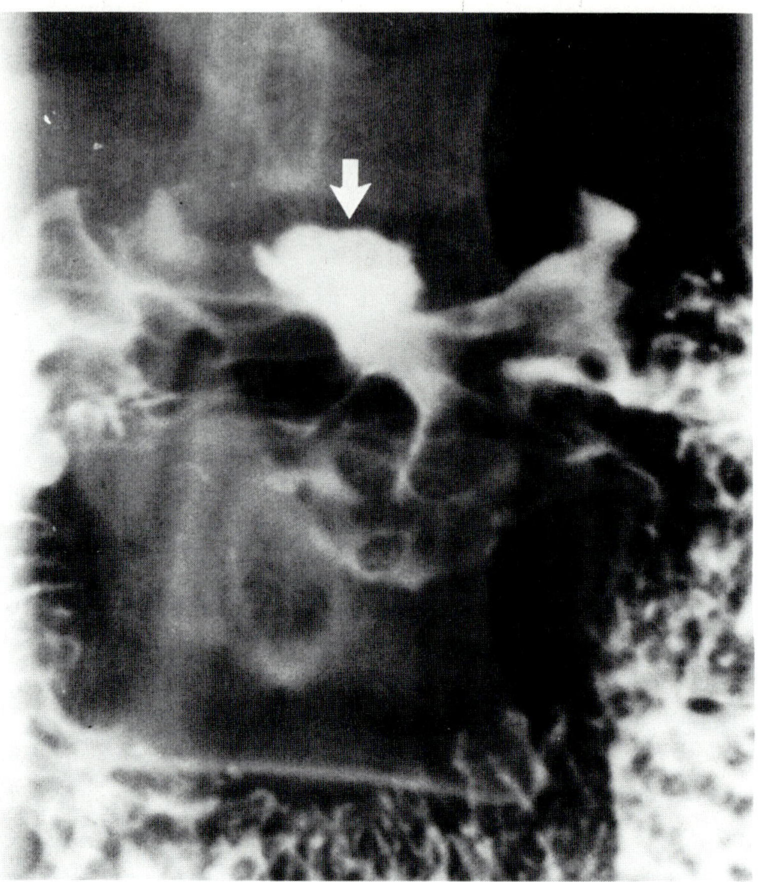

Figure 3.4. Duodenal cap ulcer: barium-filled ulcer (arrow) on superior aspect of cap; mucosal folds converge on edge of ulcer; some distortion of cap

deformity of the cap produced by fibrous scarring may be considerable; it may then be impossible to differentiate between an active ulcer and barium lying in a pocket in a scarred but healed cap. This is an important factor in the context of follow-up examination and is discussed in the next section.

A penetrating ulcer arising from the posterior wall of the cap may become walled off by adjacent tissues. As in a penetrating gastric ulcer, an ulcer of this type may appear very large and a fluid level may be seen within it on a film taken with the patient standing.

So-called 'pyloric' stenosis may develop as a complication of duodenal ulceration. This complication is discussed below.

Follow-up barium examination of patients with proven gastric and duodenal ulcers

Healing of a gastric ulcer in response to medical treatment can be readily assessed on follow-up barium examination. Evidence of healing will provide further confirmation that the original diagnosis of a benign as distinct from a malignant ulcer was correct. In view of the latter possibility it is well worth repeating the barium examination after 4–6 weeks of medical treatment. Endoscopy may also be undertaken if a tumour is suspected clinically or if the radiological findings are equivocal.

The situation is different for duodenal ulceration. As has been mentioned above, it may be impossible to distinguish radiologically between a scarred, healed duodenal cap and a cap containing an active ulcer. Furthermore, carcinoma of the duodenum is exceptionally rare, so that differentiation of a benign from a malignant duodenal cap ulcer is virtually never a practical problem. For these reasons assessment of subsequent healing or activity of a radiologically proven duodenal ulcer should be based on the patient's symptoms, and a repeat barium meal should not be carried out for this purpose. Repeat examination should be reserved for those patients in whom a complication of the ulcer—e.g. pyloric stenosis—or development of a new, different lesion—e.g. a gastric ulcer—is suspected.

Pyloric or duodenal stenosis secondary to peptic ulceration

The development of stenosis secondary to a duodenal or prepyloric ulcer is characterized by a change in the patient's clinical presentation. The symptoms of pain or severe discomfort in the epigastrium become continuous instead of being subject to periodic remissions. Sometimes the pain is colicky in nature due to increased gastric peristalsis. Vomiting of foul material containing recognizable food eaten 1 or 2 days earlier occurs. Peristaltic waves may be seen crossing the stomach from left to right. The onset may be quite insidious, and the patient may not seek medical advice until the condition has been present for a long time.

Radiologically, stenosis is characterized by the presence of a large excess of resting gastric fluid seen after overnight fasting, by slow initial emptying of the stomach after the barium meal despite vigorous peristalsis, and by slow final emptying, there being a large barium residue still present in the stomach 6 hours after the examination.

In severe cases the stomach is greatly dilated, and barium mixed with food may still be present in the stomach several days after the examination (*see Figure 3.10*, illustrating a case of gastric outlet obstruction due to antral carcinoma). It is not always possible to outline the pyloric canal or duodenum with barium, and therefore the cause and exact site of the stenosis may remain uncertain. Smooth-muscle relaxants, e.g. 20 mg intravenous hyoscine butylbromide (Buscopan), are usually given during the examination, since at least part of the obstruction may be produced by spasm.

In the absence of gross gastric dilatation or food retention it is desirable to repeat the examination after a short course of medical treatment. Successful treatment will be shown by the return of free gastric emptying, and the cause of the previous obstruction, such as duodenal ulceration, may be apparent. Obstruction that reverses in this manner is due to muscle spasm or oedema associated with the ulcer. Severe stenosis due to ulceration that does not respond to medical treatment is caused by fibrous scarring and requires surgical intervention.

Acute perforation of gastric or duodenal ulcers

The patient usually presents with a history of sudden onset of very intense, continuous abdominal pain, and he is found to have a rigid, board-like abdomen. His general condition depends on the severity of secondary peritonitis. The diagnosis of perforation can usually be confirmed readily by showing the presence of gas lying free within the abdomen below the diaphragm or below the inferior margin of the liver on a film taken with the patient standing or sitting (*Figure 3.5*). Free gas is usually identified more easily on the right side,

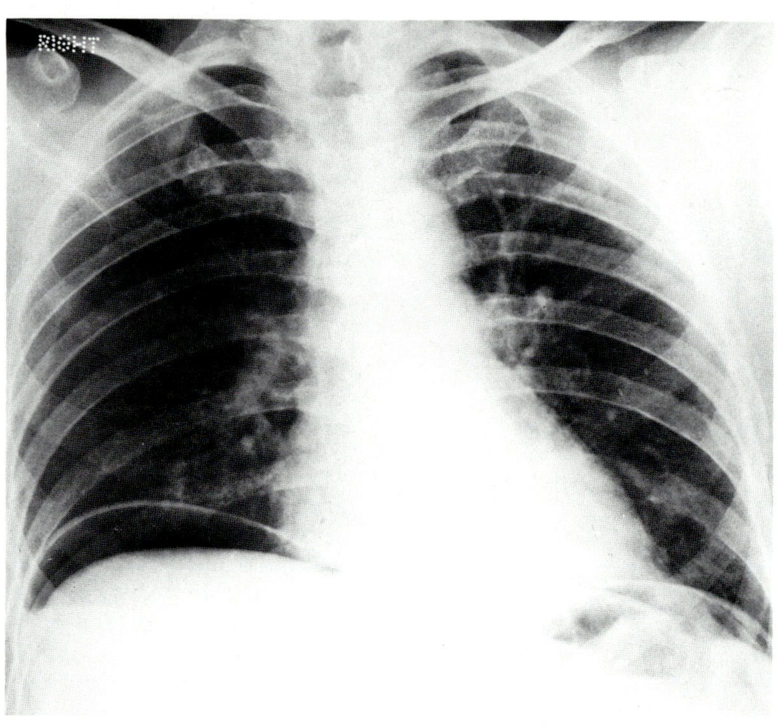

Figure 3.5. Air under diaphragm, more obvious on right side, from perforation of a duodenal ulcer; 3 hours' severe epigastric pain

between the right dome of the diaphragm and the liver, than on the left side, where free gas must be distinguished from gas contained within the fundus of the stomach or the splenic flexure of the colon. However, the hepatic flexure of the colon can at times be interposed between the right dome of the diaphragm and the liver as a normal occurrence: a loop of colon can usually be recognized by the presence of haustral folds crossing the gas shadow.

Sometimes the patient is too ill or too distressed by pain to stand or sit upright for an erect film, and it is then satisfactory to roll the patient onto his left side and to take a film of the abdomen with a horizontal X-ray beam. This is called a left lateral decubitus view. If perforation has occurred free gas will be seen between the lateral border of the liver and the lateral abdominal wall.

A large amount of free intraperitoneal gas is sometimes evident on a supine view of the abdomen. The *outside* surfaces of loops of bowel may be visible, surrounded by free intraperitoneal gas (*Figure 3.6*). Normally the outer walls of the bowel loops are invisible, and the

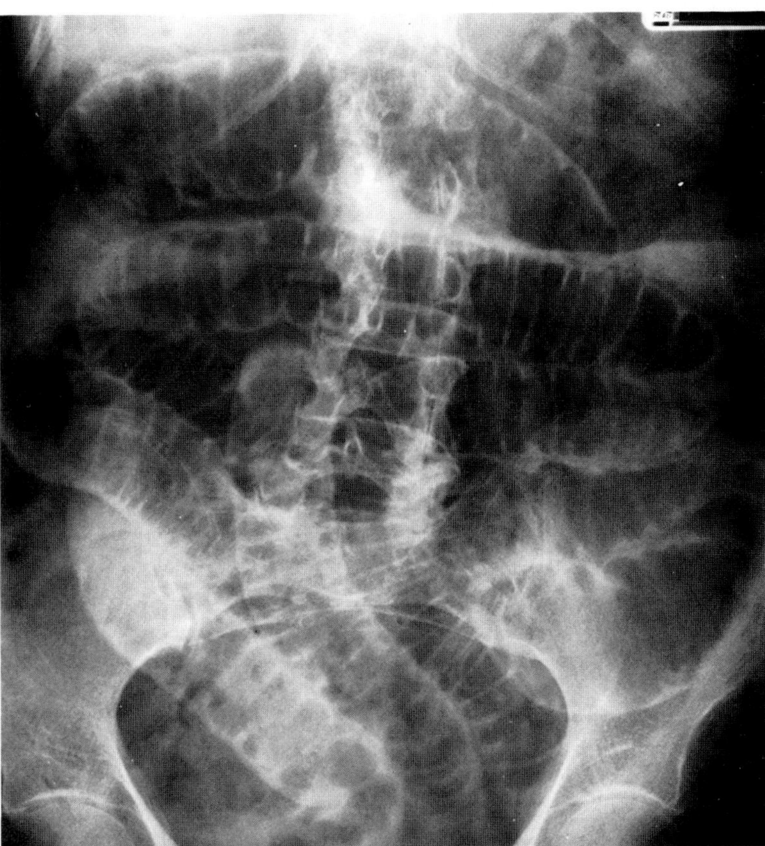

Figure 3.6. Intestinal perforation; supine film. The outer as well as the inner walls of the gas-filled jejunal loops are visible, outlined by air in the peritoneal cavity. Note valvulae conniventes of jejunum

inner walls are seen only in loops that contain air. The clinician must be aware of this feature of perforation as sometimes the clinical diagnosis is not suspected and only a supine film is requested.

On some occasions it is useful to confirm that perforation proven radiologically has been produced by a gastric or duodenal ulcer and not by a lesion sited elsewhere in the bowel, e.g. a perforated colonic diverticulum. At other times clinical evidence may suggest that the perforation has spontaneously sealed off, and it may be desirable to confirm this as surgery may thereby be avoided. In these situations the patient can be given Gastrografin by mouth (*see* page 6) and rolled onto his right side to facilitate filling of the duodenal cap. If free perforation is present a supine film taken after 15 minutes may show Gastrografin in the peritoneal cavity.

Acute peptic ulcer haemorrhage

When an upper gastrointestinal haemorrhage is suspected, endoscopy is the investigation of choice for examination of the oesophagus, stomach and duodenum. The bleeding site and the nature of the underlying lesion can usually be established by this means. The preference for endoscopy rather than radiology in this situation is

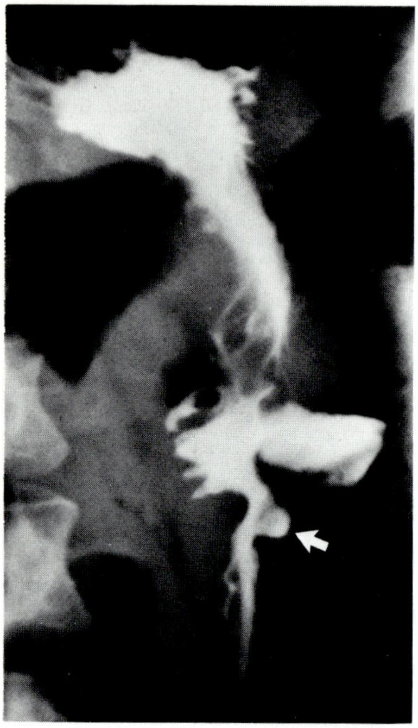

Figure 3.7. Jejunal ulcer after partial gastrectomy and gastroenterostomy. Projection of the barium-filled ulcer to the left (arrow) 1 cm below the stoma. A residue of barium was seen in the ulcer crater 1 hour later

that a barium examination may show the presence of an abnormality, such as oesophageal varices, which is not necessarily the cause of the upper gastrointestinal haemorrhage. There are, however, some quite subtle radiological changes which on occasion can indicate beyond doubt that a lesion is bleeding. For example, dilution of barium by blood may be seen in the immediate vicinity of an ulcer. Where endoscopy is not readily available therefore, barium examination is a very useful substitute. In the great majority of cases this will show the presence of an organic lesion and sometimes there will be evidence of the actual bleeding site.

The postoperative stomach

When a patient is referred for an X-ray examination after a previous operation on the stomach or duodenum, the radiologist should be informed of the nature of the operation as the altered anatomy will necessitate appropriate modification of the X-ray technique.

When a patient develops a peptic ulcer after a gastroenterostomy the new ulcer is most likely to occur at the anastomosis or in the proximal 5 cm of the efferent loop. The radiological features of filling of the ulcer crater with barium and spasm of the affected segment (*Figure 3.7*) correspond with those shown in gastric and duodenal ulceration.

Accuracy of double-contrast barium meal examination and the complementary roles of radiology and endoscopy

The double-contrast barium meal examination has an accuracy of about 90 per cent in the detection of lesions of the upper gastrointestinal tract. Several workers have found that endoscopy is of the order of 3 or 4 per cent more accurate than double-contrast barium examination in the diagnosis of upper gastrointestinal disease. This slight diagnostic superiority of endoscopy is hardly surprising, since a suspicious area can be biopsied or brushed for cytological examination during endoscopy, and colour changes in the mucosa will direct attention to a lesion. Radiology and endoscopy should be regarded as complementary rather than as competitive methods of examination. Barium examination causes little inconvenience to the patient and in the great majority of cases provides diagnostic information. Endoscopy is an invasive procedure and is substantially more time consuming than barium examination. Endoscopy is extremely valuable in assessing difficult diagnostic problems and, as discussed above, in investigating upper gastrointestinal haemorrhage.

Carcinoma of the stomach

Gastric carcinoma is a common malignant tumour, accounting for approximately 15 per cent of cancer deaths. The onset is often insidious, the patient being aware of quite minor symptoms of indigestion, anorexia, weight loss, or tiredness due to anaemia. Since the symptoms are trivial, the patient usually delays seeking medical advice. Patients presenting with a history that suggests gastric carcinoma, or in whom an epigastric mass is found, should be referred for barium meal examination. Because of the late presentation, it is common to find a large, extensively infiltrating tumour on this examination. Tumours arising in the region of the pyloric canal may produce symptoms of pyloric obstruction (*see Figure 3.10*), and tumours in the vicinity of the cardia may produce dysphagia (*see Figure 4.86*), and in these situations the patient may seek medical attention at an earlier stage of the disease. Even in these circumstances, however, a large tumour is often present at radiological investigation. In many patients, therefore, surgical resection is impossible, and the overall 5-year survival is approximately 10 per cent.

Radiological features

Approximately 50 per cent of gastric cancers arise in the antrum and pyloric region. The radiological features depend on the type of tumour present. The types found are:

1. Polypoid. An irregular, lobulated mass is seen projecting into the

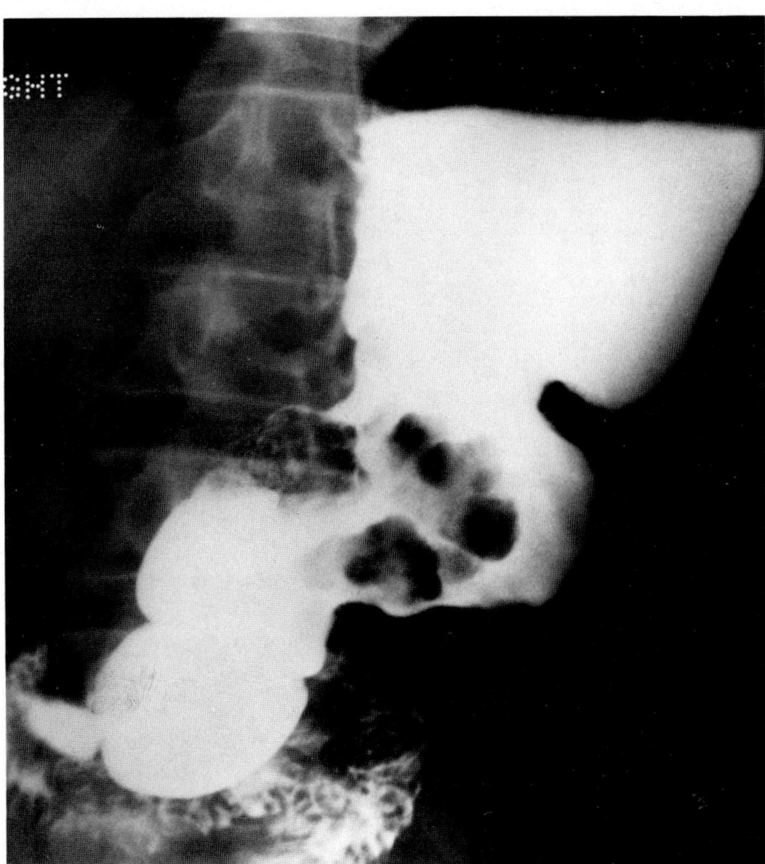

Figure 3.8. Polypoid carcinoma of body of stomach, producing large irregular filling defects in the barium-filled lumen. There is also considerable deformity of the adjacent lesser and greater curve aspects produced by surrounding tumour growth

lumen on double-contrast views, and this produces a filling defect when the stomach is filled with barium (*Figure 3.8*). The mucosa overlying the mass is destroyed, and, in place of the normal longitudinal mucosal folds of the stomach, irregular tracks of barium run over the surface of the tumour. The adjacent part of the stomach often shows rigidity and loss of peristalsis on fluoroscopy due to tumour infiltration in the wall.

2. Ulcerative. The apex of a tumour may undergo ischaemic necrosis, resulting in ulceration in the centre of the filling defect produced by the tumour (*Figure 3.9*). The radiological characteristics that distinguish benign from malignant ulcers are described below.

3. Scirrhous. The stomach becomes locally narrowed and the wall deformed and rigid. The rigidity and absence of normal distensibility is evident on fluoroscopy and on films exposed with the

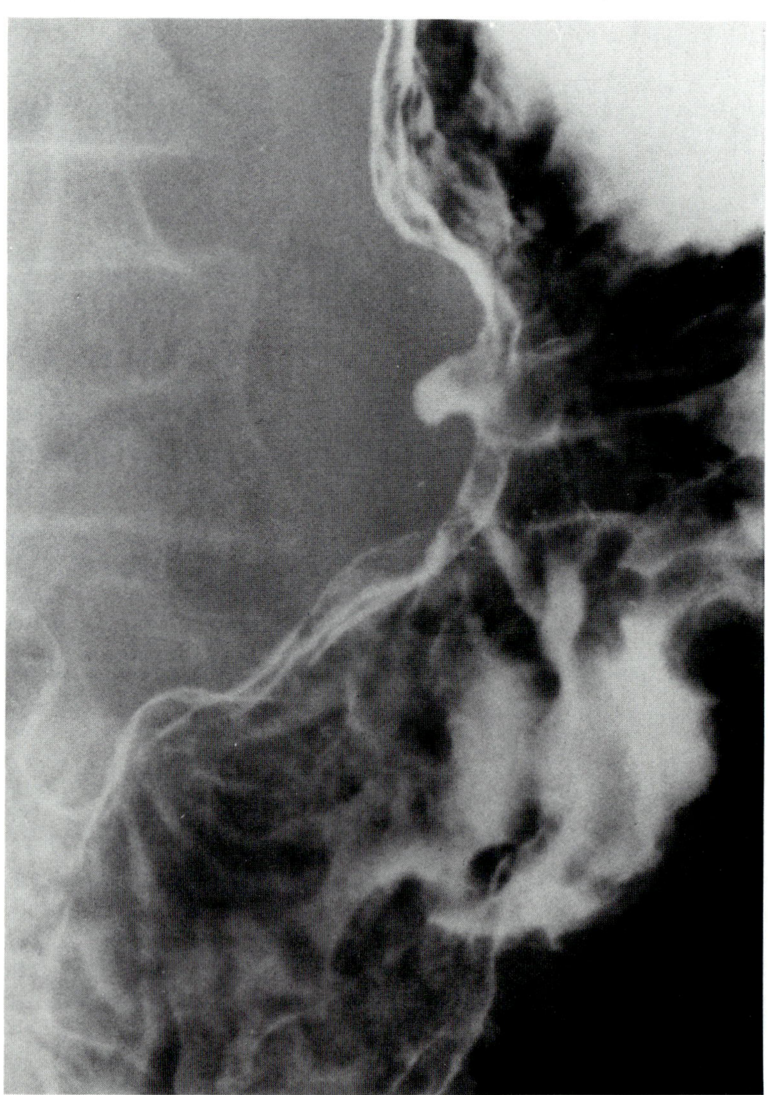

Figure 3.9. Ulcerating lesser curve gastric carcinoma, seen in profile. The ulcer has arisen at the apex of a polypoid tumour and lies within the line of the lesser curve (cf. *Figure 3.1*)

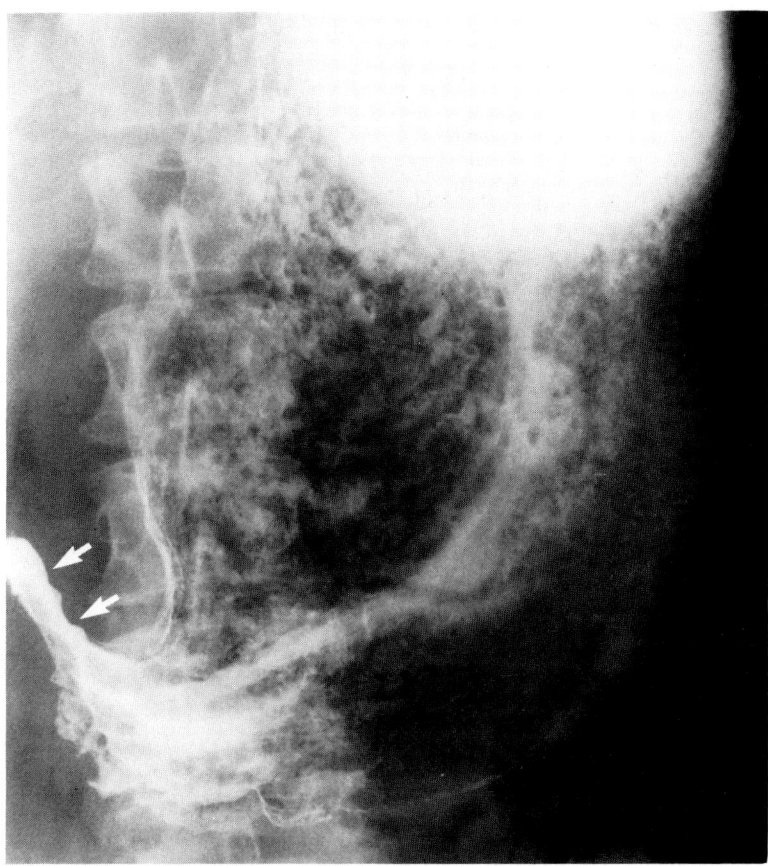

Figure 3.10. Scirrhous carcinoma of gastric antrum (arrows) producing gastric outlet obstruction. The very distended stomach contains much retained food and fluid mixed with barium

patient in different positions (*Figure 3.10*). Very extensive infiltration of this type produces a linitis plastica ('leather-bottle' stomach; *Figure 3.11*).

4. Mucosal. The occasional recognition of early gastric carcinomas, confined to the mucosa, has been rendered possible by the advent of the double-contrast examination. This technique was in fact developed in Japan, where the incidence of gastric carcinoma is very high, as a means for detecting the lesion at an early stage.

Radiological features distinguishing benign from malignant gastric ulcers

The following radiological features assist in differentiating benign from malignant gastric ulcers:

1. A gastric ulcer viewed in profile lies outside the line of the stomach (*see Figure 3.1*), while a malignant ulcer, which develops from ulceration of the apex of a tumour mass, usually lies entirely within the line of the stomach wall from which the tumour has arisen (*see Figure 3.9*).
2. On double-contrast views mucosal folds are seen to converge on and run right to the edge of benign ulcers (*see Figure 3.2*), while

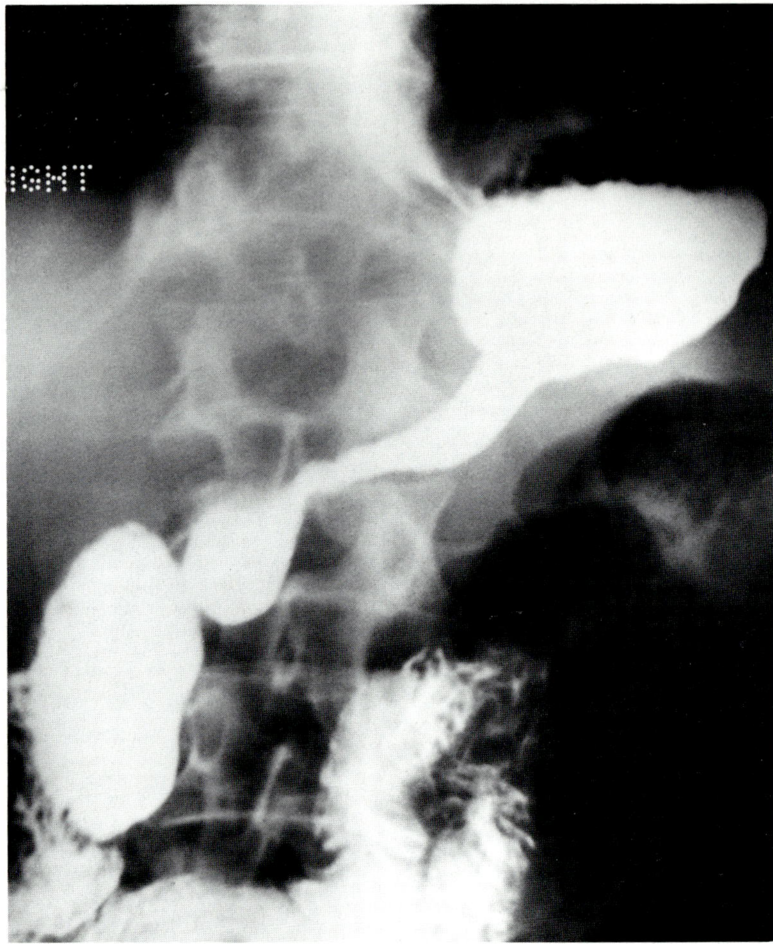

Figure 3.11. 'Leather-bottle' stomach: carcinoma of the distal two-thirds of the stomach, showing gross narrowing and deformity of the lumen

the mucosal folds of the stomach stop short of the margins of neoplastic ulcers.

3. It is rare for a benign ulcer to occur on the greater curve of the stomach, and an ulcer at this site should alert the physician to the possibility of malignancy. Nevertheless, an ulcer at this site may prove to be benign.

4. Complete healing or very substantial regression in the size of an ulcer on follow-up radiological examination after a period of medical treatment provides confirmatory evidence of a benign lesion. A malignant ulcer may decrease slightly in size but will not become substantially smaller.

Exceptions to the above generalizations do occur, and gastroscopy is of great value in cases where the diagnosis is uncertain. An area of radiographic abnormality can be viewed directly and biopsies taken. Endoscopy will sometimes show a lesion overlooked on barium examination. Benign tumours, e.g. leiomyoma, and other malignant conditions of the stomach, e.g. lymphosarcoma, may simulate the radiographic appearances of carcinoma, and endoscopy with biopsy will provide valuable information when the diagnosis is in doubt.

Radiology in relation to operability

Unfortunately, the X-ray findings are of little help in deciding whether resection of a gastric neoplasm is feasible. Occasionally, quite large growths can be successfully removed, while growths that appear to be small are often irresectible at laparotomy.

The small intestine

Supine and erect films of the abdomen show distension of and fluid levels within the small bowel in intestinal obstruction or ileus. These conditions provide the main indications for plain film investigation of the small bowel. Barium examination is the standard method for investigating most other disorders of the small intestine. The most commonly practised technique is for films to be taken at intervals of time after the patient has swallowed a liquid barium sulphate preparation: films are obtained until all segments of the small bowel have been opacified. Regions of particular interest can be assessed further with supplementary views and by fluoroscopy. As an additional or alternative investigation to the barium follow-through examination some departments now perform small-bowel barium enemas, in which barium is infused into the small intestine through a nasogastric tube positioned with its tip in the third part of the duodenum.

Crohn's disease (regional enteritis)

This condition, of unknown aetiology, is characterized histologically by chronic inflammation with non-caseating granuloma formation, oedema and fibrosis affecting all the layers of the intestinal wall. This involvement of all the walls by inflammation accounts for a number of the radiological features to be described. The condition can affect any part of the alimentary tract from the oesophagus to the anus, but by far the most common sites of involvement are the terminal ileum, caecum and adjacent ascending colon. The colon is involved in approximately 30 per cent of cases, and in about one-third of these the disease is confined to the colon. The radiological appearances of Crohn's disease of the large bowel, and the features that distinguish this from ulcerative colitis, are described in the section on the colon.

Sometimes the disease presents with the acute onset of right iliac fossa pain. The true diagnosis is established at emergency laparotomy undertaken for presumed acute appendicitis, and radiological investigation in this situation is rarely performed. If plain films of the abdomen have been obtained before surgery these will show non-specific changes consisting of a few fluid levels in the terminal loops of small bowel.

More commonly, the onset is insidious and the disease chronic. The patient presents with a history of diarrhoea, colic, anorexia and weight loss, and is found on examination to have a low-grade fever, anaemia, and sometimes a tender mass in the right iliac fossa. The barium follow-through examination may reveal disease affecting the small bowel. As already stated, the terminal ileum is the commonest site of involvement, but if other parts of the intestinal tract are affected the regions of involvement are commonly separated from each other by lengths of disease-free bowel. The presence of these 'skip areas' is a characteristic feature of Crohn's disease (*Figure 3.12*). The ulcers are typically deep, involving the mucous, sub-mucous, and muscular layers of the bowel wall, so that in profile

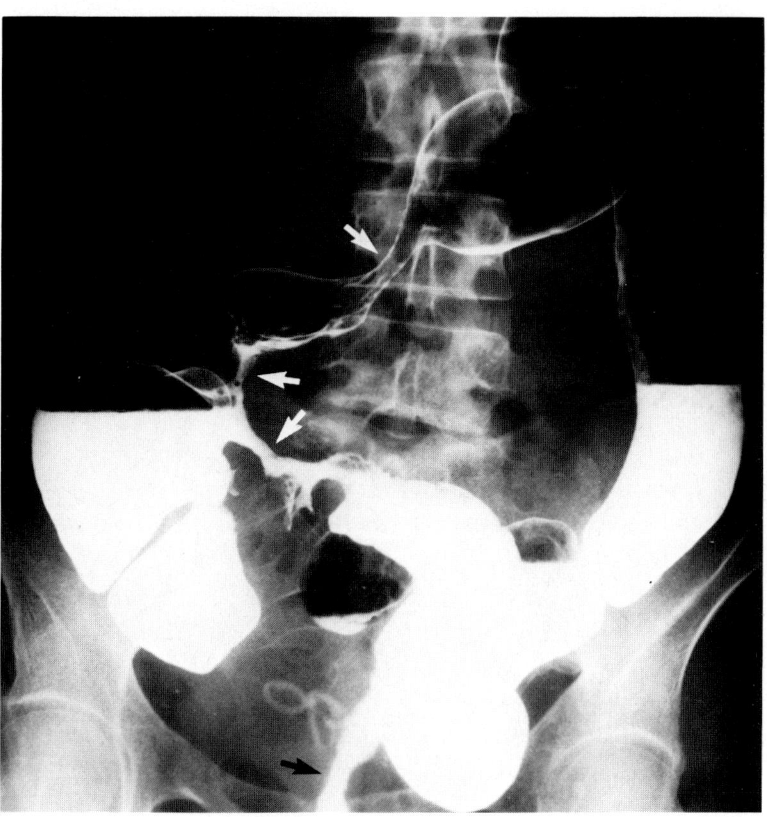

Figure 3.12. Crohn's disease: previous ileotransverse colostomy; severe strictures in the distal ileum, transverse colon and rectum (arrows) with intervening disease-free skip areas

these deep ulcers resemble rose thorns. Thorn-like ulcers of similar appearance are seen in ileocaecal tuberculosis (*see Figure 3.15*). When viewed *en face* the barium tracking in the deep, narrow, longitudinal and transverse ulcer crevices gives rise to a cobblestone appearance (*Figure 3.13*). The inflammatory involvement of all of the layers of the bowel wall produces swelling, so that affected segments become separated from adjacent loops and consequently stand out clearly.

Fibrosis is a prominent pathological feature of the disease which, together with ulceration, gives rise to rigid, narrowed, irregular tubular segments of affected bowel. This appearance in the terminal ileum (*Figure 3.14*) is sometimes referred to as the string sign of Kantor. Narrowing produces clinical features of subacute obstruction and is confirmed radiologically by dilatation of and fluid levels within small-bowel segments proximal to the stricture (*Figure 3.14*). In the advanced stages of the disease affected segments of bowel become matted together and fistulas develop between small and large bowel, or between a loop of bowel and the bladder or skin. These fistulous tracks can often be seen filled with barium.

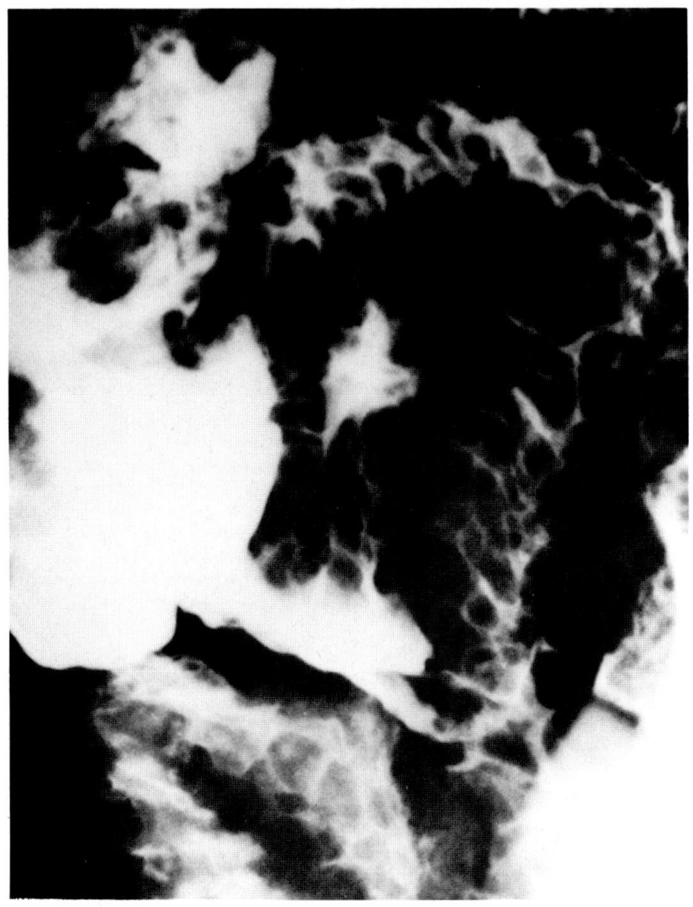

Figure 3.13. Crohn's disease. 'Cobblestone' mucosa of terminal ileum

Deformity and loss of distensibility of the caecum commonly accompany terminal ileal disease. This is best shown on barium enema examination although it may be obvious on barium follow-through.

Differential diagnosis

The radiographic features of intestinal tuberculosis may be identical with those of Crohn's disease, although there is a tendency for the caecum to become more contracted in tuberculosis (*Figure 3.15*). Since the conditions may be quite indistinguishable radiologically, tuberculosis should always be considered in a patient showing the above X-ray changes.

Intestinal malabsorption

Malabsorption may be suspected in a patient presenting with weight loss, abdominal pain and distension; a history of frequent bowel

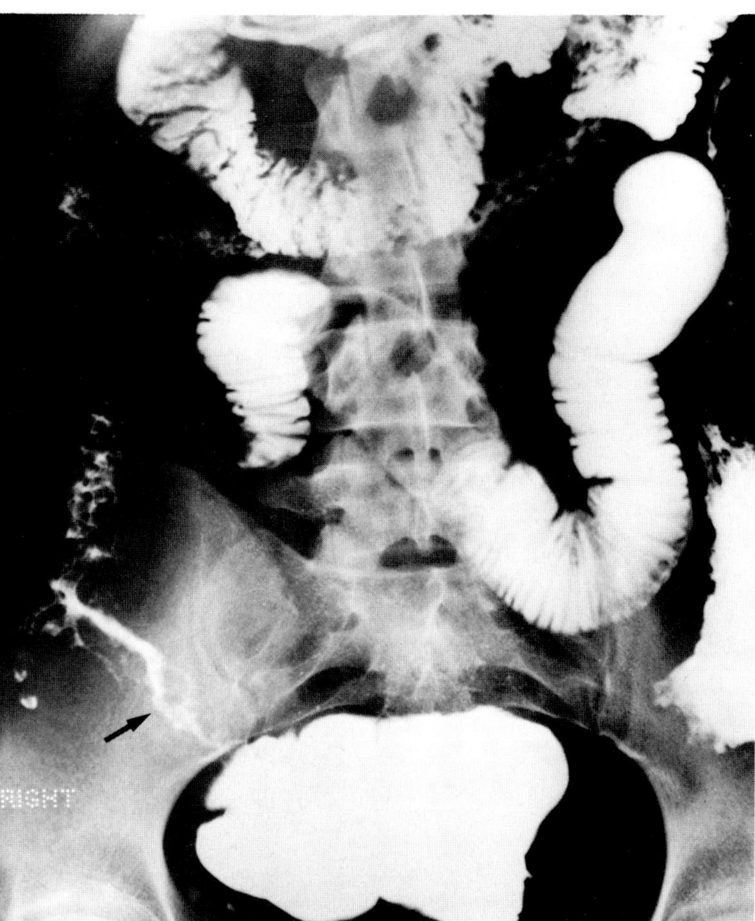

Figure 3.14. Crohn's disease in a patient aged 21: colicky right-sided abdominal pain for 2 years; narrowed, irregular terminal ileum (arrow); dilated central coil of jejunum due to partial obstruction by a narrowed, diseased mid small-bowel segment

motions with the passage of loose, pale, bulky offensive stools; or anaemia. The diagnosis can be confirmed by biochemical tests, including faecal fat estimation and the xylose absorption test. The prime function of radiological investigation by barium follow-through examination is to search for an anatomical cause for the malabsorption. In some cases of malabsorption a diagnostic radiographic abnormality will be found, while in other cases non-specific changes will be present on the barium study, which necessitate further investigation, such as jejunal biopsy, to establish the diagnosis. It is convenient to consider these two groups separately.

Conditions with specific radiographic abnormality

Bacterial contamination of the intestine is an important cause of malabsorption, and this can occur when there is an anatomical abnormality predisposing to the stagnation of intestinal contents. Barium examination may show the presence of jejunal diverticulosis (*Figure 3.16*), or chronic ileal strictures with considerable stasis of intestinal contents in distended loops proximal to the strictures (as may occur in Crohn's disease and tuberculous enteritis), or post-surgical blind loops of bowel with defective peristaltic emptying.

Intestinal fistulas can cause malabsorption by producing short circuits (e.g. directly from jejunum to colon), or by permitting retrograde passage of colonic bacteria into the small bowel. Fistulas may be seen in Crohn's disease. As mentioned in a later section, fistulas between the small bowel and colon are most reliably shown by barium enema examination. Various other abnormalities of distinctive appearance predisposing to malabsorption may be demonstrated on barium follow-through examination. These include rigidity and extensive infiltration of the small-bowel wall by lymphoma, and unexpectedly extensive previous surgical resection of small-bowel.

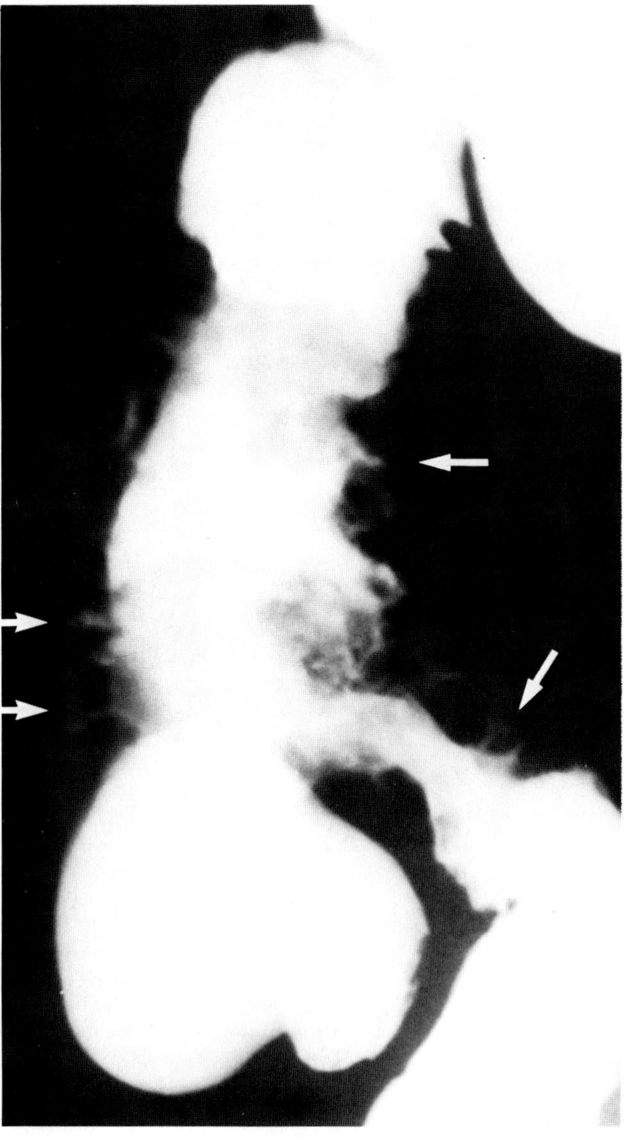

Figure 3.15. Ileocaecal tuberculosis: narrowing, deep thorn-like ulcers (arrows) and filling defects due to inflammatory swelling are present in the terminal ileum and ascending colon; deformed, shrunken caecum; patient also had active pulmonary tuberculosis

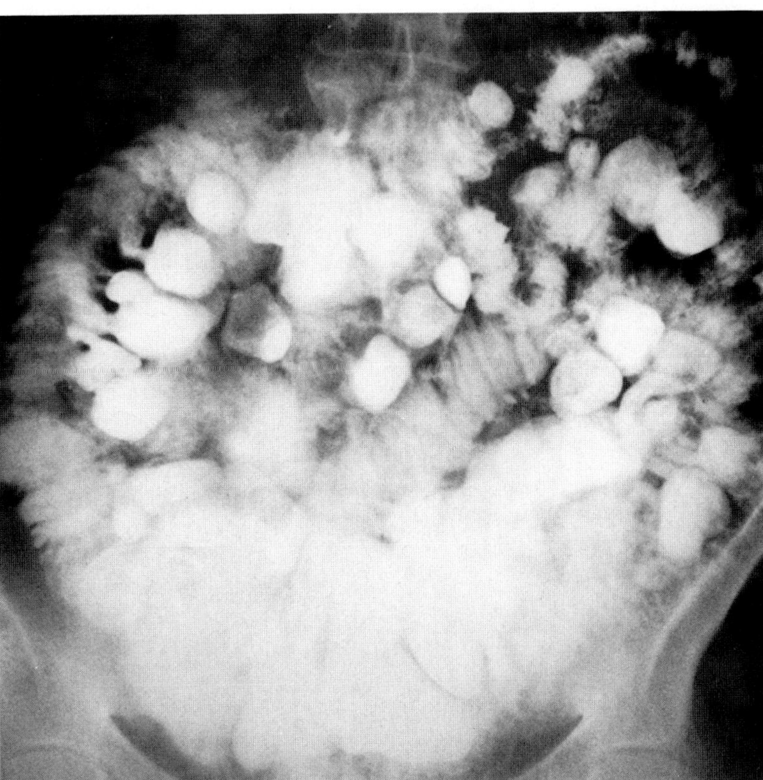

Figure 3.16. Jejunal diverticulosis; numerous round sacs with featureless walls are seen arising from loops of jejunum

Lactase deficiency is the most common of the disaccharidase-deficiency conditions and may be diagnosed by the lactose tolerance test and by estimating the enzyme activity in a sample of the jejunal mucosa obtained by biopsy. The condition produces no anatomical abnormality on barium examination but can nevertheless be diagnosed radiologically as follows. Lactose added to the barium before ingestion will be followed by excessive dilution and abnormally rapid transit of barium in the small intestine in patients suffering from this condition, while a subsequent repeat examination without added lactose will, in contrast, show normal appearances of, and a normal transit time in, the small bowel.

Conditions without specific radiographic abnormality

Dilatation of the small bowel and flocculation of barium within it are seen in gluten enteropathy, tropical sprue and Whipple's disease. The width of the small bowel may be considered to be increased above normal when three loops exceeding 3 cm in diameter or one loop exceeding 3.5 cm in diameter are present. Dilatation and flocculation are non-specific changes, and also occur, although usually to a lesser extent, in patients with malabsorption due to biliary or pancreatic disease. In this group of conditions, therefore, radiology plays little part in specific diagnosis, which must be established by other means such as jejunal biopsy and tests of pancreatic function.

Intestinal obstruction

It is convenient to consider small- and large-bowel obstruction in the same section, so that attention may be drawn to the similarities and differences. The basic radiological investigation consists of supine and erect films of the abdomen. These are valuable in showing the level of obstruction when the diagnosis is known and in confirming the diagnosis when obstruction is suspected clinically. The radiological features are of distension of, and the presence of multiple fluid levels within, the bowel proximal to the obstruction, and of empty or almost empty bowel distally. When examining radiographs, the most distal distended loop should be identified in order to determine the site of the obstruction.

In upper and mid small-bowel obstruction the jejunum is distended. Loops of jejunum are readily recognized by the characteristic appearances of the valvulae conniventes, which lie close together and tend to run across the full widths of the loops (*Figure 3.17*). On

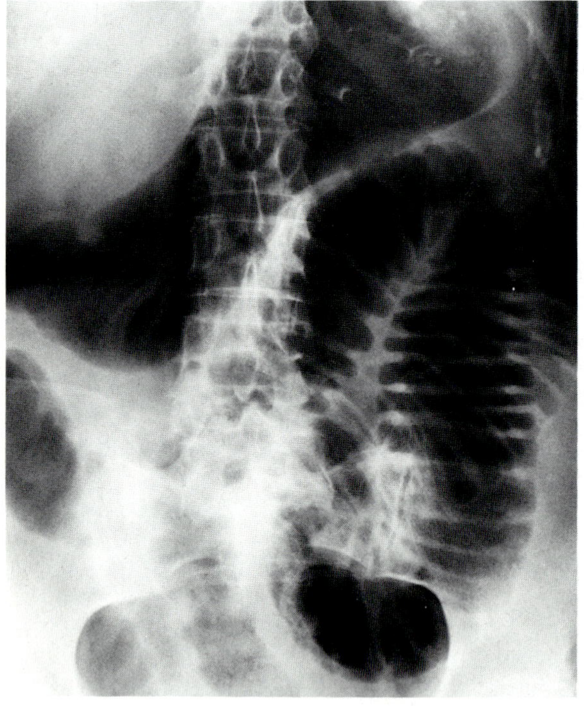

Figure 3.17. Jejunal obstruction (supine film): distended jejunal loops; valvulae conniventes lie close together and run across the full width of the loops; gas-filled stomach above

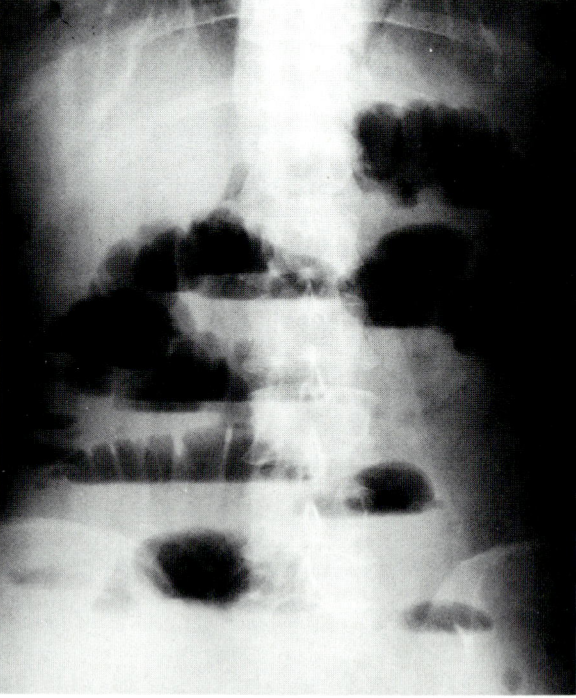

Figure 3.18. Mid small-bowel obstruction (erect film): multiple fluid levels are present in distended loops of small bowel lying centrally in the abdomen

the erect film several fluid levels are present in the distended segments, these fluid levels occupying a fairly central position in the abdomen (*Figure 3.18*).

A large number of distended loops, showing multiple fluid levels, are found in obstruction of the distal small bowel. These again occupy the central part of the abdomen, largely sparing the flanks, and the fluid levels sometimes show a cascade effect, crossing the centre of the abdomen from the left upper quadrant to the right iliac fossa. In contrast to the characteristic appearance of the valvulae conniventes of the jejunum, the terminal ileal loops are featureless. Gas is absent from, or present in only a very small quantity in, the undistended colon.

The features described are readily distinguished from those of lower colonic obstruction. In this condition the colon is distended and occupies a predominantly peripheral position in the abdomen. The mid-portion of the transverse colon may, however, lie comparatively low in the central part of the abdomen, but this is readily distinguished from distended small bowel by the fact that this single loop can be followed and seen to be in continuity with the ascending and descending segments. In contrast to the appearances of the valvulae conniventes of the jejunum, the haustra of the colon are fewer in number and only partially cross the widths of the bowel loops (*Figure 3.19*). If the ileocaecal valve is competent the caecum may be

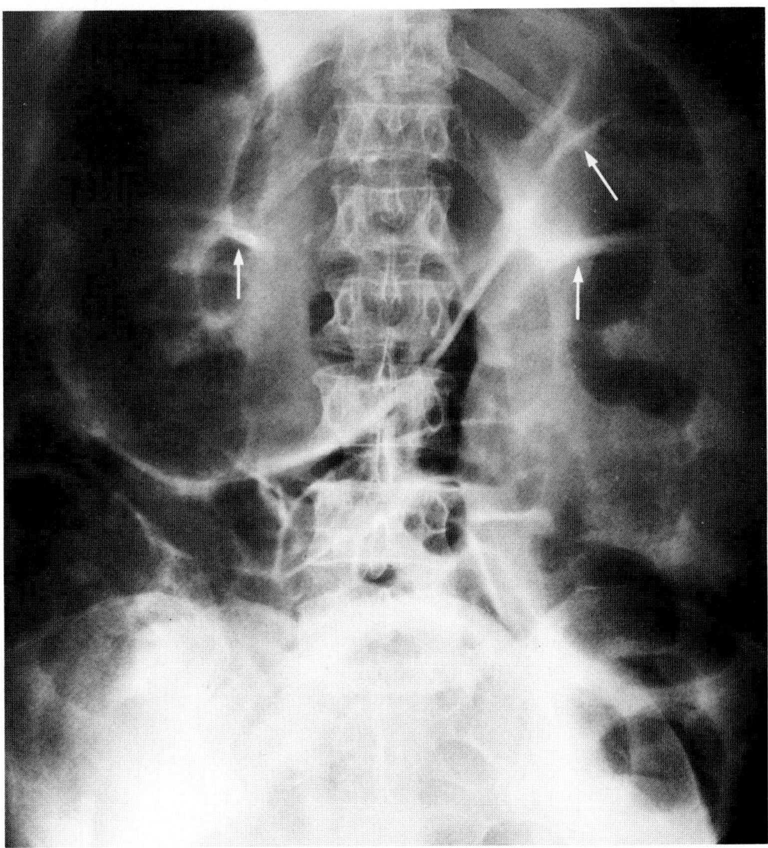

Figure 3.19. Lower large-bowel obstruction (supine film). Distended, gas-filled colon, occupying predominantly the periphery of the abdomen, although the transverse colon loops downwards as far as the level of the third lumbar vertebra to the right of the midline. Note sparse haustral folds, only partially crossing the width of the bowel (three are arrowed). Some distension of small-bowel loops also. Small- and large-bowel fluid levels were present on erect film

Table 3.1 Differences between small-bowel and large-bowel obstruction

Small-bowel obstruction	*Large-bowel obstruction*
Many distended loops, involving central abdomen. Colon empty, or almost empty	Distended colon around periphery of abdomen with or without prominent changes of small-bowel obstruction
Valvulae conniventes close together and seen crossing width of jejunum	Haustra fewer in number, more separated, and folds only partially cross colon

grossly distended. Commonly, however, the valve is incompetent and distension of the caecum less marked. Features of small-bowel obstruction are present to a variable extent.

Table 3.1 summarizes the main differences between small- and large-bowel obstruction.

Differential diagnosis

1. Ileus. Distension of small and large bowel with multiple fluid levels in the bowel loops characterizes this condition. In contrast to obstruction, however, gas-filled loops are usually shown throughout the bowel to the sigmoid segment and rectum. Sometimes difficulty can arise in the clinical and radiological differentiation between partial obstruction and ileus in the early postoperative period. This can be resolved by the subsequent clinical course and by serial follow-up radiographs.
2. Multiple small-bowel fluid levels without distension are a feature of gastroenteritis, and an unusually gaseous bowel without abnormal distension or multiple fluid levels arises from excessive air swallowing in the presence of pain.
3. Features of obstruction occur in bowel ischaemia from mesenteric thrombosis or embolization. In the acute stage filling defects simulating multiple thumb impressions are sometimes seen silhouetted against the gas-filled lumen (*see Figure 3.30*). These are produced by haemorrhage and oedema in the bowel wall.

The colon

Supine and erect plain films of the abdomen are used in assessing colonic obstruction, sometimes supplemented by limited barium enema examination to establish the nature of the obstructing lesion. Plain films should be obtained in cases of suspected toxic dilatation complicating ulcerative colitis, and in the presence of this complication barium enema examination is contraindicated because of the considerable risk of colonic perforation.

For most conditions of the large bowel, however, barium enema examination is the standard method of radiological investigation. A barium enema provides an incomplete examination of the colon on its own, and sigmoidoscopy should also be performed: this allows for direct inspection and biopsy of lesions in the rectum and distal colon and is therefore complementary to the barium study. Sigmoidoscopy should precede barium enema examination, since a barium enema is contraindicated in the presence of a fungating mass in the rectum because of the risk of perforation leading to barium peritonitis (*see Chapter 1*). If a biopsy has been performed the barium enema is usually deferred for at least 3 days, and sometimes longer, from the time of sigmoidoscopy, because of the potential risk of perforation of the bowel during biopsy. If there is any suspicion of perforation being present from any cause, water-soluble contrast media are used instead of barium (*see* page 6).

Double-contrast barium enema examinations (*see* page 6) are performed in most radiology departments nowadays, since there is considerable evidence that these are superior to single-contrast studies in demonstrating small neoplasms (polyps and carcinomas) and in investigating inflammatory conditions of the bowel.

Sometimes both barium meal and barium enema examinations are required in investigating a patient with, for example, unexplained anaemia or unexplained rectal bleeding. Without any clinical features pointing to a possible source of blood loss (e.g. chronic duodenal ulcer), the barium enema is given preferably before the barium meal, since barium confined to the colon can be removed fairly quickly with laxatives and enemas, thereby allowing the barium meal to be carried out without undue delay on an abdomen cleared of contrast material.

The presence of colonic diverticula is a common and often incidental barium enema finding in the elderly. If shown, a patient's rectal bleeding or anaemia should not be attributed too readily to this condition. Unless the clinical features suggest this diagnosis it is often wise to proceed to a barium meal examination, at which time a symptomless paraoesophageal hernia or peptic ulcer, representing the real cause of the bleeding, may be discovered.

Arteriography can be useful in demonstrating the source of bleeding during a gastrointestinal haemorrhage in patients with recurrent intestinal haemorrhage and with repeatedly normal barium studies.

Crohn's disease (regional enteritis)

The features of Crohn's disease of the small intestine have been described in an earlier section, in which it was mentioned that the large bowel is affected in approximately 30 per cent of cases, sometimes without associated small-bowel involvement. Many of the radiological features seen in the colon on barium enema examination are similar to those already described for disease affecting the small bowel. Thus involvement of the colon tends to be patchy, with 'skip areas' of healthy bowel intervening between inflamed segments (*see Figure 3.12*). In addition to this patchy distribution along the length of the bowel, there is a tendency for the condition to affect one side of the bowel wall only, the opposite side being spared. This can cause considerable distortion of the lumen when fibrosis ensues. While any part of the colon can be affected, involvement of the caecum and ascending colon is most common. Inflammation of the rectum is found on histological examination in approximately 50 per cent of patients with Crohn's disease of the colon, but this is less often evident radiologically.

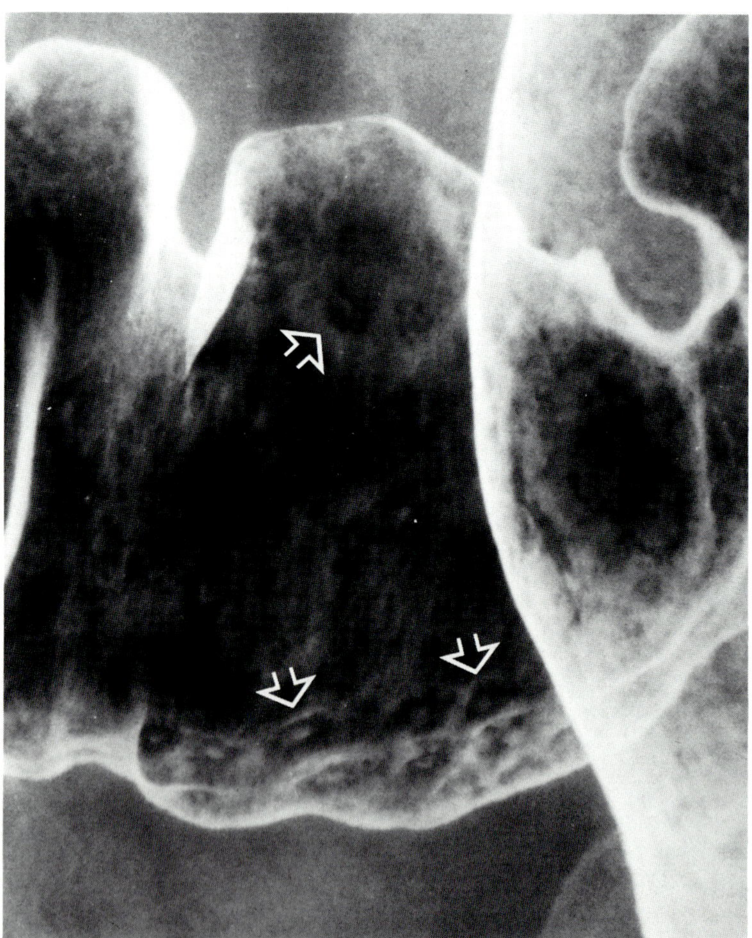

Figure 3.20. Crohn's disease of colon. Aphthous ulcers (several shown, three arrowed), each consisting of a central speck of barium surrounded by a translucent halo, giving a target or bull's eye appearance

Deep ulceration is common, reflecting the in
layers of the bowel wall, and produces the t
ulceration and cobblestone appearance already
section on the small intestine. Aphthous ulcers m
colon on double-contrast barium enema examir
appears as a small spot of barium surrounded by a transradiant halo
resembling a target or bull's eye (*Figure 3.20*). Aphthous ulcers are
occasionally seen in other forms of colitis, including amoebic colitis.

Fibrous scarring with stricture formation is common during
healing (*see Figure 3.12*), but unlike the strictures in ulcerative colitis
those in Crohn's disease are almost invariably benign. Fistulas and
paracolic abscesses are other important complications.

Ulcerative colitis

The inflammation in this disease of unknown aetiology primarily
involves the mucosa, in contrast to the transmural inflammation
that characterizes Crohn's disease. Diarrhoea is the predominant
symptom, the patient passing between two and 20 loose, blood-
stained stools per day. The disease sometimes follows an acute
fulminating course, rapidly endangering the patient's life. More
commonly the condition is chronic, and subject to partial or
complete remissions alternating with periods of relapse. Ulcerative
colitis first affects the rectum and may remain confined to this region
or may extend proximally from the rectum to affect the colon to a
variable extent. Regardless of the extent of colonic involvement an
important feature of this condition, which can be shown radiologically, is that the involved segments of the colon are in continuity
with each other. These aspects assist in differentiation from Crohn's
disease, which most commonly affects the terminal ileum and right
side of the colon and, when more extensive, is usually patchily
distributed.

Radiological appearances

Granularity of the mucosa is the earliest manifestation of ulcerative
colitis and can be shown on double-contrast barium enema examination (*Figure 3.21*).

Mucosal ulcers may be small or they may penetrate through the
mucosa to reach the submucosa. Ulcers reaching the submucosa
spread out in this layer, and these fill with barium to produce a
collar-stud appearance, characteristic of ulceration in this condition
(*Figure 3.22*). Pseudopolyps represent small remnants of inflamed
oedematous mucosa surrounded by ulcers and may be seen on the
radiological examination as rounded filling defects (*Figure 3.21*).

Normally the posterior wall of the rectum lies 1 cm or less in front
of the sacrum. This post-rectal space is clearly visible on a lateral

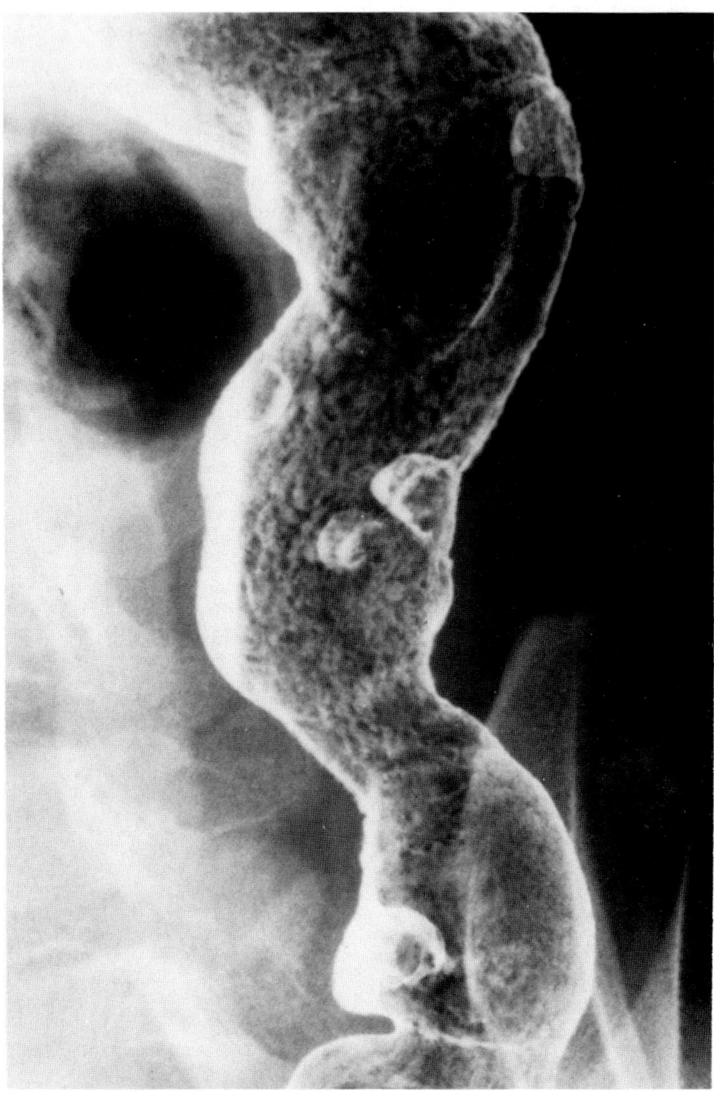

Figure 3.21. Ulcerative colitis; inflammatory pseudopolyps; characteristic granular appearance of mucosa

view of the barium filled rectum and may be considerably widened by inflammation.

In contrast to Crohn's disease, ulceration does not occur in the terminal ileum in ulcerative colitis. Sometimes reflux of colonic contents through an incompetent ileocaecal valve leads to some dilatation and loss of peristalsis in the terminal ileum (*Figure 3.23*) but this is quite different from the ulceration, narrowing and rigidity found in the terminal ileum in Crohn's disease.

The colon may revert to normal during remissions of ulcerative colitis. In chronic cases, however, there is a tendency for stricture formation to occur, which may be localized or may involve the whole colon. In the latter situation the narrowing and shortening of the colon that result from widespread fibrosis produce a characteristic 'hose-pipe' appearance (*Figure 3.23*).

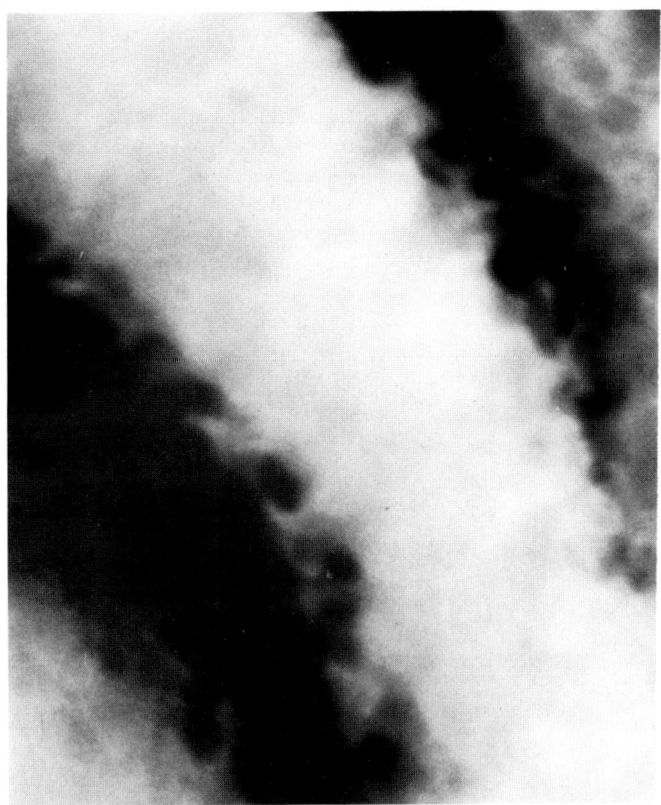

Figure 3.22. Ulcerative colitis: collar-stud ulcers

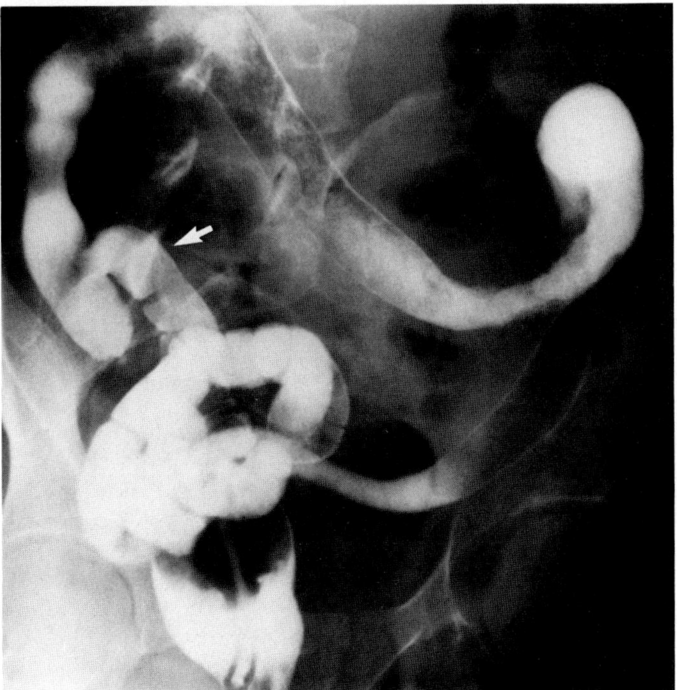

Figure 3.23. Chronic ulcerative colitis: hose-pipe appearance of colon due to narrowing and shortening from fibrosis; slightly dilated but otherwise normal terminal ileum (arrow); ulcerative colitis for 35 years

The major complications of ulcerative colitis are toxic dilatation of the colon and predisposition to colonic carcinoma. Toxic dilatation occurs when inflammation spreads to involve all of the layers of the bowel wall and can be rapidly followed by perforation of the bowel. The patient with toxic dilatation is critically ill with pyrexia, tachycardia, severe diarrhoea and hypokalaemia. On radiographs the dilatation is usually most clearly seen in the transverse colon. It is unusual for this segment to exceed a diameter of 5.5 cm in health, and in toxic dilatation the diameter is commonly 7 or 8 cm. The normal haustral markings of the colon are lost, and severe inflammation produces areas of irregular swelling of the mucosa, seen silhouetted against the gas-filled lumen (*Figure 3.24*). In addition to a supine view an erect view or, in a critically ill patient, a left lateral decubitus view should be obtained to investigate possible perforation.

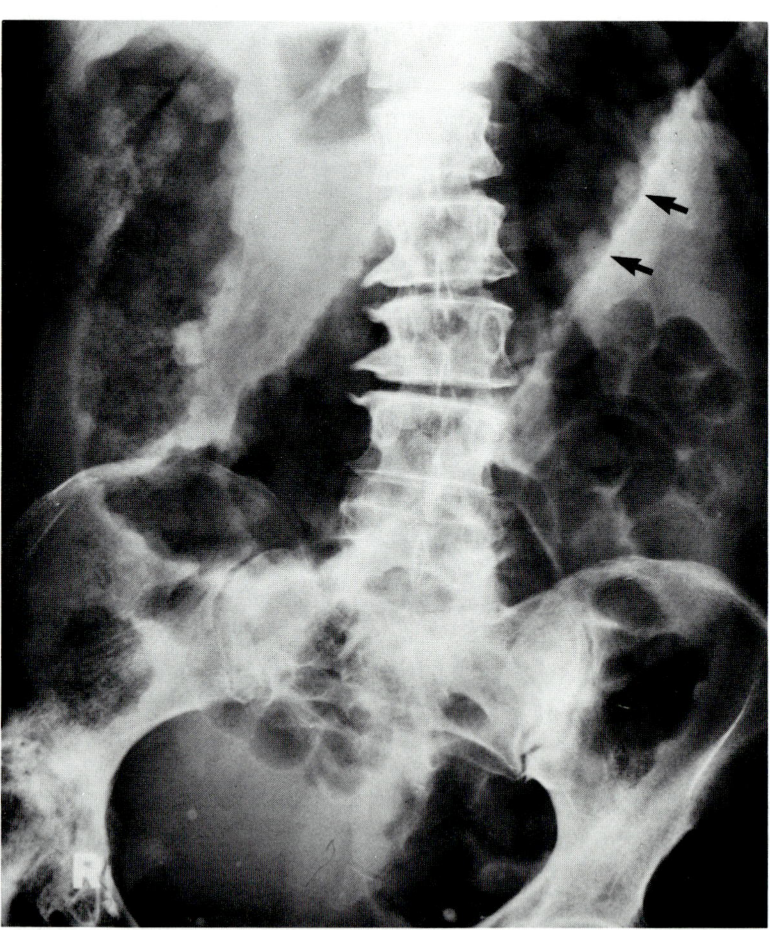

Figure 3.24. Ulcerative colitis—acute toxic dilatation: female aged 52 years; 19 years' diarrhoea with blood and pus in stools at times; recent exacerbation; dilated transverse colon showing loss of normal haustra and polypoid swellings of mucosa (two areas arrowed)

The incidence of carcinoma of the colon is significantly increased in patients with ulcerative colitis. The risk of this complication depends on the duration and extent of the disease. Between 30 and 40 per cent of patients with widespread colitis eventually develop this complication. Carcinomas arising in colitic patients are usually annular, producing circumferential narrowing of the lumen. These are often asymmetrical but may be indistinguishable radiologically from benign strictures.

Radiological examination, and complementary roles of radiology and endoscopy

The diagnosis of ulcerative colitis is usually made by sigmoidoscopy combined with rectal biopsy. The main value of barium enema examination is to determine the extent of the colitis. Double-contrast barium examination is of established superiority to single-contrast studies in this disease. It is usually safe to prepare the colon in the standard manner for radiological examination. In a very ill patient, however, it may be considered advisable to forgo bowel preparation with colonic washouts, lest this causes perforation of the inflamed bowel. In this situation a limited barium examination without prior bowel preparation can be of value. Faeces will normally be expelled from an inflamed segment of bowel. Barium run gently into the unprepared colon will give an approximate indication of the extent of the colitis by showing the point at which barium starts to mix with faeces. This is, however, only a rough guide to the extent, since an empty segment of colon is not necessarily inflamed.

Difficulty is sometimes experienced in establishing a definite diagnosis of ulcerative colitis from rectal biopsy, and in these circumstances consideration of the combined clinical, radiological and pathological aspects is of value.

Colonoscopy can be of great value in patients with ulcerative colitis in the further investigation of radiologically demonstrated strictures of the colon.

Differential diagnosis

The main differential diagnosis is from Crohn's disease. The distinguishing features, which have been mentioned in the text, are summarized in Table 3.2.

Table 3.2. Differential diagnosis of ulcerative colitis from Crohn's disease

	Ulcerative colitis	*Crohn's disease*
Sites	Rectum, and extension of disease proximally without interruption from rectum to involve colon to variable extent. No ulceration or narrowing of terminal ileum	Especially terminal ileum, caecum, and ascending colon. Any part of gastrointestinal tract may be involved. Lesions not in continuity
Mucosa	Granular; pseudopolyps	Cobblestone
Ulcers	Collar stud	Rose thorn; aphthous
Complications	Benign strictures sometimes occur. Carcinoma. Toxic dilatation and perforation	Benign strictures common. Fistulae. Abscess formation

Diverticular disease of the colon

Diverticula are seen on barium enema examination as small, almost spherical barium filled sacs with narrow necks protruding from the wall of the colon (*Figure 3.25*). After evacuation of the barium enema, or of barium from an upper gastrointestinal contrast examination, isolated rounded opacities 2–5 mm in diameter may be visible on plain radiographs, produced by barium retained in the diverticula. These may persist for several days or weeks, so that the demonstration of colonic diverticula is sometimes an incidental finding on an abdominal film taken after a recent barium meal examination. Considerable narrowing of the colon due to spasm may be present in

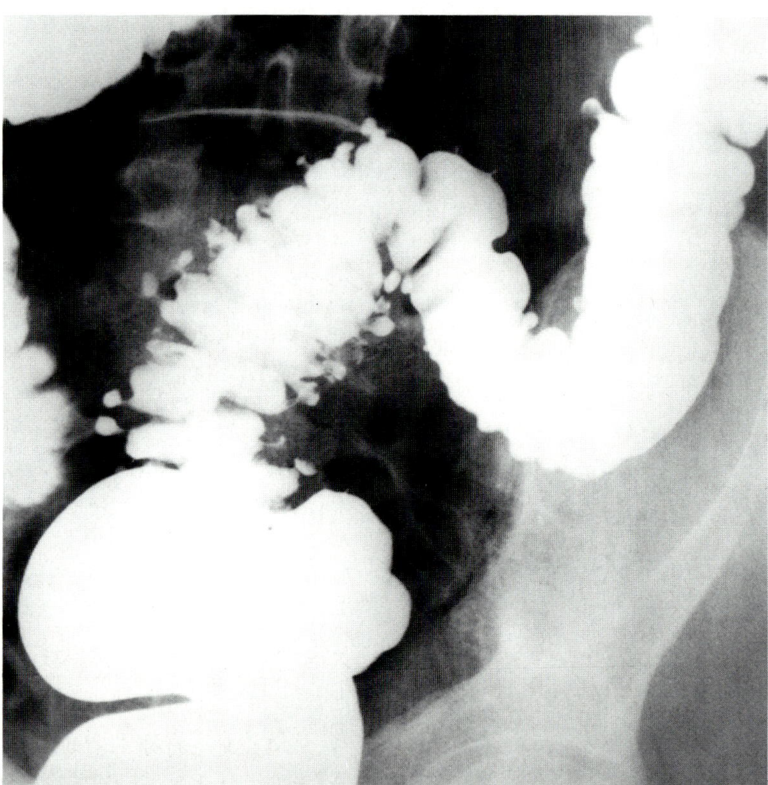

Figure 3.25. Diverticulosis of the colon: small, almost spherical barium-filled sacs with narrow necks are shown arising from the pelvic colon

areas affected by diverticulitis, and it is important to distinguish between narrowing due to this cause and that due to colonic carcinoma (*see* page 133). It is also important that the demonstration of diverticula is not used to account for a patient's symptoms when these are in fact due to some other condition. Diverticula are common in elderly people, and patients with colonic neoplasms often have coexisting diverticular disease. The radiographic changes of diverticular disease may to some extent obscure the presence of a coexisting colonic carcinoma. Occasionally it is impossible to distinguish with certainty between a paracolic abscess in a patient with diverticulitis and a colonic neoplasm.

No difficulty should be experienced in differentiating between round, flask-shaped diverticula of the colon and the flattened, collar-stud ulcers of ulcerative colitis (*see Figure 3.22*).

Carcinoma of the colon

Sigmoidoscopy and barium enema examination should be performed whenever a patient is suspected on clinical grounds of having a carcinoma of the colon. Barium enema examination on its own provides an incomplete examination of the large bowel. 75 per cent of large-bowel carcinomas occur in the pelvic colon and rectum, and tumours of the lower pelvic colon and rectum can be missed on barium examination but are nearly always seen on sigmoidoscopy. Few neoplasms in other parts of the colon should pass undetected on double-contrast barium enema examination provided that the colon has been thoroughly cleared of faeces before the examination. Occasionally a neoplasm in its early stages is not demonstrated on X-ray examination, and in cases of doubt the clinician should have no hesitation in referring the patient for a repeat examination after an interval of 2 or 3 months. If a tumour of the lower bowel is found

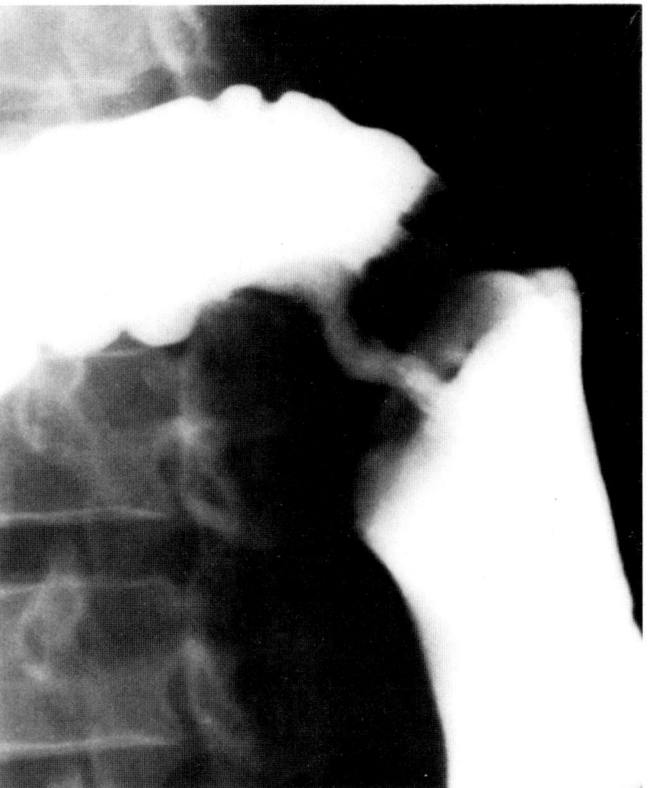

Figure 3.26. Annular carcinoma of colon at splenic flexure; typical 'apple-core' deformity

on sigmoidoscopy the barium enema examination should still be performed (provided that there is no risk of perforating the rectum in doing so), since colonic neoplasms are multiple in 5 per cent of cases.

Carcinomas of the colon are seen on barium examination as annular or polypoid masses. Ulceration may be a prominent feature in either form of tumour. Carcinomas of the left side of the colon are usually of the annular type. Polypoid tumours are commonly found in the caecum and ascending colon.

The characteristic features of an annular carcinoma are shown in *Figure 3.26*. The tumour surrounding the bowel produces an irregular rigid stricture. The mucosa in the strictured segment is entirely destroyed, and irregular filling defects representing the lobulated inner margin of the tumour are visible in profile and *en face* along the length of the stricture. Characteristically the circumferential tumour

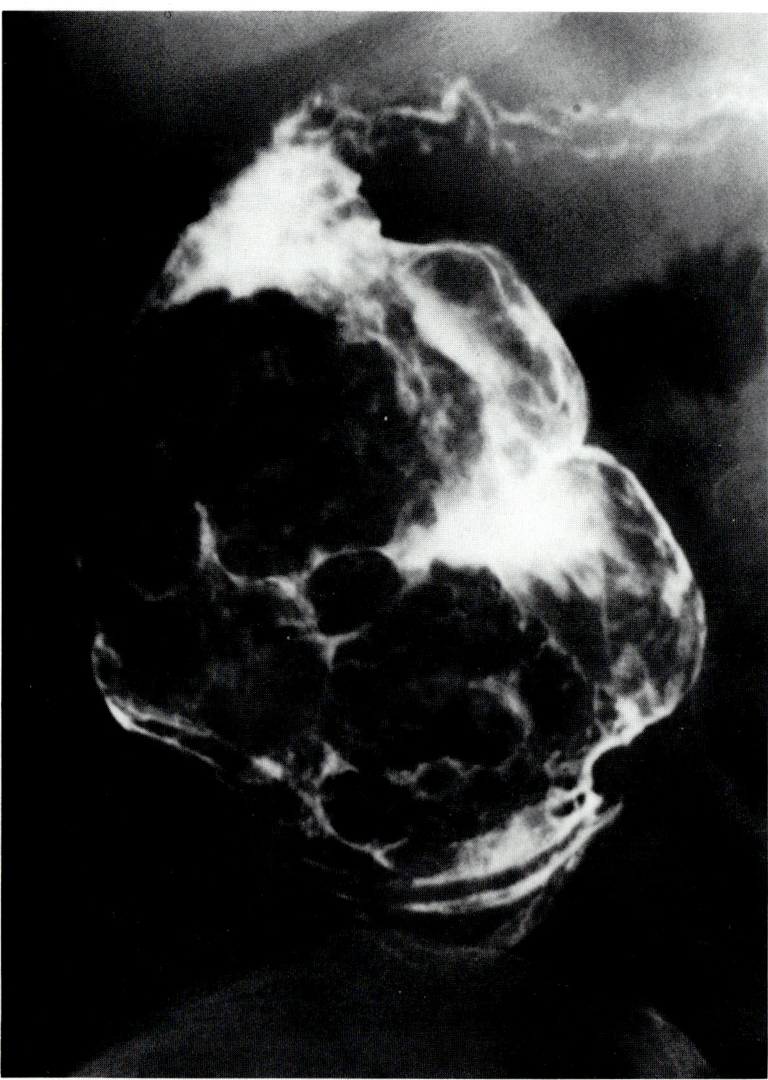

Figure 3.27. Polypoid carcinoma of ascending colon; post-evacuation barium enema film. Barium is tracking in grooves on the surface of a huge polypoid mass filling and distending the lumen of the ascending colon

produces an abrupt, almost right-angle demarcation between the diseased and adjacent normal segments, this giving rise to a shouldered appearance at each end of the tumour. The term 'apple-core deformity' is often applied to this characteristic barium appearance, which resembles the discarded core and ends of an apple from which the fruit has been eaten.

Polypoid or encephaloid carcinomas produce filling defects in the barium column. These tumours can grow to a considerable size in the caecum and ascending colon, where the faeces are liquid, before obstruction is produced (*Figure 3.27*). Double-contrast or post-evacuation films show barium tracking in irregular grooves on the lobulated surface of the tumour. Sometimes faeces in the inadequately prepared colon produce a similar appearance, but the two conditions can usually be differentiated since a mass of faeces can generally be made to alter its position during the course of the examination, and this will be evident on the series of films obtained. This possible source of confusion and the fact that faeces can obscure a small tumour emphasizes the importance of adequate bowel preparation before the barium examination, and it is sometimes necessary to subject the patient to the inconvenience of a repeat examination when the bowel has been imperfectly cleared with laxatives or washouts before the procedure.

Sometimes a polypoid tumour of the colon may produce intussusception, with characteristic barium appearances as described below.

Extensive ulceration of a colonic carcinoma can lead to perforation with paracolic abscess formation, generalized peritonitis or fistula formation. Fistulas can develop between the colon and other hollow intra-abdominal viscera such as the stomach or bladder, or between the colon and skin. Suspected fistulas between the colon and the stomach or small intestine should be investigated by barium enema rather than by barium meal and follow-through examination, since the greater intraluminal pressure in the colon will usually result in barium entering the fistula from the colon.

Involvement of the ureters by direct extension of a pelvic carcinoma of the colon can be assessed preoperatively with an intravenous urogram. Ultrasound and isotope liver scanning are the investigations of choice for the investigation of possible liver metastases.

Differential diagnosis

1. Benign strictures (due, for example, to Crohn's disease, tuberculosis, and strictures of the pelvic colon resulting from irradiation of pelvic organs). In contrast to the features of annular carcinoma of the colon, benign strictures are characteristically smooth and have gradually tapering proximal and distal ends merging with adjacent normal bowel (*see Figure 3.12*).
2. Spasm. Narrowing of the colon due to spasm is seen most commonly in diverticulitis. In this condition there is no massive hold-up of faeces proximal to the stricture, as commonly occurs in the presence of an organic lesion, and spasm can be confirmed

diagnosing the condition, the barium examination can often be used to reduce the intussusception. Barium is run into the colon at moderate hydrostatic pressure, and progressive reduction can be observed under fluoroscopy during the procedure. Sometimes infarction of the intussuscepted portion occurs, and this will not be evident on the X-ray examination. Surgery should not be withheld if this complication is suspected, even though the intussusception has been successfully reduced with barium.

Ischaemic colitis

Ischaemia of the colon is most common in elderly patients, who typically present with abdominal pain and bloody diarrhoea. The most common sites to be affected are the caecum and terminal ileum in superior mesenteric occlusion, and the colon in the region of the splenic flexure. The occlusion may be arterial or venous, but in most cases it is probably a combination of the two.

In acute vascular occlusion supine and erect plain films of the abdomen will commonly show the features of intestinal obstruction, with dilated small- and large-bowel loops containing multiple fluid

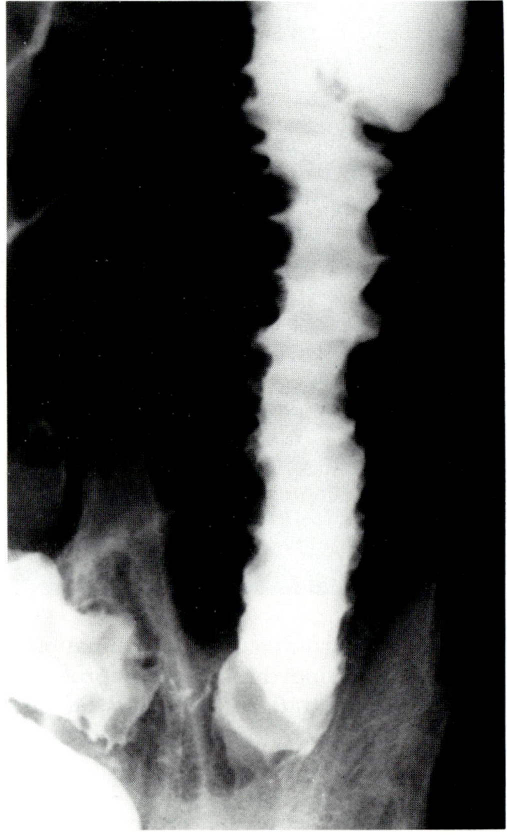

Figure 3.30. Ischaemia of descending colon; barium enema examination. 'Thumbprint' defects seen in profile and *en face* in the descending and sigmoid portions produced by haemorrhage and oedema in the submucosa

levels. Since these changes are non-specific, the possibility of this diagnosis should be borne in mind when examining an elderly patient with the above symptoms and with radiographic features of obstruction.

In addition to the changes of obstruction, changes indicating ischaemic necrosis of a segment of bowel may be present. This may be manifest by gas in the wall of the bowel, or free gas in the peritoneum indicating that perforation has occurred, or gas in the portal veins. Gas in the wall of the bowel appears as linear translucent streaks parallel with the gas-filled lumen. Gas in the portal veins indicates an exceedingly bad prognosis and is shown by linear streaks of gas in the region of the liver periphery.

In subacute vascular occlusion filling defects may be seen encroaching on the gas-filled lumen of the colon from the mucosal surface. This appearance is aptly termed 'thumb printing', since it may be imagined to resemble the distortion of the colon that would be brought about by numerous thumb impressions on the bowel wall. This characteristic appearance can be confirmed on barium enema examination (*Figure 3.30*) and is produced by haemorrhage and oedema in the submucosa.

Revascularization of an ischaemic segment sometimes occurs by development of a collateral circulation or by recanalization of occluded vessels, and the colon may revert to normal. At other times a permanent stricture develops. This stricture resembles that of other benign conditions (e.g. Crohn's disease), with a smooth narrowed segment through which the mucosa is preserved, and with tapering margins blending with the adjacent normal bowel.

Subphrenic abscess

An abscess may form in the subphrenic region after abdominal or pelvic surgery or following peritonitis (e.g. from appendicitis or perforation of the gastrointestinal tract). The patient may present with localizing symptoms of pain, tenderness or a palpable swelling, but more commonly presents with evidence of systemic sepsis without localizing signs. The untreated condition carries a high mortality, so that recognition and localization of a subphrenic abscess are essential in order that effective surgical drainage can be carried out.

The initial radiological investigation comprises an erect chest film and supine and erect films of the abdomen. In the presence of a subphrenic abscess the chest film commonly shows elevation of the corresponding hemidiaphragm, a pleural effusion, and consolidation with or without some associated atelectasis at the lung base on the affected side. These findings are not specific for subphrenic abscess, since they also occur with lung infection and pulmonary embolism, and all three conditions are common postoperative sequelae. Subphrenic abscesses may contain gas, and the chest film and more particularly the erect film of the abdomen may then show the presence of a fluid level within an abscess beneath one or other

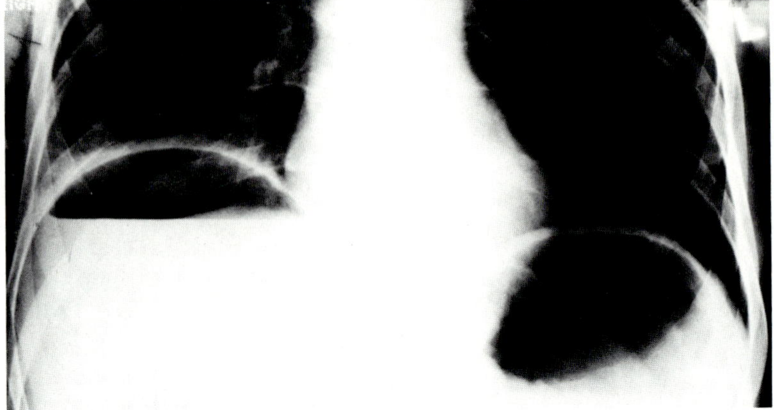

Figure 3.31. Right subphrenic abscess. The abscess contains gas, so that a fluid level is seen beneath the right dome of the diaphragm on the erect film (The gas shadow on the left is swallowed air in the stomach.)

hemidiaphragm (*Figure 3.31*). Alternatively an intra-abdominal abscess may be seen to contain multiple small pockets of air. The cluster of small gas pockets in this condition can usually be distinguished from gas within the bowel.

A subphrenic abscess containing no air may be apparent on the abdominal film as a mass of soft-tissue density, sometimes displacing the air-containing stomach or flexures of the colon.

Reduced movement of the diaphragm on the affected side, shown on fluoroscopy, is a common but non-specific manifestation of subphrenic abscess. When the erect abdominal film shows an obvious fluid level within an abscess an erect lateral film is a useful supplementary view to establish whether the abscess lies anteriorly or posteriorly.

In practice, doubt can often arise as to whether a fluid level in the upper abdomen indicates the presence of an abscess or simply air and fluid within a loop of gut. This can be resolved with appropriate limited barium investigation of the intestine, either by barium follow-through examination or barium enema. When a barium study is required for this purpose this may show displacement of the opacified stomach or intestine, further aiding localization of an abscess. Ultrasound and computed tomography can be of great value in diagnosing this condition when the results of conventional radiological investigation are equivocal.

The liver and pancreas

Gall stones and bile duct calculi

A common clinical problem for which radiological assistance is often sought is to determine whether a patient has gall stones. The symptoms and physical signs of cholecystitis are varied and often indefinite. Pain is commonly felt near the right costal margin, or referred to the right scapular region. This may be a dull ache or stabbing pain, and if a small calculus has entered the cystic duct severe colic may be experienced. There is often tenderness on palpation in the region of the lower right costal cartilages. Sometimes the symptoms resemble those of gastric dyspepsia, with a feeling of fullness or distension in the epigastrium and some intolerance to fatty foods.

Radiological investigation

A plain film of the gall bladder region is usually obtained in the first instance. Gall stones, however, calcify in only 20 per cent of cases, so

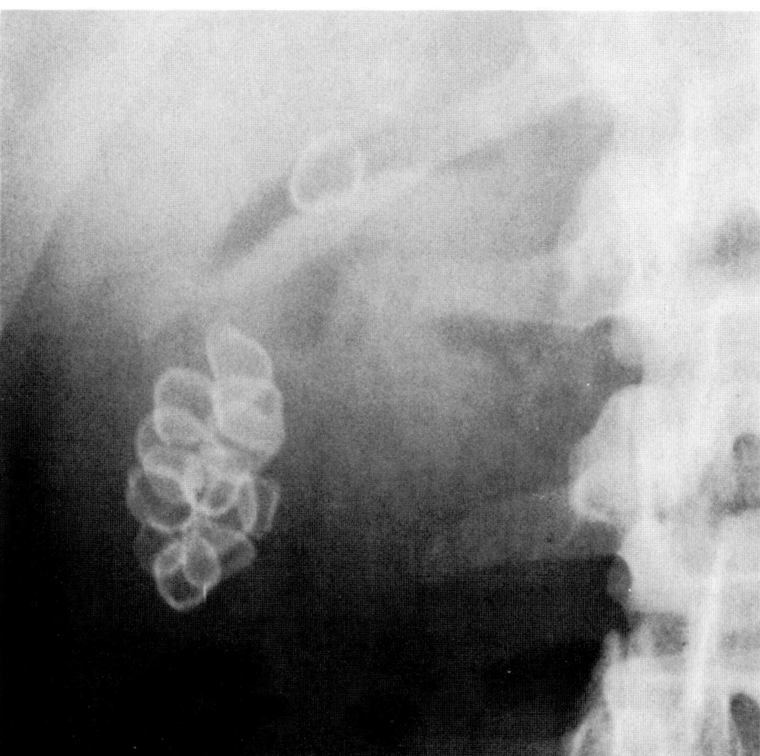

Figure 3.32. Calcified spherical and faceted gall stones, the majority lying free within the gall bladder but one at a higher level, lodged in the gall bladder neck or cystic duct

that the plain film alone constitutes an inadequate investigation. Calcified gall stones may show as single or multiple spherical or faceted opacities; they may calcify in layers, giving a laminated appearance, or only the rims may calcify (*Figure 3.32*). Sometimes the appearances are less characteristic, and in these situations calcified gall stones must be distinguished from calcifications that can occur within other structures in the right upper abdomen, such as costal cartilages, lymph glands, and renal calcification.

The oral cholecystogram is the standard investigation for gall stones. The evening before the examination one of several suitable iodine-containing preparations is taken by mouth. In order to opacify the gall bladder, this compound requires to be absorbed by the small intestine, excreted by the liver, passed with the bile through the cystic duct to the gall bladder, and concentrated by the gall bladder. When this sequence of events proceeds normally the concentrated contrast medium in the gall bladder may show filling

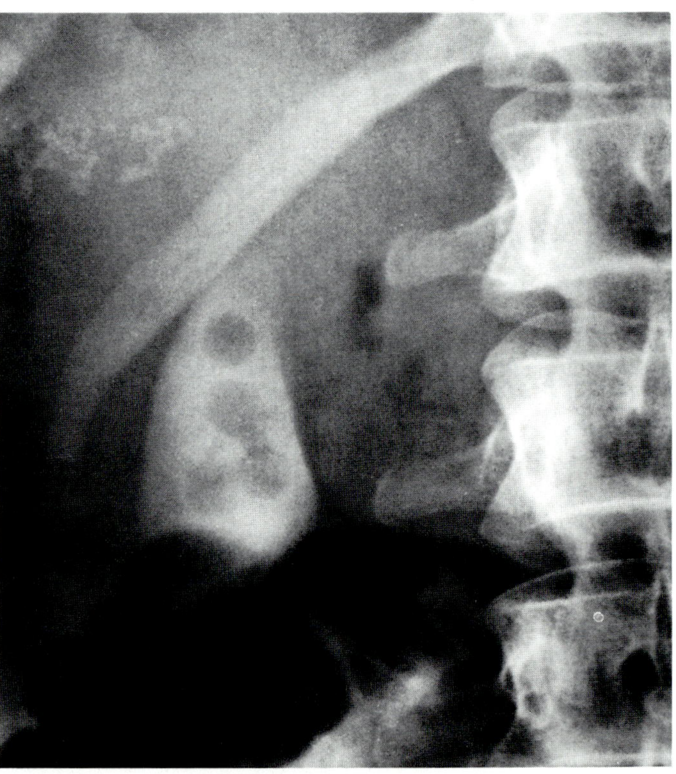

Figure 3.33. Gall stones; oral cholecystogram: the gall bladder has been opacified with contrast medium, and filling defects produced by several spherical gall stones are shown

defects due to radiolucent stones (*Figure 3.33*). It will also establish whether calcifications of uncertain nature shown on the plain film represent stones within the gall bladder.

Failure of the gall bladder to opacify on oral cholecystography may be due to obstruction of the cystic duct by a stone or to inflammation of the gall bladder mucosa preventing concentration of the contrast medium in the gall bladder. Since oral cholecystography requires a number of physiological processes, it is clear from the above that the gall bladder will also fail to opacify if the contrast medium is not absorbed from the small bowel (in the presence of diarrhoea or vomiting, for example) or if there is impaired hepatic function preventing the normal excretion of the contrast agent by the liver. Good liver function is vital for the success of this examination and it is generally fruitless carrying out cholecystography if the serum bilirubin concentration exceeds 35 μmol/ℓ (2 mg/100 ml) since the gall bladder will very rarely opacify in these circumstances.

Ultrasound examination is highly accurate in detecting gall stones and is the next examination of choice in those patients in whom the gall bladder has failed to opacify on cholecystography. Ultrasound is also of great value in confirming the presence of gall stones in patients presenting with a clinical diagnosis of acute cholecystitis and for whom emergency surgery is planned.

It should be remembered, however, that gall stones are a common incidental finding in elderly people. Demonstration of gall stones on cholecystography or ultrasound does not necessarily imply that these are the cause of a patient's symptoms, and the significance of the radiological findings must be considered in the full context of the clinical presentation.

The common bile duct can be investigated in detail with ultrasound or intravenous cholangiography. For the latter investigation a suitable iodine-containing contrast agent is injected intravenously. The agent is both excreted and concentrated by the liver and is not dependent on the gall bladder for the latter function. As with oral cholecystography, however, the examination depends on good liver function and will rarely show opacification of the common bile duct if the serum bilirubin concentration exceeds 35 μmol/ℓ (2 mg/100 ml). Situations in which this examination is useful are the examination of stones in the common bile duct in patients who have had a recurrence of symptoms after cholecystectomy, or in patients with a history of obstructive jaundice of undetermined cause. Intravenous cholangiography is also useful as an alternative to ultrasound examination to confirm a preoperative diagnosis of acute cholecystitis when emergency surgery is planned. The diagnosis will be virtually certain if there is opacification of the common bile duct but not of the gall bladder, implying obstruction of the cystic duct by a stone.

Further radiological examination of the biliary tree is commonly undertaken for possible biliary tract calculi during and shortly after a cholecystectomy. The examinations that can be carried out are operative cholangiography and postoperative (T-tube) cholangiography.

Operative cholangiography is performed by injecting a water-soluble iodine-containing contrast agent directly into the cystic duct during surgery. Films are taken in theatre after injection of approximately 3 ml, 7 ml, and 10 ml of contrast. These may show direct evidence of calculi (rounded filling defects in the opacified biliary tree) or evidence of obstruction at the lower end of the common bile duct (abnormal distension of the common bile duct or failure of passage of the contrast to the duodenum). The surgeon can then proceed directly to explore the common bile duct if a radiographic abnormality is shown.

When a T-tube is left in the bile duct for drainage of bile postoperatively, T-tube cholangiography can be performed 7–10 days after surgery, before the tube is removed, as a final check that stones in the bile duct have not been overlooked. A water-soluble contrast agent is injected into the tube, and the same observations of the biliary tract are made as in operative cholangiography. In the event of stones being shown on this examination the T-tube can be left in position for several weeks to establish a fistulous track, and an attempt can then be made to snare the stones under fluoroscopic control with a Dormia basket passed through the fistula to the bile duct. If successful this eliminates the need for reoperation.

Obstructive jaundice

As mentioned above, oral cholecystography and intravenous cholangiography usually fail if the serum bilirubin concentration exceeds 35 µmol/ℓ (2 mg/100 ml), so that these examinations are not of use in investigating the jaundiced patient.

Ultrasound is now generally accepted as the initial imaging procedure of choice in investigating this condition. Dilated bile ducts can be readily seen, so that this technique is extremely accurate in distinguishing between hepatocellular (medical) jaundice and jaundice produced by extrahepatic obstruction (surgical jaundice). The level of the obstruction can usually be deduced by ultrasound examination of the gall bladder and common bile duct, since these structures will be dilated above an obstruction. Furthermore, the nature of an obstructing lesion (e.g. carcinoma of the head of the pancreas, gall stones) can be accurately ascertained by ultrasound in approximately 70 per cent of cases. In those patients with non-obstructive jaundice, ultrasound examination can readily show focal liver disease (e.g. hepatic metastases—*see Figure 1.4*) and, in many instances, diffuse liver disease (e.g. cirrhosis, severe hepatitis). In many patients, therefore, this simple painless non-invasive investigation provides a complete diagnostic investigation, obviating the need for more unpleasant invasive procedures.

The accuracy of computed tomography in investigating obstructive jaundice appears, from data currently available, to be similar to that of ultrasound. Computed tomography is therefore valuable in those patients in whom the cheaper, more readily available ultrasound study is inconclusive.

Percutaneous transhepatic cholangiography (PTC) and endoscopic retrograde cholangiopancreatography (ERCP) can also provide more definitive information on the site and nature of biliary obstruction in those patients in whom ultrasound examination is inconclusive or unavailable. In PTC a very fine gauge needle is passed percutaneously into the liver, and a small amount of contrast medium is injected under fluoroscopic observation while the needle is slowly withdrawn. When the contrast injection shows the needle tip to lie in a dilated bile duct further contrast is injected to opacify

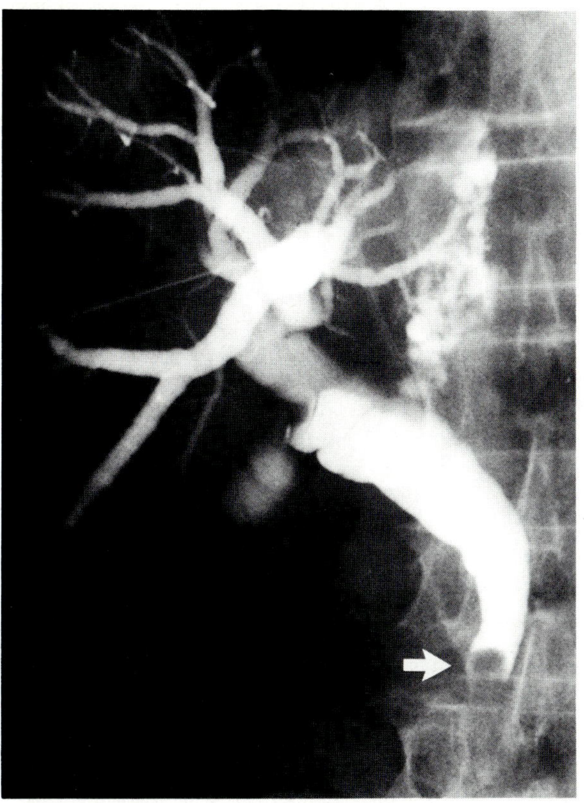

Figure 3.34. Jaundice due to stone at lower end of common bile duct: percutaneous transhepatic cholangiogram. Characteristic smooth, rounded, central filling defect (arrow) produced by large stone at lower end of grossly dilated (obstructed) common bile duct

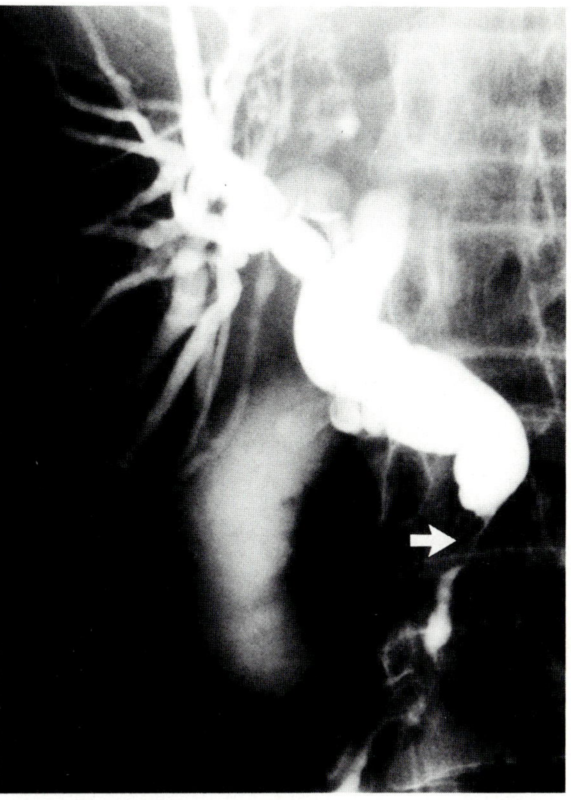

Figure 3.35. Jaundice due to carcinoma of head of pancreas; percutaneous transhepatic cholangiogram: irregular, very tight stricture of lower end of common bile duct (arrow) due to tumour invasion by pancreatic carcinoma; grossly dilated (obstructed) biliary system proximally

the biliary tree and to outline the obstructing lesion (*Figures 3.34 and 3.35*). With a very fine Chiba needle there is a small risk of producing biliary peritonitis due to leakage of bile into the peritoneum from the puncture site in the liver. This examination should therefore be performed only when there are facilities available for urgent surgery in the event of this complication arising.

In ERCP examination the fibreoptic endoscope is positioned with its tip in the second part of the duodenum and a catheter is threaded through this and into the ampulla of Vater. Contrast medium is injected to opacify the bile duct and pancreatic duct. This technique has the advantages over PTC of allowing for opacification of both the bile duct and the pancreatic duct, and for biopsy of any abnormality seen in the region of the ampulla. ERCP has the disadvantages, however, of being a lengthy and technically more difficult procedure.

The liver

Plain films are of very limited value in assessing liver disease. The relationship of the inferior border of the liver, which is often visible, to the lower costal margin can only be roughly assessed since the costal cartilages are commonly uncalcified. An enlarged liver may depress the gas-filled hepatic flexure of the colon, cause some elevation of the right diaphragm, and indent the lesser curve aspect of the stomach. In the presence of these changes, however, liver enlargement will usually be quite obvious clinically. Thin rims of calcification may be seen on plain films in the walls of hydatid cysts after death of the parasites, and amorphous calcification occurs in old tuberculous liver abscesses.

The two most useful and widely used imaging techniques for the liver are isotope liver scanning and ultrasound. In certain situations examination by one or other technique will provide diagnostic information, while in other situations it will be useful to carry out both procedures. Since an ultrasound examination must be performed by a skilled, highly trained person, an isotope scan, which is technically less exacting, is usually performed first when investigating disease of the liver parenchyma. Sufficient information is often obtained from this single investigation.

The principles of isotope scanning have already been mentioned (*see Chapter 1*). This technique has been variously reported as having an accuracy of between 72 and 90 per cent in the detection of hepatic metastases. Cysts, abscesses and tumours show as 'cold' spots on technetium-labelled sulphur colloid scans (*see Figure 1.3*). Since the appearances of these conditions are similar, interpretation of the scan requires to be made in the context of the particular clinical problem.

A primary hepatoma can be diagnosed in the following manner. This tumour will show as a 'cold' area on the technetium–sulphur colloid scan, but if the patient is rescanned using the isotope selenomethionine a high uptake of the isotope by this liver-cell carcinoma will usually occur.

Ultrasound is particularly indicated to assess a known or suspected hepatic mass, or to provide further information on the nature of a 'cold' area on an isotope scan. Completely transonic cysts can usually be distinguished without difficulty from liver tumours (*see Figure 1.4*). Abscesses (*see Figure 1.5*) also can often be differentiated from tumours. In cases of doubt, a change in size of a liver mass on repeat examination after an interval of 1 week almost invariably indicates the presence of an abscess. Ultrasound has a further value in assessing the liver when an equivocal isotope scan has been obtained. Carefully performed ultrasound examination is likely to detect over 90 per cent of hepatic lesions greater than 1 cm in diameter. Fine needle aspiration biopsy of hepatic lesions for cytological examination can be facilitated by using ultrasound for guidance of the needle to areas of abnormality within the liver.

Computed tomography (CT) has an accuracy similar to isotope scanning and ultrasound in the detection of liver disease, and there is presently no evidence that CT offers a significant advantage in this field over the cheaper, simpler methods of examination.

In cases where further diagnostic information is required hepatic angiography may be valuable in showing, for instance, an obvious malignant tumour circulation within a hepatic mass. Portal venography, performed by puncturing the spleen percutaneously with a needle and then injecting contrast medium directly into the substance of the spleen, provides a means of opacifying the portal vein and of demonstrating oesophageal varices in portal hypertension (*see* page 273).

The pancreas

The pancreas has traditionally been one of the most difficult organs of the body to image. Nowadays this can be investigated non-invasively by ultrasound and computed tomography.

The diagnosis of acute pancreatitis is usually made on the basis of the clinical findings together with the presence of a serum amylase activity above 1000 IU/ℓ. Plain films of the abdomen in this condition may show the presence of a gas-distended loop of duodenum or proximal jejunum or transverse colon produced by a local ileus in the vicinity of the inflamed pancreas. Acute pancreatitis is commonly a sequel of biliary lithiasis, so in some cases calcified biliary tract stones will be visible. Plain films obtained on initial presentation of the patient are valuable in excluding an alternative cause of the patient's acute abdomen, e.g. acute perforation of a peptic ulcer with free gas beneath the right dome of the diaphragm. Calcification across the upper abdomen in the line of the pancreas is sometimes seen in patients with chronic pancreatitis.

Ultrasound is the examination of choice for investigating suspected mass lesions of the pancreas, and diffuse abnormalities of the pancreas (as may be produced by chronic pancreatitis) can sometimes be detected with this procedure. With careful examination using grey scale display (*see* Chapter 1) visualization of the head and body of the pancreas is possible in 80–90 per cent of cases, and pseudocysts can be detected with nearly 100 per cent accuracy (*Figure 3.36*). Occasional difficulties arise in distinguishing carcinoma of the head or body of the pancreas from chronic pancreatitis,

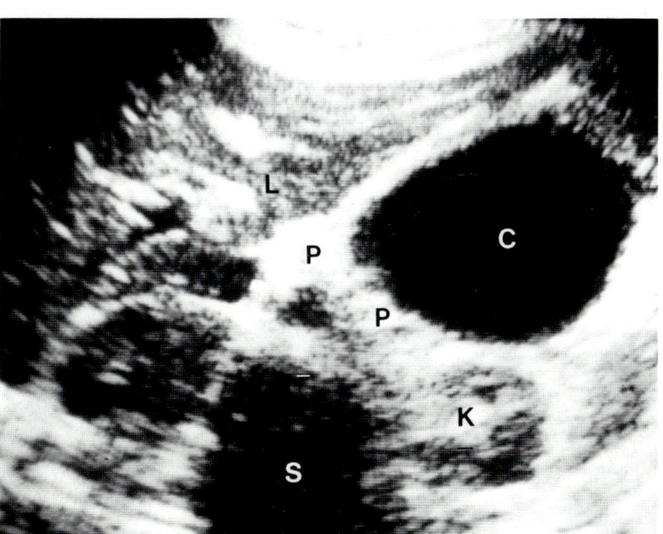

Figure 3.36. Pancreatic pseudocyst. Ultrasound examination; transverse scan of abdomen at level of pancreas: smooth-walled, well-defined, echo-free area represents cyst arising from tail of pancreas; C, pseudocyst; K, kidney; L, liver; P, pancreas; S, spine

and in some instances the two conditions coexist. The tail of the pancreas is less easy to examine than the head and body.

CT has an accuracy similar to that of ultrasound in the detection and diagnosis of pancreatic lesions. In general, therefore, the simpler, cheaper investigation of ultrasound should be performed initially, and CT reserved for those patients in whom the ultrasound examination is equivocal or at variance with the clinical diagnosis.

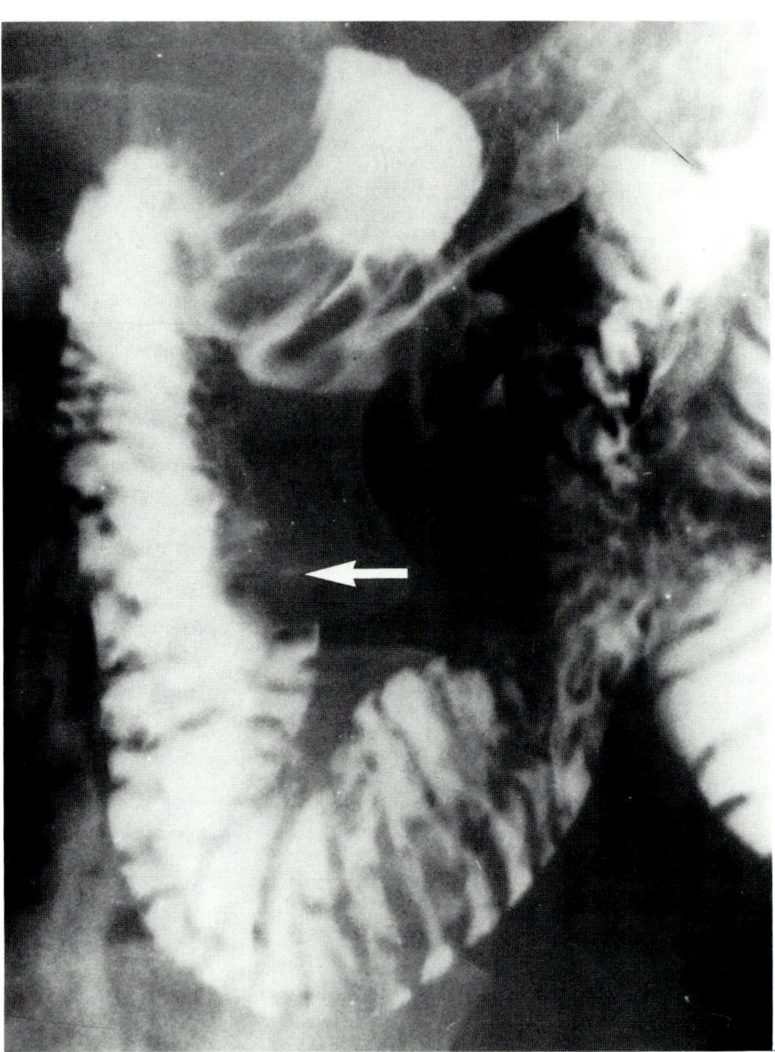

Figure 3.37. Carcinoma of ampulla of Vater, producing obstructive jaundice: large filling defect (arrow) due to tumour at site of ampulla on inner aspect of second part of duodenum

Space-occupying lesions of the ampulla of Vater and of the head of the pancreas can often be seen on barium examination of the duodenal loop or, more particularly, on hypotonic duodenography. This is a modification of the standard barium meal examination in which hyoscine butyl bromide (Buscopan) is given intravenously to relax and allow for distension of the duodenal loop during the examination. A tumour of the ampulla may produce a local indentation of the second part of the duodenum on the medial side

(*Figure 3.37*), while a mass in the head of the pancreas may stretch the duodenal loop and flatten the mucosa on the inner aspect of the loop. A tumour of the head of the pancreas may also invade directly into the loop to produce an irregular filling defect. Hypotonic duodenography is a simple examination to perform and is a useful preliminary examination when ultrasound is not readily available.

When the results of non-invasive investigations are inconclusive, or more detailed information is required, endoscopic retrograde cholangiopancreatography (*see* section on liver above) may be undertaken to investigate lesions of the ampulla and pancreas, while percutaneous transhepatic cholangiography can be performed to investigate tumours of the head of the pancreas and ampulla that are obstructing the common bile duct (*see Figure 3.35*). Selective arteriography is sometimes extremely helpful and may provide the only evidence of small tumours within the pancreas. A characteristic tumour circulation may be seen in vascular tumours of the pancreas (e.g. cystadenomas and islet-cell tumours), while displacement of normal vessel branches can indicate the presence of avascular or poorly vascularized space-occupying lesions.

The abdominal lymph nodes

Lymphography is the traditional radiological examination for detecting involvement of the abdominal lymph glands by malignant disease. The procedure entails injecting oily contrast medium (ultra-fluid lipiodol) into a lymphatic on the dorsum of each foot: the pattern and distribution of uptake of the contrast in the lymph glands is then studied on subsequent X-rays of the abdomen and pelvis. Lymphography is used in the staging of lymphomas and to investigate lymphatic dissemination by various other neoplasms such as testicular tumours and carcinomas of the female genital tract.

Lymph node infiltration is manifest by glandular enlargement or displacement, areas of non-filling in individual glands, and lymphatic obstruction leading to failure of filling of whole groups of glands with opacification of collateral drainage pathways (*Figure 3.38*). Although glands involved by lymphoma often have a foamy appearance it is impossible in practice to make a firm pathological diagnosis from the lymphographic features. Inflammation also produces lymph node enlargement, usually with preservation of the glandular outline.

A major limitation of lymphography is that the internal iliac and other pelvic lymph nodes, which may be involved by tumour, are not opacified, and cannot therefore be assessed, after the injection of contrast medium into the foot.

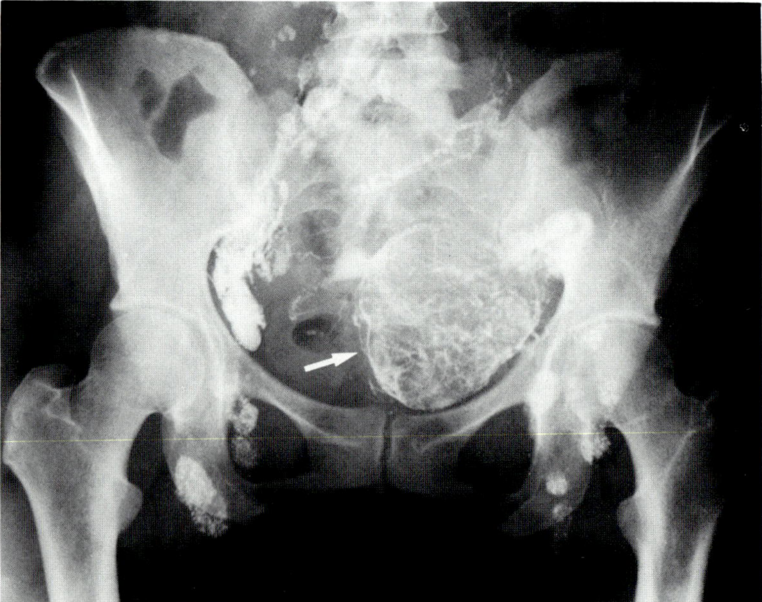

Figure 3.38. Hodgkin's disease; lymphangiogram. The pelvic lymph nodes are enlarged and foamy in appearance. There is a huge glandular tumour mass (arrow) in the left side of the pelvis

CT provides an important alternative method for detecting lymph node disease: glandular enlargement can be recognized; certain pelvic and mesenteric nodes that cannot be shown by lymphography can be demonstrated; and tumour deposits in bone and liver can be disclosed. CT is unfortunately unreliable in detecting splenic involvement by lymphoma, so that laparotomy is still required for this purpose. Furthermore, CT does not distinguish neoplastic from inflammatory glandular enlargement, although massive glandular enlargement usually denotes malignant disease.

Both lymphography and CT have important roles in assessing tumour response to treatment. Lipiodol remains within diseased lymph glands for 6–12 months, so that repeat films of the abdomen can be taken at selected intervals of time and the appearances of the glands compared with those shown on the initial investigation. CT can likewise be repeated and the presence and distribution of enlarged glands compared with the findings of earlier investigations.

one of the renal arteries or in the aorta above the renal arteries. Contrast medium is then injected through the catheter. Assessment of renal artery stenosis and of renal tumours (*see Figure 3.50*) provide the main indications for this examination.

Venography

Extension of a renal carcinoma into the renal veins or inferior vena cava can be assessed accurately by injecting contrast medium through a catheter introduced into the venous system from the femoral vein and positioned with its tip in either the lower inferior vena cava or a renal vein.

Ultrasound

Ultrasound is of prime value in determining whether a renal mass, shown on IVU examination, is due to a tumour or a cyst (*see* page 165). Ultrasound is also of value in assessing a kidney that has failed to opacify on an IVU, and since ultrasound is non-invasive this is the next examination of choice in this situation. Ultrasound can be performed as an alternative to an IVU examination in the initial assessment of a patient presenting with renal failure: hydronephrosis due to obstruction can be rapidly and reliably confirmed or excluded. In experienced hands, ultrasound can provide useful information on the extent of spread of bladder tumours within the pelvis.

Radioisotope scanning

In patients with unilateral renal disease the function of the two kidneys can be compared by radioisotope scanning. An intravenous injection of a radioisotope that is excreted by the kidneys is given. Serial gamma-camera images of the two kidneys are obtained during the ensuing 20 or 30 minutes. The isotope present in each kidney at specified times after injection can also be recorded and plotted graphically. Renograms performed in this manner provide an accurate comparison of function of the two kidneys. They do not, however, provide good detail of renal anatomy. The main indication for renography, therefore, is to assess renal function in patients with known renal disease (e.g. after surgical relief of ureteric obstruction).

Radioisotope scanning is a safe procedure and may at times be an adequate substitute for intravenous urography in patients with a previous severe reaction to contrast medium.

Computed tomography

CT will differentiate solid from cystic renal masses, will accurately demonstrate the extent of spread of renal carcinoma, and can be used to assess patients with renal failure. These conditions are, however, usually investigated with the simpler, cheaper techniques of intravenous urography and ultrasound, supplemented when necessary by cyst puncture or arteriography. The role of CT in modifying this traditional scheme of investigation is not yet established.

Needle aspiration of renal masses

A cyst shown on ultrasound can be confirmed and a solid renal mass can be biopsied by passing a fine needle directly through the skin of the patient's back and into the mass. Ultrasound is commonly used to assist correct positioning of the needle.

Normal appearances of the urinary tract

The outlines of the kidneys are visible on IVU films taken after the injection of contrast and are sometimes seen on plain films of the abdomen. Measurement of the lengths of the kidneys should be made after careful identification of the upper and lower poles. The normal range in adults is from 11 to 15 cm, and the difference between an individual's two kidneys should not exceed 2 cm. The normal renal outlines are smooth and the long axes of the kidneys are parallel with the lateral psoas margins. The tips of the calyces are separated from the renal margins by a thickness of parenchyma of approximately 1.5–2 cm. The calyces vary considerably in number from individual to individual but in any one person the number of calyces tends to be fairly similar on the two sides. The normal calyces appear cup shaped with sharp, pointed lips to the cups (*Figure 3.39*). The renal pelvis commonly lies predominantly within the kidney but sometimes it forms a large extrarenal sac as a normal variant. The pelvis tapers smoothly to the pelviureteric junction.

The ureter lies in front of and approximately in line with the tips of the transverse processes of the lumbar vertebrae, but on entering the pelvis it descends more laterally to enter the posteroinferior portion of the bladder. The ureter is normally only partially opacified with contrast at any one time due to ureteric contraction, and the diameter of the ureter is approximately 4 mm. The bladder may be indented by adjacent bowel, and this extrinsic compression should not be mistaken for a tumour within the bladder itself. The bladder should be almost empty of contrast on a film taken after micturition.

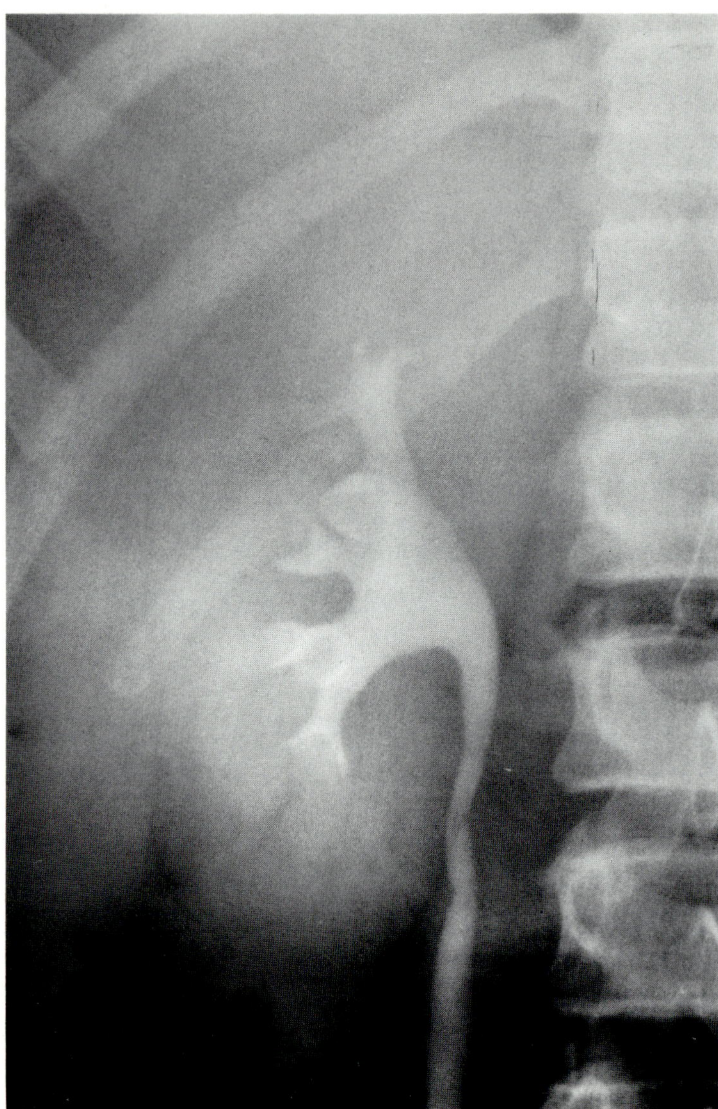

Figure 3.39. IVU film of normal kidney: long axis parallel with lateral psoas margin; smooth renal outline; cup-shaped calyces facing outwards; calyces all roughly equidistant from renal margin

Calcified renal tract calculi can readily be concealed by contrast medium in the collecting system. No attempt therefore should be made to interpret films of the opacified renal tract without reference to the accompanying preliminary plain film of the abdomen.

Congenital variations

The possibility that a patient has a congenital single kidney must always be remembered, and it is essential before removing one kidney to demonstrate radiologically that there is a normal kidney on the other side.

When an IVU shows opacification of only one kidney on the full-length film, the possibilities are that the opposite kidney is non-functioning, congenitally absent or has been removed. The last possibility can usually be reliably confirmed or refuted by the patient, and ultrasound is valuable in determining whether a non-functioning kidney is present. In cases of doubt, aortography will show the presence or absence of a renal artery and associated kidney.

Ectopic kidney

The kidney forms in the pelvis, and migrates during fetal development to its normal position in the upper abdomen. This normal

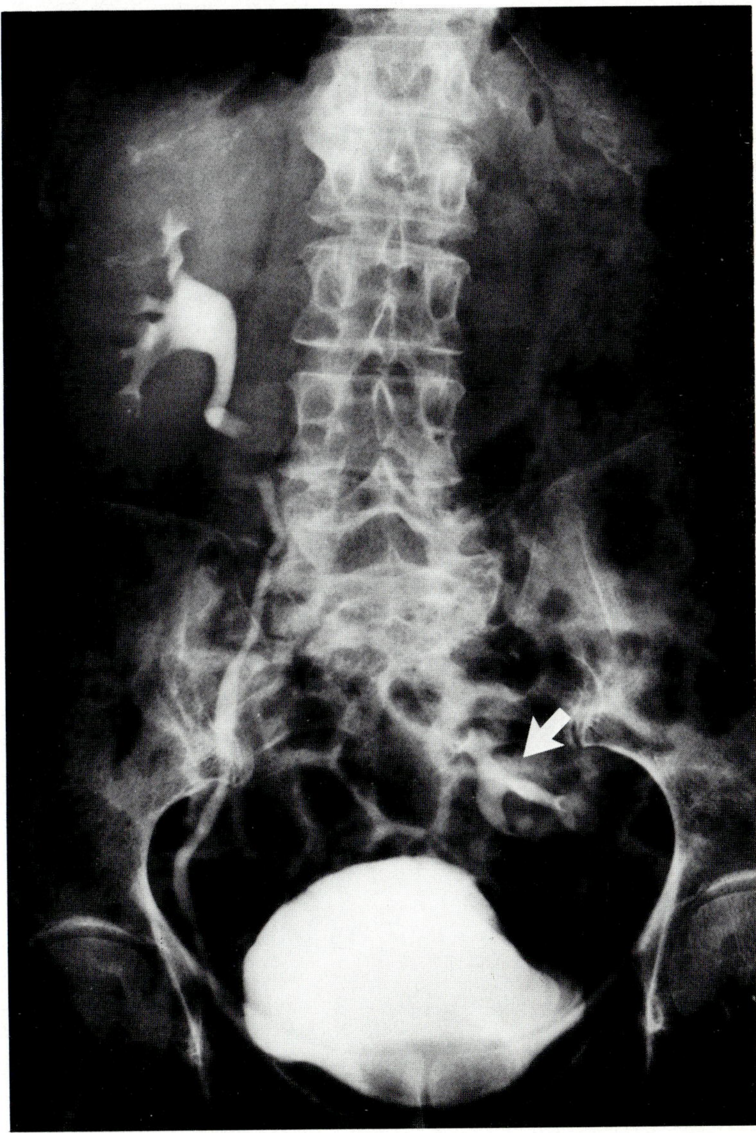

Figure 3.40. IVU film of left pelvic kidney (arrow). Careful inspection of the abdomen for an ectopic kidney should be made when a kidney is not seen in the normal position

movement may become arrested, with the result that the kidney remains within the pelvis or lower abdomen. From the practical standpoint failure of opacification of a kidney in its expected position in the upper abdomen on an IVU examination must not be attributed to a non-functioning or absent kidney until a full-length film has been carefully examined for an ectopic kidney (*Figure 3.40*).

Horseshoe kidney

In this congenital variant a bridge of renal tissue joins the two kidneys, usually by their lower poles. Sometimes the kidneys and associated bridge are visible as a central abdominal soft-tissue mass on plain films. The characteristic features are clearly seen on the IVU. The long axes of the kidneys lie vertically, parallel with the spine (instead of in a normal alignment parallel with the lateral psoas margins). Each kidney is commonly rotated about its long axis, so that the pelvis lies anteriorly and many of the calyces point medially.

A horseshoe kidney is more vulnerable to injury from direct abdominal impact than is a normally sited kidney, and patients with this variant are more prone to urinary tract infection and urinary calculus formation.

Double renal pelvis and ureter

Duplication of the renal pelvis and ureter, whereby the upper pole of the kidney drains separately from the middle and lower poles, is a common variant of normal. This feature may be unilateral or bi-lateral, and if unilateral the affected kidney will usually be 2–3 cm longer than its opposite number. The two ureters may join before reaching the bladder or may enter the bladder separately. In the latter situation the ureter draining the upper pole enters the bladder below and medial to the ureter draining the middle and lower poles. There is a tendency for vesicoureteric reflux to occur into the ureter draining the middle and lower poles, since this ureter passes less obliquely than normal through the bladder wall.

Pelviureteric junction obstruction

Obstruction at the pelviureteric junction may have an obvious organic cause (calculus, tumour, etc.), but often no organic cause is shown and the obstruction is attributed to a functional failure of co-ordinated renal pelvic and ureteric contractions. The condition may present in childhood or adulthood, the patient complaining of recurrent loin pain, sometimes after a large fluid intake. During an attack an IVU will show the characteristic features of pelviureteric junction obstruction, i.e. hydronephrosis together with a normal undistended ureter. When the IVU is carried out during remission the typical radiological features may be confirmed by injecting a diuretic intravenously during the examination to induce a diuresis.

Adult polycystic disease of the kidneys

A patient with adult polycystic disease of the kidneys usually first presents in his forties, with haematuria or with symptoms resulting from hypertension or renal failure. Alternatively, the patient may be aware of a swelling in his abdomen, or renal enlargement may be discovered during examination by his physician.

An IVU is usually sufficient to establish a diagnosis, but in doubtful cases renal arteriography and ultrasound provide further information. Characteristically, both kidneys are enlarged, and cysts projecting from the surfaces of the kidneys produce lobulation of the borders. Since the cysts do not opacify with contrast, films taken shortly after injection show a non-homogeneous blotchy opacification of the enlarged kidneys. On later films, cysts within the substance of the kidneys give rise by compression to characteristic stretching, narrowing and displacement of the calyces.

Urinary calculi and nephrocalcinosis

It is useful to distinguish between urinary calculi (stones within the calyces, renal pelves, ureters or bladder) and nephrocalcinosis (calcification within the parenchyma of the kidneys).

Urinary calculi

Conditions known to cause the formation of urinary calculi are:
1. Urinary infection.
2. Stasis of urine, e.g. in pelviureteric junction obstruction and bladder diverticula.
3. Dehydration.
4. Conditions causing hypercalcaemia or hypercalciuria, e.g. hyperparathyroidism and idiopathic hypercalciuria.
5. Conditions causing deposition of urate crystals, e.g. gout and polycythaemia.

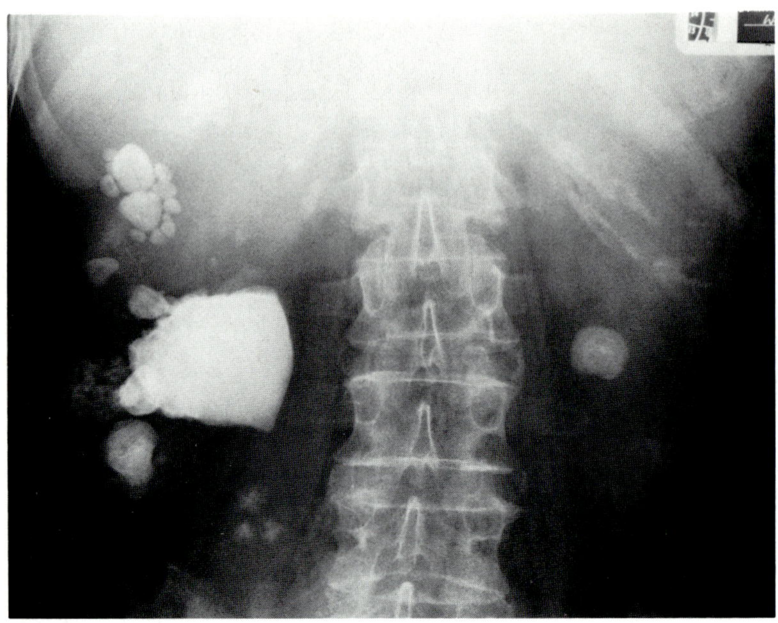

Figure 3.41. Bilateral renal calculi; plain film. Huge laminated calculus filling right renal pelvis. This has produced obstruction, and clusters of calculi are shown lying free in the grossly hydronephrotic upper-, middle-, and lower-pole calyces. Smaller laminated calculus in left renal pelvis. Linear calcification present in left lower costal cartilages

6. Renal papillary necrosis, in which a sloughed papilla may act as a nidus for calcium deposition.
7. Cystinuria.

The great majority of urinary calculi are radio-opaque (*Figure 3.41*). These may range in size from tiny opacities to calcified casts of the pelvicalyceal system (staghorn calculi). Urinary calculi are sometimes seen on X-ray to be laminated (*Figure 3.41*) or to have spiculated margins resembling mulberries. Pure urate stones are radiolucent.

Plain films of the abdomen are extremely valuable in the diagnosis of urinary calculi, since the majority are opaque. While there is no difficulty in recognizing renal staghorn calculi or large stones in the bladder, smaller stones must be distinguished from other causes of calcification that may overlie the urinary tract. These include calcification in costal cartilages or gall stones overlying the kidney, or in lymph glands or pelvic veins lying in the line of the ureter. Differentiation between renal calculi and calcification in structures overlying the kidneys can usually be made on oblique views (*see* page 150).

An intravenous urogram will confirm that an opacity lies within the collecting system of the urinary tract, will show non-opaque calculi, and will establish whether a calculus is obstructing the collecting system. This examination is therefore undertaken in the initial assessment of patients with known or suspected calculi. Plain films are often sufficient for follow-up. A calculus producing obstruction of the collecting system will produce a characteristic appearance of delayed opacification and then persistence of opacification of the parenchyma of the affected kidney and dilatation of the renal pelvis and affected ureter to the point of the obstruction (*Figure 3.42*). Since the flow of urine through the obstructed kidney and ureter may be exceedingly slow, delayed films taken up to 24 or 48 hours

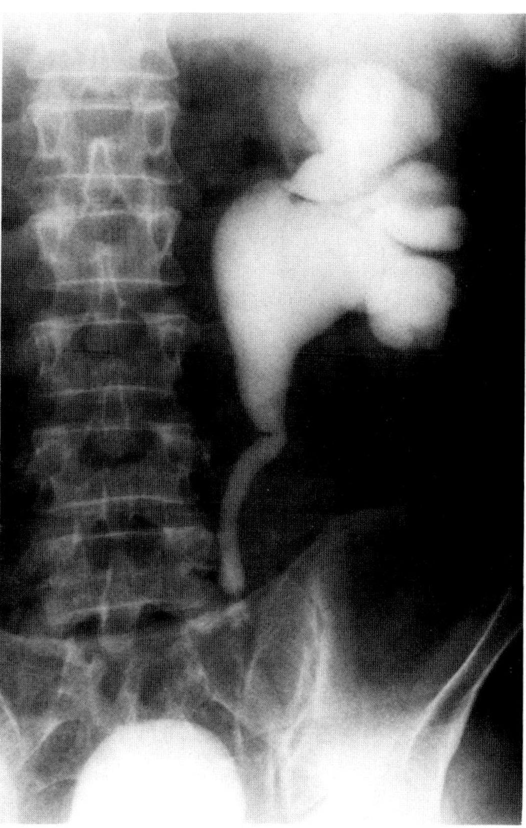

Figure 3.42. Hydronephrosis and hydro-ureter due to a ureteric calculus obstructing the ureter at the pelvic brim. 30-minute IVU film

after the injection of contrast are sometimes required to show the level of obstruction.

Occasionally an obstructed kidney may fail to opacify on an IVU, and in this situation ultrasound will readily confirm that hydronephrosis is present, while antegrade or retrograde pyelography will, if necessary, provide further information on the precise site, and sometimes the nature, of the obstructing lesion.

Nephrocalcinosis

The following conditions can give rise to small, round, calcified opacities in the renal parenchyma:

1. Conditions causing hypercalcaemia or hypercalciuria: hyperparathyroidism, renal tubular acidosis, idiopathic hypercalciuria, Cushing's syndrome, steroid therapy, multiple myeloma and carcinomatosis, sarcoidosis, hypervitaminosis D (*Figure 3.43*), and milk alkali syndrome.
2. Medullary sponge kidney. Calculi form in the dilated collecting tubules which characterize this condition. These calculi may be discovered by chance on X-ray examination of the abdomen for an unrelated reason, or the condition may present with recurrent bouts of renal colic produced by intermittent passage of small stones.

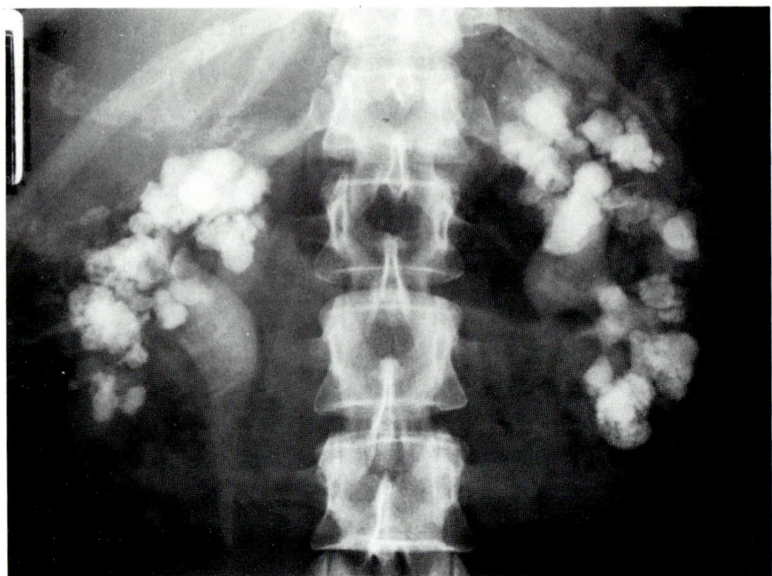

Figure 3.43. Nephrocalcinosis. There is particularly gross calcification in the renal parenchyma. The renal pelves are seen to be free of calculi on this 5-minute IVU film, although some calcification could be present in the calyces. The patient had had a massive vitamin D intake over several years

Extensive calcification of the cortex of the kidney can occur in renal cortical necrosis resulting from antepartum haemorrhage, and localized areas of calcification can occur in renal tuberculosis, renal carcinoma, and in simple and hydatid cysts.

Urinary tract trauma

Early radiological examination is indicated in suspected trauma of the urinary tract and this may reveal the need for prompt surgical intervention. Loss of definition of the psoas margin or renal outline on plain films will suggest the presence of a perirenal haematoma, although these landmarks may simply be obscured by overlying bowel shadows.

An immediate IVU, without preparation of the patient, may show displacement and distortion of the calyces and bulging of the renal outline by an intrarenal haematoma, or leakage of contrast into the renal substance or perirenal tissues due to a laceration of the collecting system. Total failure of opacification of the kidney will suggest an acute vascular lesion, and angiography should then be carried out urgently to establish whether the renal artery is thrombosed. Renal angiography also provides an accurate indication of the extent of renal parenchymal injury, and in patients with severe trauma who require surgery the information obtained from angiography is useful in preoperative planning.

One of the prime functions of an IVU is to confirm the presence of a normally functioning contralateral kidney, since emergency resection of the traumatized kidney may be required.

Urinary tract infections

Acute infections of the urinary tract

Intravenous urography should be performed in children with proved urinary infections, since a correctible cause may be found and progressive renal damage thereby prevented. It is common practice for IVU to be undertaken in the investigation of urinary infections in adults. This is rarely warranted in the presence of an isolated infection but is probably justified in troublesome recurrent infections, particularly if these are accompanied by loin pains suggesting an upper urinary tract abnormality. The examination in these situations is usually normal, but occasionally a factor predisposing to infection is found, such as a urinary calculus or stasis from obstruction at some point of the collecting system.

A kidney affected by acute suppurative pyelonephritis may show virtually no excretion of contrast on intravenous urography. Urography and ultrasound can be used to demonstrate the presence and position of a renal abscess.

Chronic pyelonephritis

The radiographic appearances of this condition are characteristic (*Figure 3.44*). The disease is patchy in distribution, and calyces in affected regions lose their normal cup shapes and instead assume the appearances of clubs. The normal smooth renal outline is lost over the affected calyces, and deep depressions occur from scarring of the underlying parenchyma, so that in severely affected areas the indented renal margins and underlying clubbed calyces approximate closely to each other. A grossly diseased kidney will be abnormally small. The hallmark of the disease is the patchy distribution, certain areas showing more pronounced changes than others. The radiographic abnormality is sometimes accentuated by compensatory hypertrophy of unaffected regions of the kidney, or more particularly by compensatory hypertrophy of the unaffected or less affected opposite kidney.

While these changes can be seen on urography performed on children or adults, it is believed that scarring represents the effects of disease occurring in early childhood. It is exceptionally rare for scarring to develop *ab initio* in adulthood, and although the above features may be seen for the first time when an adult has an intravenous urogram for repeated urinary infections the changes almost invariably stem from early childhood.

Since there is a strong association between vesicoureteric reflux and chronic pyelonephritis, micturating cystography plays an important part in establishing whether appreciable reflux is present. This is particularly valuable in children, in whom surgical intervention to correct reflux may be required to prevent irreparable renal damage. Radioisotope studies to assess reflux can be carried out as an alternative to micturating cystography.

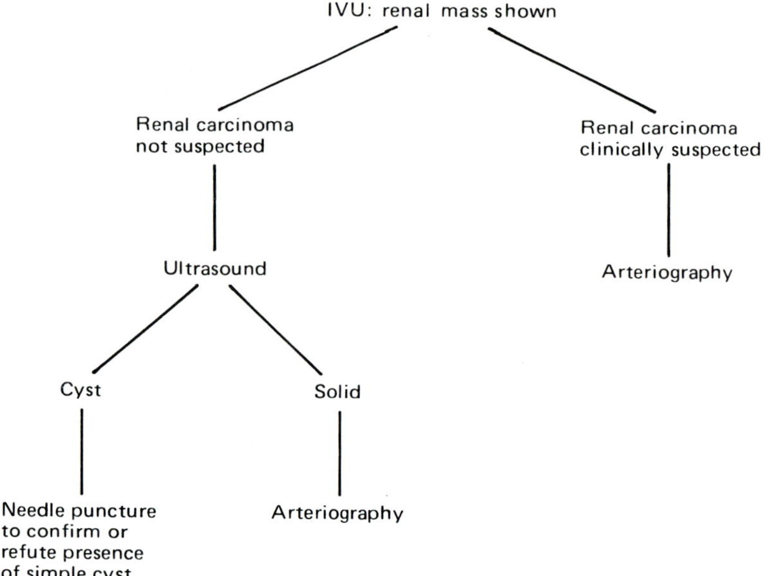

Figure 3.51. Investigation of a renal mass

Dilatation of the urinary tract collecting system

Bilateral dilatation of the calyces, pelves and ureters

The most common cause of dilatation of the collecting system bilaterally is lower urinary tract obstruction, often due to benign prostatic hypertrophy but also found in other conditions producing bladder outflow obstruction (e.g. urethral valves in children, or post-traumatic or postinflammatory strictures of the urethra).

The ureters will be seen to be dilated (hydroureter) on the IVU. The normal cup-shaped appearance of the calyces (*see Figure 3.39*) is lost, these being rounded and distended (hydronephrosis, *see Figure 3.42*). The severity of the changes in bilateral hydronephrosis may be very different on the two sides. All of the calyces of a particular kidney, however, are affected to a very similar extent. This feature aids in differentiating hydronephrosis from chronic pyelonephritis or renal tuberculosis, in which the calyces are usually affected to an unequal degree and some calyces may be normal. The IVU in obstruction shows delayed, persisting opacification of the renal tract, the extent of this change depending on the severity of the obstruction. Bladder trabeculae and diverticula may be seen as manifestations of bladder outflow obstruction.

Urethrography is indicated for the investigation of a suspected urethral stricture.

Bilateral hydronephrosis and hydroureter occur in conditions other than those producing mechanical obstruction of the lower urinary tract. They are seen in urinary obstruction due to neurological causes, either congenital (e.g. meningomyelocele) or acquired (e.g. traumatic, vascular or neoplastic lesions of the spinal cord). Bilateral hydronephrosis and hydroureter also occur in the presence of severe bilateral vesicoureteric reflux.

Unilateral dilatation of the calyces, pelvis and ureter

Obstruction is also the commonest cause of unilateral dilatation of the urinary collecting system. As a general rule the lower point of the dilatation indicates the level of obstruction, although occasionally the ureter is dilated distal to a ureteric calculus without a second obstructing lesion being present. The causes of ureteric obstruction are as follows:

1. Stones, blood clot, etc., lying free within the lumen itself.
2. Organic lesions of the wall of the ureter, e.g. post-traumatic or postinflammatory strictures, ureteric tumours.
3. Extrinsic disease compressing or invading the ureter, e.g. retroperitoneal fibrosis due to methysergide, or retroperitoneal or pelvic tumours.
4. Neuromuscular incoordination may be the cause of incomplete obstruction at the junction of the pelvis and ureter when none of the above factors is present. The obstruction in this condition can sometimes be shown dramatically after the intravenous administration of a diuretic during intravenous urography.

Vesicoureteric reflux is an important cause of ureteric dilatation, particularly in children. The changes may be unilateral or bilateral. Any child suspected of this condition should have a micturating cystogram performed, since gross reflux can cause progressive, irreversible damage to the growing kidney, and reimplantation of the ureter into the bladder may be required on this account. Unexplained dilatation of the collecting system on an IVU, or recurrent urinary infections and a normal IVU, are indications for micturating cystography in children.

The right ureter is commonly found to be dilated on an IVU performed after pregnancy. The overdistensibility of the ureter, brought about by a combination of obstruction and hormonal influences during pregnancy, may become a permanent change.

Hypertension due to renal or adrenal disease

The great majority of patients with high blood pressure suffer from essential or primary hypertension, for which no cause can be found. In a small number the hypertension is due to renal disease, a tumour of the adrenal gland, or coarctation.

In a very small proportion of patients with severe progressive hypertension a unilateral renal lesion may be found which can be dealt with surgically and the hypertension relieved. Predominantly unilateral chronic pyelonephritis is one such condition and renal artery stenosis is another. It is common practice to examine the kidneys for a potentially correctable unilateral lesion in young hypertensive patients, and in older patients in whom medical treatment has been unsuccessful. On intravenous urography renal artery stenosis is manifest by:

1. A reduction in length of the affected kidney of more than 1.5 cm compared with the opposite kidney. It is unusual to find a disparity of this magnitude in healthy kidneys, except in the presence of a unilateral duplex kidney which may be 2–3 cm longer than its partner.
2. Delayed opacification of the collecting system of the affected kidney.
3. A greater density of the subsequently opacified pelvicalyceal system on the affected side.

These disparities between the two sides are shown on rapid-sequence films of the two kidneys, usually taken at 1-minute intervals for the first 5 minutes after the contrast injection. The above changes will not be seen, and the IVU will appear normal, in 20 per cent of patients with renal artery stenosis. If therefore the condition is strongly suspected in a young patient with a normal IVU, this should be investigated further by renal angiography. If a stenosis is shown on angiography, the question arises as to whether this is an incidental finding or is responsible for the hypertension. Sampling of the renal veins for renin concentrations through a catheter introduced into the venous system from the femoral vein and positioned with its tip in each renal vein in turn provides further biochemical data concerning the significance of a renal lesion in the production of hypertension.

The adrenal glands may be implicated in the production of hypertension in Cushing's syndrome, Conn's syndrome and phaeochromocytoma. While adrenal hyperplasia is much commoner than an adrenal tumour in the first condition, Conn's syndrome is usually produced by an adrenal cortical tumour and phaeochromocytoma by a tumour in the medulla. A large adrenal tumour is often shown on an IVU examination (when it is seen as an extrarenal mass displacing the kidney downwards) and on ultrasound. These examinations, however, rarely demonstrate a small tumour of the adrenal gland, and CT is the most sensitive of the non-invasive imaging techniques for detecting adrenal tumours. Adrenal venography and in certain instances adrenal arteriography are sensitive but invasive techniques, which can be carried out when CT is unavailable, or the results of non-invasive investigation are equivocal.

Renal failure

The prime functions of radiology in the investigation of renal failure are:

1. To establish if renal obstruction is the causative factor.

2. To assess renal size.
3. To establish whether pulmonary oedema due to fluid retention is present.

The first two factors can usually be ascertained with an IVU. Generally twice the normal dose of contrast medium is injected. The uraemic patient should on no account be dehydrated in preparation for the examination, as this may cause further harm to the kidneys.

The fundamental importance of establishing whether urinary tract obstruction is present is that this condition can be relieved. In renal failure due to obstruction the dilated calyces, pelves and then ureters slowly become opacified, and it may be necessary to take films for 24 hours or more after the injection of contrast to determine the level of obstruction. A carefully monitored IVU examination will usually establish whether obstruction is present, but ultrasound will produce an equally reliable and much more rapid answer. If ultrasound is performed as the initial investigation, a plain film of the abdomen should still be obtained to determine whether calculi are the possible cause of the renal failure.

The importance of estimating renal size on the IVU is that bilateral, small, shrunken kidneys usually indicate the presence of irreversible end-stage renal disease (e.g. chronic glomerulonephritis or chronic pyelonephritis), while kidneys of normal or increased size may be affected by a potentially reversible condition. In some cases a specific diagnosis can be made from the altered appearances of the kidneys,. e.g. in polycystic disease (*see* page 157).

Although shrunken kidneys usually imply irreversible end-stage renal disease, it is nevertheless important when they are found to exclude the additional presence of obstruction, since this reversible condition may precipitate acute superimposed on chronic renal failure.

The bladder

Plain films of the abdomen may show opaque bladder calculi. These most commonly arise in the presence of bladder outflow obstruction. Curved wavy lines of calcification in the wall of the bladder are seen in bilharzia and occasionally in tuberculosis.

The IVU is a sensitive examination in the detection of renal disease but is insensitive in detecting lesions of the bladder. A bladder tumour may be visible on an IVU producing a filling defect in the contrast-filled bladder, but small tumours will readily pass undetected and it is essential to remember that a normal IVU examination does not exclude a bladder carcinoma. Cystoscopy therefore must supplement the IVU in any patient presenting with haematuria in whom a tumour of the bladder is suspected.

It is customary to conclude the IVU examination with a film of the bladder area taken after the patient has micturated. In the presence of severe lower urinary tract obstruction bladder diverticula or an abnormally large bladder may be seen and, as discussed above, the pelvicalyceal system may be dilated. The significance of a contrast-filled bladder of normal volume and normal appearance on the post-micturition film requires guarded interpretation. This is commonly due to a psychological difficulty in micturating when requested to do so.

Prostatic hypertrophy is the commonest cause of lower urinary tract obstruction in elderly males. The enlarged prostate often produces an indentation of the base of the bladder.

Obstetrics and gynaecology

Obstetrics

Ultrasound has acquired a role of prime importance in the investigation of the fetus, and in recent years has largely eliminated requirements for radiological examination. The advantages to the fetus of a technique carrying no known biological risk are obvious. The following are the main uses of ultrasound in obstetrics.

The gestational age of the fetus can be assessed accurately between the eighth and twelfth weeks of pregnancy by measuring the crown–rump length, and up to the twenty-fourth week by measuring the biparietal diameter of the fetal skull. Measurements are less accurate during the last trimester. Determination of the gestational age is of value when the mother cannot recall the date of her last menstrual period or has an irregular cycle.

Multiple pregnancies and certain fetal abnormalities can also be determined by ultrasound examination early in pregnancy (*Figure 3.52*). Anencephaly can be diagnosed within the first 3 months. Ultrasound can provide accurate localization of the fetus and placenta when amniocentesis is being undertaken for possible chromosomal or metabolic abnormality. The amniocentesis should be carried out immediately after the ultrasound examination since the fetal position can alter rapidly. Alternatively, the amniocentesis needle can be passed through a special ultrasound probe, enabling the needle to be positioned under direct imaging control.

The fetal heart can be recorded reliably by ultrasound after the seventh or eighth week of gestation. Ultrasound therefore has an

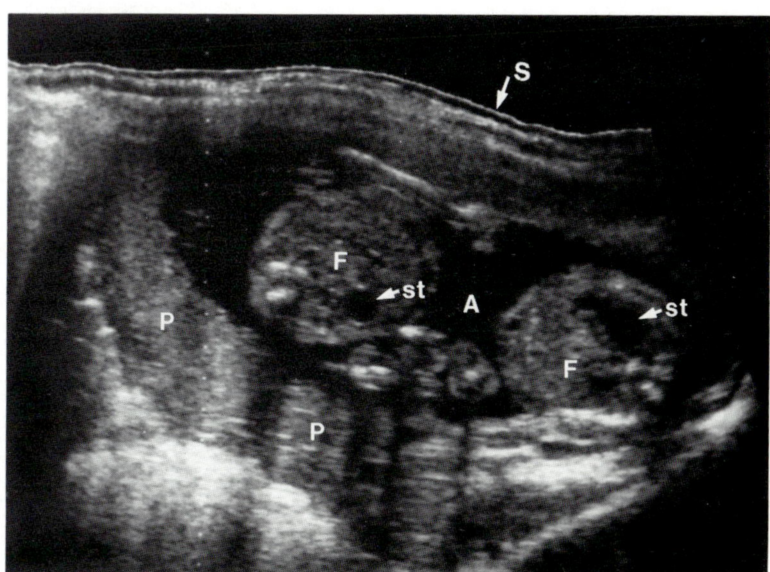

Figure 3.52. Twins at 20 weeks' gestation; transverse ultrasound scan through uterus. Scan shows transverse sections of the bodies of the twins. There is a posterior-wall placenta. The image of the placenta is interrupted by transverse acoustic shadows from the fetal limbs and spines. A, amniotic fluid; F, fetus; P, placenta; S, skin line; st, fetal stomach

important role in determining fetal viability in patients presenting with threatened abortions. Ultrasound is now established as the foremost investigation for determining the position of the placenta and has replaced traditional radiological techniques for placental localization, which involved considerable irradiation of the fetus.

One of the prime functions of ultrasound in the later stages of pregnancy is in the investigation of the female whose uterine fundal height is at variance with that predicted from the presumed gestational age. A high fundus may be shown to be due to an obstetric cause, e.g. multiple pregnancy (*Figure 3.52*) or to a gynaecological cause, e.g. ovarian cyst. Measurement of the biparietal diameter does not in itself provide reliable confirmation of failure of fetal growth in a female who is small for dates, since the development of the brain is less affected than that of other organs in intrauterine growth retardation. Cephalometry is nevertheless usually performed in this situation, but in addition it has been found useful as an indicator of growth retardation to measure cross-sectional diameters of the fetal abdomen at the level of the liver. Because of the safety of ultrasound, examinations can be repeated as required during pregnancy to monitor the progress of fetal development.

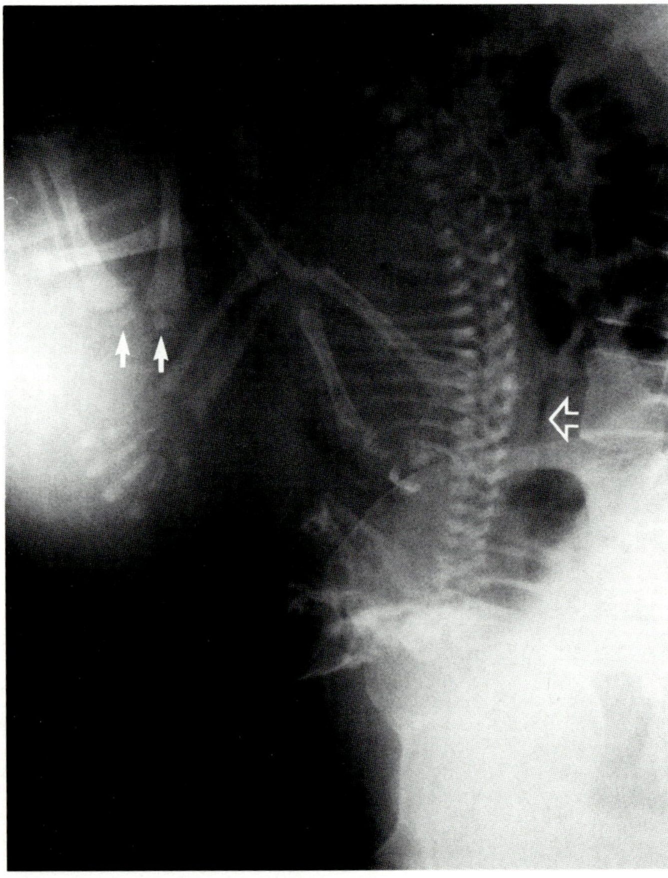

Figure 3.53. Fetus at term. Well-developed lower femoral and upper tibial epiphyses (arrows) and conspicuous subcutaneous fat line over fetus's back (open arrow)

There are very few situations in which X-ray examination of the fetus is required when ultrasound facilities are available. In the late stages of pregnancy gestational age can be assessed from a plain X-ray film of the abdomen. If the patient has had ultrasound carried out early in pregnancy there is clearly no requirement for an abdominal film for this purpose during the last few weeks. Situations in which plain films are useful are when a gravid female presents for the first time late in pregnancy, or when a decision is made to induce or perform a Caesarean section on a patient close to term and ultrasound has been omitted in the earlier stages of pregnancy. Assessment of fetal age close to term is most readily made radiologically from the state of development of the epiphyses of the knee. The lower femoral epiphysis becomes visible at 37 weeks' gestation and the upper tibial epiphysis can usually be seen at 38 weeks (*Figure 3.53*). In addition a dark line representing subcutaneous fat is often present over the fetus's back in the last month of pregnancy.

There is a wider range of indications for X-ray examination in centres where ultrasound is not available. X-rays can be used to confirm fetal death. One sign of this is over-riding of the bones of the skull vault due to shrinkage of the skull contents (*Figure 3.54*). If the

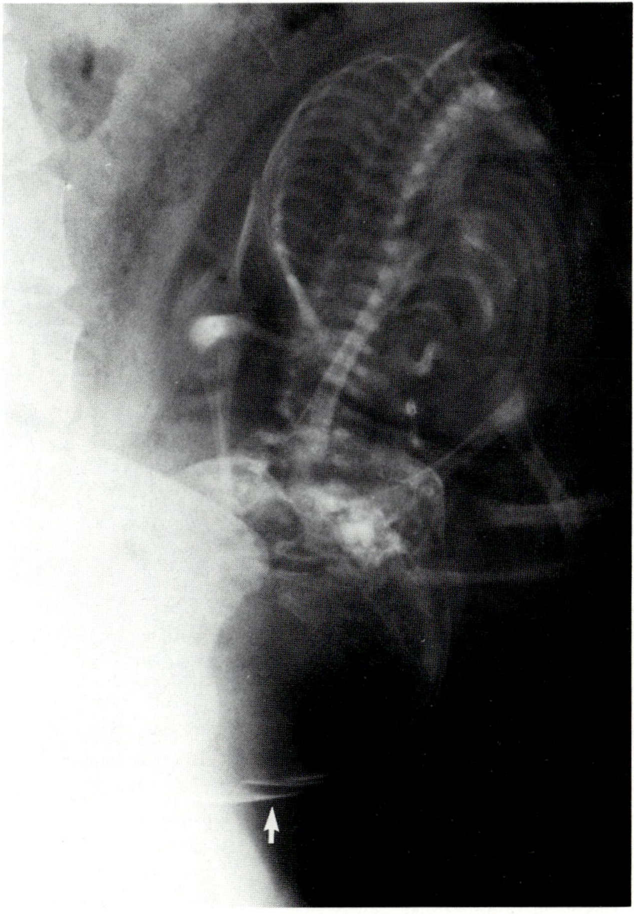

Figure 3.54. Fetal death, shown by over-riding of bones of skull vault (arrow)

X-ray finding is equivocal the examination can be repeated after 2 weeks, when the over-riding may be found to be more pronounced. This sign is not of value after engagement of the fetal head in the pelvis, when over-riding is a common normal finding. Sometimes translucencies due to gas in the fetal heart and blood vessels are seen, and these represent certain evidence of fetal death. In addition, a dead fetus may show extreme flexion of the spine.

Parts of the fetal skeleton first become visible on X-ray at approximately 16 weeks' gestation, but it is only later, when the skeleton is widely ossified, that multiple pregnancies and fetal abnormalities, e.g. anencephaly and spina bifida, can be detected. The soft-tissue shadow of the placenta or calcification within the placenta can sometimes be seen, and this information may be useful in cases of suspected placenta praevia. Ultrasound, however, should be performed wherever possible for placental localization because of the greater accuracy and safety of this method.

In suspected cephalopelvic disproportion, measurements of the internal diameters of the maternal pelvis can be made from anterior and lateral-view radiographs.

Gynaecology

A pelvic tumour or cyst may show on the plain abdominal radiograph as a shadow of soft-tissue density within, or rising up out of, the pelvis, and gas-filled loops of bowel may be displaced by the

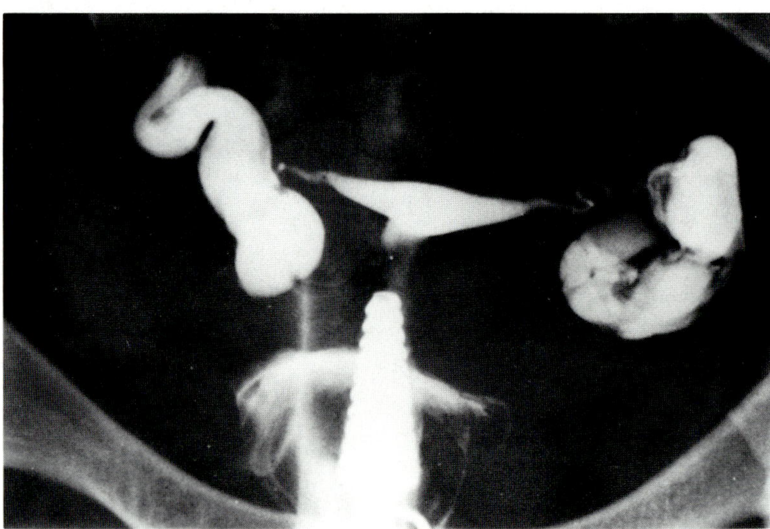

Figure 3.55. Bilateral hydrosalpinx; hysterosalpingogram. Normal cone-shaped uterine cavity and narrow medial ends of Fallopian tubes. The lateral portions of the tubes are grossly dilated and are occluded, preventing contrast from reaching the peritoneal cavity

mass. Uterine fibroids may be heavily calcified. In patients with known malignant disease of the pelvis intravenous urography can be performed to assess for obstruction or invasion of the lower urinary tract. Ultrasound provides a simple non-invasive means of determining whether a pelvic mass is cystic or solid. When more extensive investigation is required arteriography can be undertaken to examine for a tumour circulation.

Hysterosalpingography is important in the investigation of the infertile patient. For this procedure a cannula is positioned in the cervical canal, or a special suction cap applied to the canal, and water-soluble contrast medium is injected to fill the body of the uterus and Fallopian tubes. The normal uterine cavity presents as a V-shaped shadow with a smooth outline. The normal Fallopian tubes are also smooth in outline, and have a calibre of about 0.5 mm adjacent to the uterus, widening to about 5 mm at the ovarian ends. In the normal patient contrast medium should spill from the lateral ends of the Fallopian tubes and spread out freely in the adjacent peritoneal cavity. The examination may show abnormalities of the uterus, e.g. a bicornuate uterus, or of the Fallopian tubes. Occlusion with or without gross dilatation of the tubes (hydrosalpinx, *Figure 3.55*) may be found as a cause of infertility following pelvic inflammation.

4 Radiology of the chest

The indications for radiology of the chest are many and cover a wide field of clinical medicine. Those pertinent to each type of chest lesion are briefly described in the following sections. To generalize, patients needing radiography of the chest fall into three main groups:

1. Those included in schemes of routine chest radiography, e.g. miners and tuberculosis contacts.
2. Those with symptoms and signs directly indicative of an intrathoracic lesion.
3. Those with general constitutional symptoms, or with a disease in some part of the body other than the chest, which may be caused by or associated with an intrathoracic lesion (e.g. fever of unknown origin, or a malignant tumour with possible secondary deposits in the lung).

The need for chest radiography is not always obvious, and the selection of patients often depends on the skill and experience of the physician. Typical chest symptoms, such as cough or pain in the chest, may be caused by extrathoracic conditions for which radiography is useless, while large thoracic lesions may be present with very inconspicuous physical signs.

In all chest conditions the initial X-ray examination is carried out as soon as convenient, but the timing of subsequent examinations requires judgement. The changes of silicosis, for instance, only appear some years after the worker has been subjected to the particular industrial hazard, while a lung abscess may develop or resolve so rapidly that further radiographs are often required in a matter of days.

Radiography

The standard practice in adult chest radiography is to take a posteroanterior (PA) radiograph, with the patient standing with his chest pressed against the flat, light-tight film container (cassette), and the X-ray tube positioned behind the patient at a distance of 2 m (6 ft) from the film. With this arrangement very little magnification of the heart occurs (*Figure 4.1a*), so that a fairly accurate assessment of the true cardiac diameter can be obtained from the radiograph. In a correctly exposed radiograph the disc spaces between the dorsal vertebrae should just be discernible behind the heart shadow.

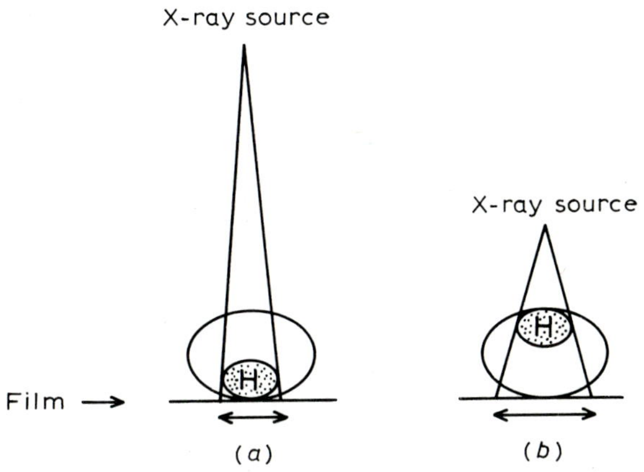

Figure 4.1. Cross-section of chest at level of heart H. (a) Standard posteroanterior radiograph: X-ray tube 2 m (6 ft) from film, patient facing film; very little magnification of heart. (b) Anteroposterior ward radiograph: tube about 1 m (3 ft) from film, patient facing tube; magnified image of heart

Variations from the standard procedure should be indicated, since these may influence interpretation of the film. For example, it is necessary to place the film behind an ill patient examined in bed, and it may be impossible in this anteroposterior (AP) view to position the X-ray tube more than 1–1.2 m (3–4 ft) from the film. In this situation the cardiac image is considerably magnified on the film (*Figure 4.1b*), so that accurate assessment of cardiac size cannot be made.

The radiograph should always be viewed in a proper light—that is, before a special X-ray viewing box—and not just held up to the nearest lamp or window.

Order of inspection of the chest X-ray and criteria for normality

In most cases the chest X-ray is normal, and this information is of great value to the clinician. In order to avoid mistakes and to gain the maximum amount of information from the image, it should be inspected methodically. The following routine of inspection is recommended. Reference should be made to the normal examination shown in *Figure 4.2*.

Preliminary observations

Posteroanterior or anteroposterior film?

This information is required since assessment of heart size cannot be made on an AP film (*see* above). It is very difficult to tell from the

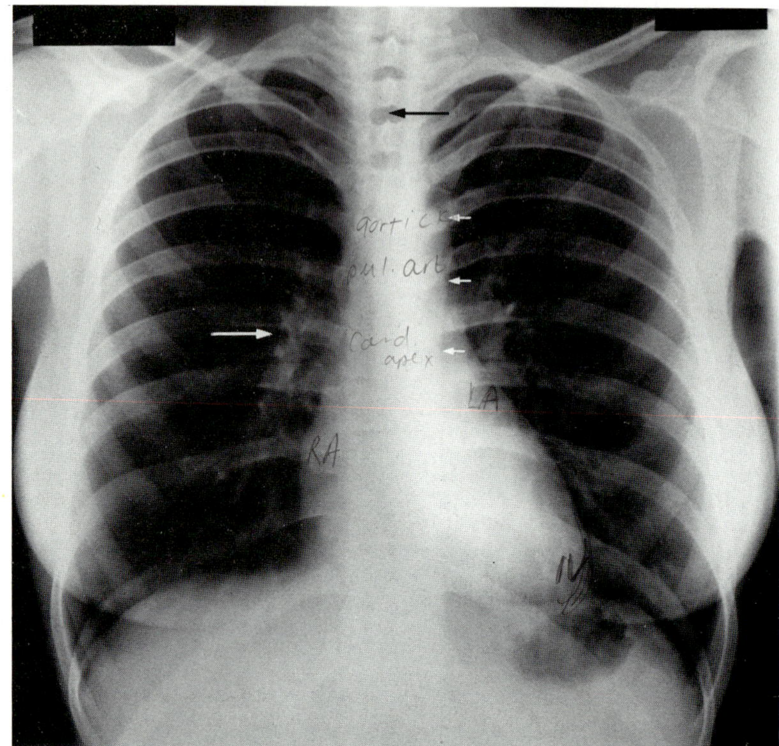

Figure 4.2. Normal posteroanterior chest radiograph. Female patient. See text. Note central position of trachea (black arrow); midpoint of V-shaped right hilum (large white arrow) at level of 6th rib in midaxillary line; left hilum a little higher than right hilum; shadow of aortic arch and lateral border of descending thoracic aorta (small white arrows); acute costophrenic angles

appearances of the chest whether the examination is PA or AP. While the labelling of films with the patient's name, date of examination, etc. varies from hospital to hospital, it is usually possible to tell from simple knowledge of the method of labelling of a particular hospital how a patient has been examined. Furthermore, AP films are commonly labelled AP or with a letter P (indicating a portable ward examination).

Is the patient straight with the chest shown symmetrically?

Slight rotation will produce unequal transradiancy of the two sides of the chest due to asymmetry of the chest wall, and such inequality should not be mistaken for lung disease. Rotation can also make a normal hilum appear unduly prominent. Confirmation that the patient is straight can be made by comparing the respective positions of the medial ends of the clavicles on the two sides (anterior structures) with the lateral margins of the bodies of the dorsal vertebrae lying behind them (posterior structures). If rotation is present there will be a space between the clavicle and vertebral body on one side while the medial end of the clavicle will overlie the vertebral body on the other side.

Is the film adequately penetrated?

This is important, since lesions can be obscured behind the heart and the hila on an underpenetrated film. As already mentioned, the disc spaces between the dorsal vertebral bodies should just be visible behind the heart on an adequately penetrated film.

Diaphragm

The medial (highest) portion of the diaphragm normally lies at the level of the fifth or sixth intercostal space anteriorly. The right diaphragm is normally 1–2 cm higher than the left. The diaphragms are convex and the costophrenic angles acute.

Heart

It is very unusual for the maximum cardiac transverse diameter to exceed 15.5 cm in healthy adults, so that this figure can be regarded as the upper limit of normal. Usually between two-thirds and three-quarters of the diameter of the heart lies to the left of the midline (as assessed on the radiograph from the centre of the dorsal vertebral bodies).

Trachea

The trachea is visible as a vertical translucent band and should be centrally situated in the neck and at the thoracic inlet, but its lower third may deviate slightly to the right.

Hila

The normal hilar shadows are produced entirely by blood vessels. Hilar glands are not visible unless they are pathologically enlarged. The normal hila can often be seen forming the shape of a letter V lying on its side, the upper limb representing the upper-lobe veins crossing the hilum to reach the left atrium, and the lower limb representing the branch of the pulmonary artery to the lower lobe. The midpoint of the hilum, representing the apex of the V, can usually be identified. The midpoint of the right hilum lies at the level of the horizontal fissure and of the sixth rib in the axillary line. The midpoint of the left hilum lies 1–1.5 cm higher than that of the right hilum.

Horizontal fissure

This is visible in approximately 80 per cent of chest X-rays as a fine line running horizontally to the sixth rib in the axillary line.

Lungs

As with the hilar shadows, the branching linear shadows seen crossing the lungs are due entirely to blood vessels. The walls of normal bronchi are too thin to cast shadows on the radiograph. The upper, middle and lower thirds of each lung should be carefully examined in turn and compared with the corresponding areas of the opposite lung. Any alteration of the normal vessel pattern or any abnormal shadows should be carefully noted.

Thoracic cage

The skeleton of the thorax should be examined for bony abnormalities such as fractures or areas of destruction due to bone metastases. The shoulder girdles are usually visible on a chest film and sometimes disorders of the shoulder joints, such as changes from rheumatoid arthritis, can be detected.

Soft-tissue shadows

A search should be made for asymmetry or other abnormality, such as an absent breast shadow following a mastectomy in a female patient. Sometimes nipple shadows appear as 0.5–1.5 cm diameter opacities overlying the lower lung fields on X-rays either of male or of female patients. These can be mistaken for pulmonary lesions. The true nature of such a shadow can sometimes be established by seeing a similar shadow at approximately the same position on the opposite side. When doubt arises the patient can be re-examined after attaching a small radio-opaque marker to the nipple with adhesive tape. If the opacity lies separate from the marker on the second film then it clearly does not represent the nipple shadow. When doubt still arises the uncertainty is simply resolved by rotating the patient under fluoroscopic observation to establish whether the shadow can be projected entirely clear of, and anterior to, the lung.

This basic analysis can be performed quite rapidly and will define the normal chest. It should be carried out even when obvious abnormal shadows are present, since further abnormality contributing to the assessment of the case, or even to the diagnosis, may be detected.

Figures 4.3–4.5 illustrate the value of a routine scheme of analysis. They all show a homogeneous opacity of the left hemithorax, but in *Figure 4.3* the heart and trachea are displaced to the right by a very large left pleural effusion. In *Figure 4.4* there is no heart or tracheal displacement; the patient has lobar pneumonia and there is no change in lung volume. In *Figure 4.5* the heart and trachea are displaced to the left in a case of atelectasis of the lung due to obstruction of the left main bronchus; the air in the alveoli is rapidly absorbed, and the alveolar space is collapsed. In all three cases the X-ray diagnosis depends on a correct assessment of the position of the heart and trachea, and this can be made only if the patient is straight and not rotated.

A lateral view of the chest is taken when further characterization or localization of a lesion shown on the anterior view is required. In general the patient should be examined with the side of interest next

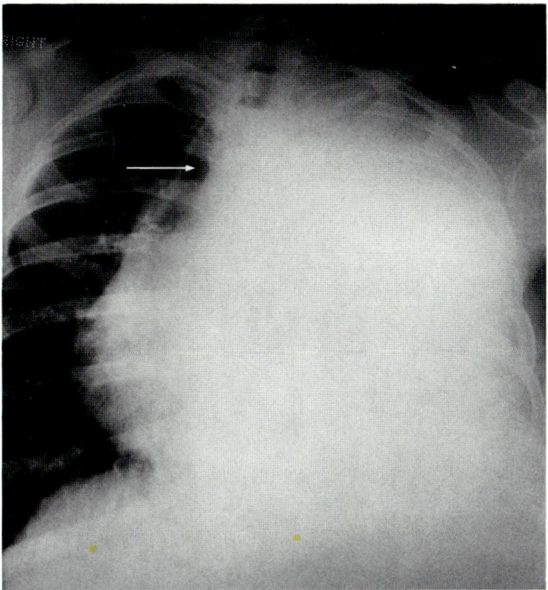

Figure 4.3. Large left pleural effusion, displacing the heart and trachea (arrow) to the right

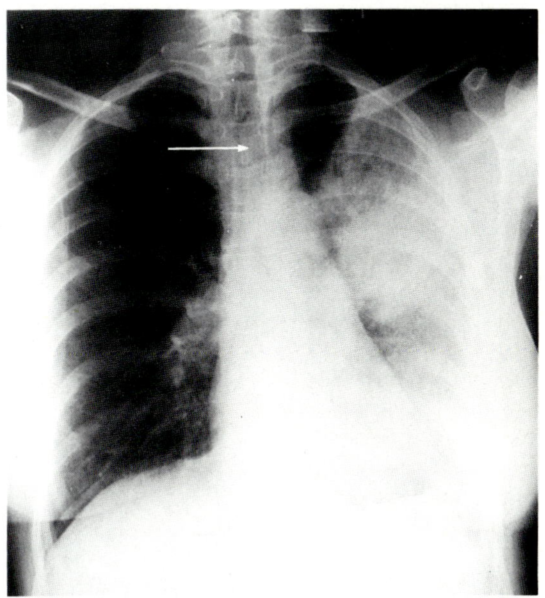

Figure 4.4. Extensive pneumonia of the left lung; no cardiac or tracheal (arrow) displacement

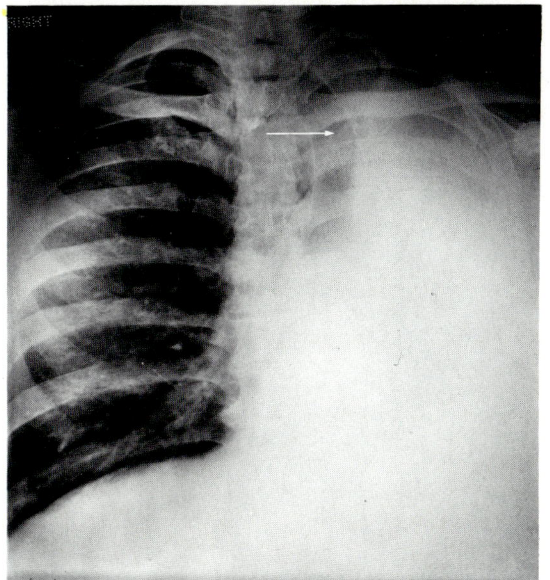

Figure 4.5. Collapse of the left lung, with displacement of the heart and trachea (arrow) to the left. There was obstruction of the left main bronchus by a carcinoma. Absorption of alveolar air resulted in the loss of lung volume

to the film, but it is unnecessary to obtain both lateral views when bilateral pulmonary lesions are present as visualization of the side away from the film is also quite adequate. A left lateral film signifies that the patient has been examined with his left side placed against the film. A lateral film should also be obtained when an abnormality such as a bronchial carcinoma is suspected clinically but no abnormality is seen on the anterior view. In a small proportion of cases a lesion can be seen on a lateral view only.

A lateral view is less easy to analyse than an anterior view since the two lungs are superimposed and cannot be compared with each other. Nevertheless a similar routine scheme can usefully be employed and the following points should be borne in mind. *Figure 4.6* should be used for reference.

Both of the diaphragms are normally visible. It is sometimes necessary in the presence of an adjacent abnormality to establish

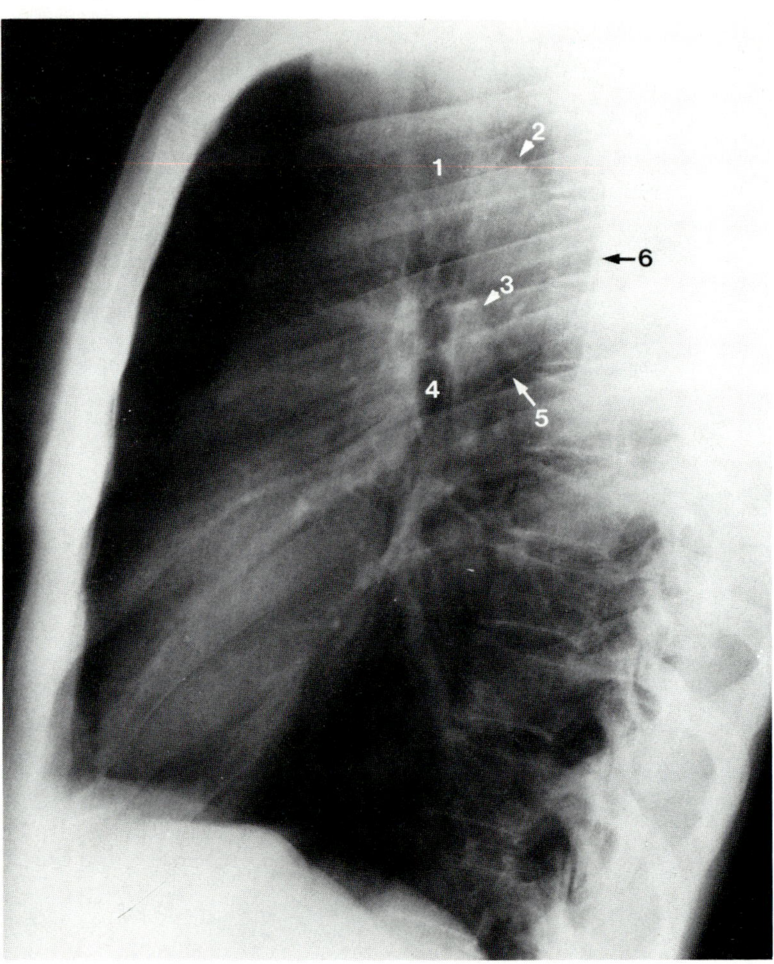

Figure 4.6. Normal lateral view radiograph; see text. Note retrosternal and retrocardiac transradiancies; vertical transradiancy of trachea (1) crossed by shadows of aortic arch (2) and left pulmonary artery (3); left main bronchus (4); part of oblique fissure (5); and edges of scapulae (6)

which diaphragm is which. In most patients some air can be seen within the fundus of the stomach, and the left diaphragm can thereby be identified as the diaphragm situated immediately above the air-filled fundus.

The heart is clearly visible lying behind the sternum and adjacent to the diaphragm.

The trachea is seen on the lateral film as a broad translucent band running downwards from the thoracic inlet and crossed in the upper chest by the shadow of the arch of the aorta and at its bifurcation by the shadow of the pulmonary artery. The arch of the aorta can be seen to be continuous with the shadow of the ascending aorta in front and the descending aorta behind.

The hila are superimposed on the lateral film. While minor abnormalities of the hila may therefore be overlooked on the lateral film this view can often be of considerable use in confirming a hilar abnormality suspected on the anterior view.

The horizontal fissure is visible running forwards from the hilar shadow in most lateral chest radiographs, and in this view also parts of the right oblique and left lung fissures are usually shown, running downwards and forwards from the level of the disc space between the fourth and fifth dorsal vertebrae posteriorly to reach the diaphragms approximately 4 cm behind the plane of the sternum anteriorly.

Detail of the pulmonary vascular markings is difficult to see on the lateral film due to the superimposition of the two lungs, but a careful search should be made for any added shadowing that may be present in the lung fields. On the normal lateral film there is an area of transradiancy between the sternum and the anterior border of the ascending aorta, produced by apposition of the left and right lungs anteriorly. The retrocardiac area should be of similar transradiancy. Normally the dorsal vertebrae become progressively more transradiant from top to bottom, until one of the diaphragms is reached. Slight increase in density of the lower dorsal vertebrae compared with the upper vertebrae may be the only indication on the lateral film of collapse of one of the lower lobes or of a lesion within a lower lobe (*see Figure 4.37*).

The bodies of the dorsal vertebrae are clearly defined on the lateral view radiograph, but apart from these the skeleton is not well shown on this view.

The exact anatomical site of a pulmonary lesion is often not evident from the anterior radiograph, although principles of localization such as the silhouette sign (*see* page 197) may provide this information. When the site is not known and a lateral film is not available to furnish this information it is convenient for descriptive purposes to be able to say that a lesion lies within the upper, middle or lower zones of the lung. The upper zone refers to the region from the apex of the lung to the lower border of the second rib anteriorly, the middle zone extends from the lower border of the second to the lower border of the fourth rib anteriorly, and the lower zone constitutes the portion of lung below this level.

Investigation of chest diseases

The following investigations are normally carried out within an X-ray department. The more sophisticated or costly of these are available only in larger hospitals or specialist chest units. Adequate radiological assessment of the great majority of patients with chest disorders is obtained from PA or PA and lateral chest films, and only a small proportion of patients require investigation by supplementary techniques. As in the investigation of any system of the body, careful consideration should be given in each case to the selection of examinations which will be quickest, least uncomfortable or least painful to the patient, and cheapest to perform, and which will also provide the required information. The following summarises the investigations which are useful in chest disease in order of increasing complexity or discomfort to the patient.

Standard PA and lateral chest films

As discussed above.

Supplementary views

These include an expiration film when a pneumothorax is suspected but not shown on the standard film (*see Figure 4.17*), and an apical view taken with the patient leaning back to project the clavicles above the level of the lungs to display more clearly disease affecting the lung apices.

Fluoroscopy

This quick, simple procedure is extremely useful in confirming and localizing the intrapulmonary position of a lesion shown on one standard view radiograph only, e.g. on the PA but not the lateral film. Fluoroscopy also confirms paralysis of a hemidiaphragm, the whole of the diaphragm on the affected side moving sharply upwards instead of downwards on sniffing.

Tomography

Ribs and other structures that overlie and obscure detail of a pulmonary lesion can be blurred out by tomography, permitting clear delineation of the margins of the lesion contrasted against the air-filled lungs. Detail of the outline of the opacity, and the presence of cavitation, contained calcification, or shadows in the surrounding lung can be obtained.

In some patients with pulmonary metastases whole-lung tomography will reveal the presence of metastases when these are not evident on the chest X-ray. The technique involves making several tomographic cuts of both lungs at regularly spaced intervals. This can be a most useful procedure when a decision to resect a primary carcinoma depends on exclusion of demonstrable metastases.

Barium swallow examination

The applications in the investigation of lung disease include demonstration of a pharyngeal pouch (*see* page 298) or other cause for recurrent aspiration pneumonia, and demonstration of extrinsic compression on the oesophagus by enlarged glands in a patient with bronchial carcinoma, indicating glandular spread of the tumour to the mediastinum (*see Figure 4.65*).

Isotope scans

Lung perfusion scans, supplemented when necessary by ventilation scans, provide the main radiographic means of investigating pulmonary thromboembolism (*see* page 232). Bone, liver and brain scans are important in examining for metastases in patients with malignant primary tumours of the thorax.

Other contrast studies

An oily contrast medium, e.g. lipiodol, can be injected into the pleural space through a drainage tube to outline the extent of an empyema cavity and the relationship of the cavity to the tube (*see Figures 4.13 and 4.14*). Abnormalities of the aorta, superior vena cava, or pulmonary arteries or veins can be investigated by angiography. For demonstration of the pulmonary arteries and veins in pulmonary angiography a catheter is inserted into the venous system from the femoral vein or a vein in the cubital fossa, is advanced under fluoroscopic control through the right side of the heart, and is positioned with its tip in the main pulmonary artery. Bronchography, involving the instillation of oily contrast media into the bronchi, is undertaken chiefly in the investigation of bronchiectasis (*see* page 224).

Biopsy techniques under fluoroscopic guidance

Transbronchial biopsy of pulmonary lesions that lie beyond the range of direct vision with the fibreoptic bronchoscope (i.e. in the subsegmental or distal bronchi) can be biopsied by passing a special brush or pair of fine forceps through a central channel in the bronchoscope and directing the biopsy instrument under fluoroscopic control to the region of interest (*see Figure 4.62*). This technique can be used for diffuse pulmonary lesions, e.g. to confirm a suspected diagnosis of pulmonary infiltration by sarcoidosis, or for a localized lesion, e.g. to obtain a histological diagnosis for management planning in a case of peripheral bronchial neoplasm. The success rate of the procedure in obtaining a histological diagnosis in patients with subsequently proved peripheral bronchial carcinoma is approximately 70 per cent. The morbidity is exceptionally low.

Alternatively, biopsy of a well-defined peripheral opacity can be obtained by passing a needle through the chest wall into the lesion, and a satisfactory position of the needle tip can be confirmed by fluoroscopy supplemented if necessary by radiographs. Various types of needle can be used, although cutting needles have been replaced largely by fine needles of approximately 19 gauge. The success rate is high, of the order of 90 per cent in the diagnosis of peripheral bronchial carcinoma. Since the procedure involves the passage of a needle through the pleura the induction of a pneumothorax is not infrequent, and approximately 5 per cent of patients require active management of a pneumothorax by intercostal drainage.

Success with both of these techniques requires the services of a skilled cytologist. A specimen that shows inflammatory cells only without evidence of malignancy should not lead to a false sense of reassurance and comfort, since an area of inflammation surrounding a tumour may have been biopsied rather than the tumour itself. The findings should be considered in the full clinical context in each case.

Computed tomography

Computed tomography (CT) can sometimes provide useful information in the diagnosis or assessment of the extent of thoracic disease. However, neither the absolute indications for, nor accuracy of, CT in the investigation of thoracic disease have yet been established. It is recognized that CT will detect small pulmonary nodules in patients with malignant disease in a greater proportion of cases than can be achieved with whole-lung tomography. However, reports have shown that the nodules detected are by no means always malignant, and so the role of CT in this situation also is still unclear.

The pleural cavity

Pleural effusion

Indications for radiology

The symptoms and physical signs of a pleural effusion are usually sufficiently well defined to establish the diagnosis. A radiological investigation of the chest is valuable as a check, especially if for one reason or another the physical signs are not quite typical or the effusion is small, when the diagnosis may be less certain.

Radiographs are also useful to demonstrate the position of the effusion and to show whether there are abnormal shadows in the part of the lung visible above the fluid shadow or in the opposite lung. It is not easy to judge accurately from the radiographs how much fluid it will be possible to withdraw by needle drainage, but a rough idea of the size of the effusion can be obtained. It cannot be forecast from the radiographs whether the fluid will be serous, purulent or haemorrhagic. It is desirable to obtain a chest X-ray before paracentesis is performed. This will show the position of the effusion and whether it is encysted owing to local adhesions between the visceral and parietal pleura. This information will enable the clinician to introduce the aspirating needle in the correct position without unnecessary and possibly fruitless trial punctures.

X-ray appearances

In a moderate-sized free pleural effusion (*Figure 4.7*) the homogeneous opacity caused by the fluid is seen to be highest in the axilla. The upper margin, which runs downwards and medially with a superior concave curvature, is not distinctly outlined.

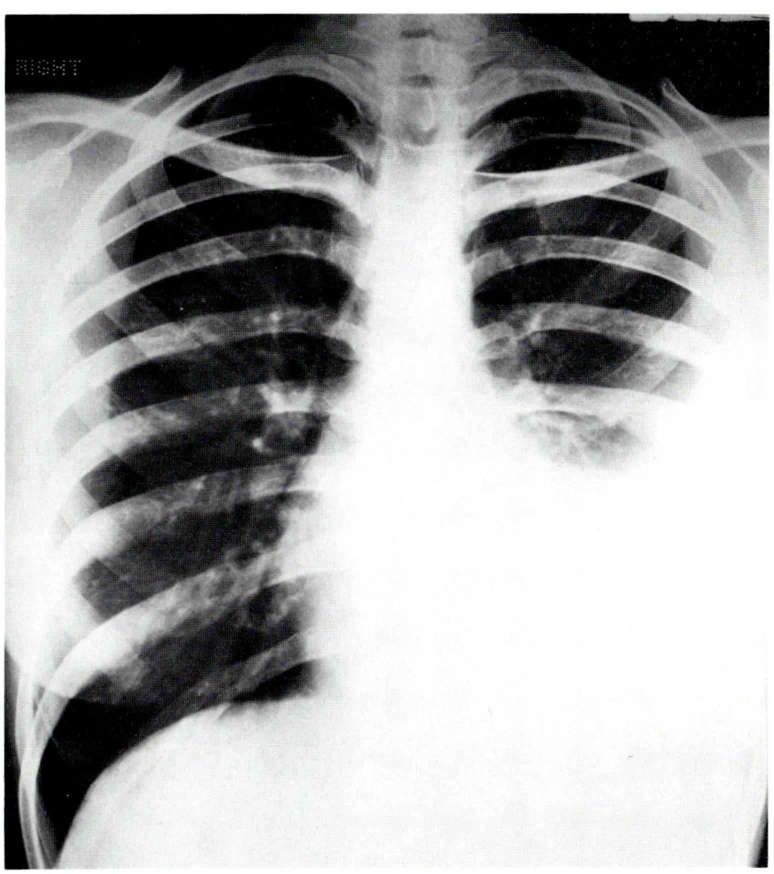

Figure 4.7. Moderate-sized left pleural effusion: homogeneous shadow with ill-defined superior concave margin, highest in the axilla

If the effusion is large the lung may be completely obscured, and there is considerable displacement of the heart and trachea to the opposite side (*see Figure 4.3*). A small effusion is seen as a homogeneous opacity filling in the normally acute costophrenic angle in the axillary line on the anterior view, and the posterior costophrenic angle in the lateral view. If it is very small it will often be visible only in a lateral view.

The exact degree of heart or tracheal displacement can be observed if the patient is correctly positioned (with the ribs, clavicles etc. symmetrical). The larger the effusion, the more the heart and trachea are displaced to the opposite side, but the degree of displacement in relation to the amount of fluid is very variable. There is much individual variation in the mobility of the mediastinal contents; in some patients there is no displacement unless the effusion reaches nearly to the apex, while in others there is considerable displacement with only a moderate amount of fluid.

In a hydropneumothorax the fluid level marking the junction between the pleural fluid and the air in the pleural cavity is, as would be expected, horizontal (*see Figure 4.15*).

Differentiation between effusion and consolidation

When there is much associated lung consolidation, it is sometimes impossible to tell which part of the shadow is due to pleural fluid and which to solid lung, but a careful study of both PA and lateral views will usually suffice to make the distinction. The shadow of a consolidated lobe, or segment of a lobe, will be seen in a position more or less corresponding to the position of that lobe or segment when normal, whereas fluid will tend to accumulate in the costophrenic region or interlobar fissure.

Encysted pleural effusion

The X-ray appearances of an encysted effusion vary according to its size and position. When it is in the axilla, it casts a characteristic shadow with a well-defined medial convex margin (*Figure 4.8*). If it lies posteriorly it may cause a poorly defined shadow in the PA view which is easily mistaken for an area of solid lung; but in the lateral

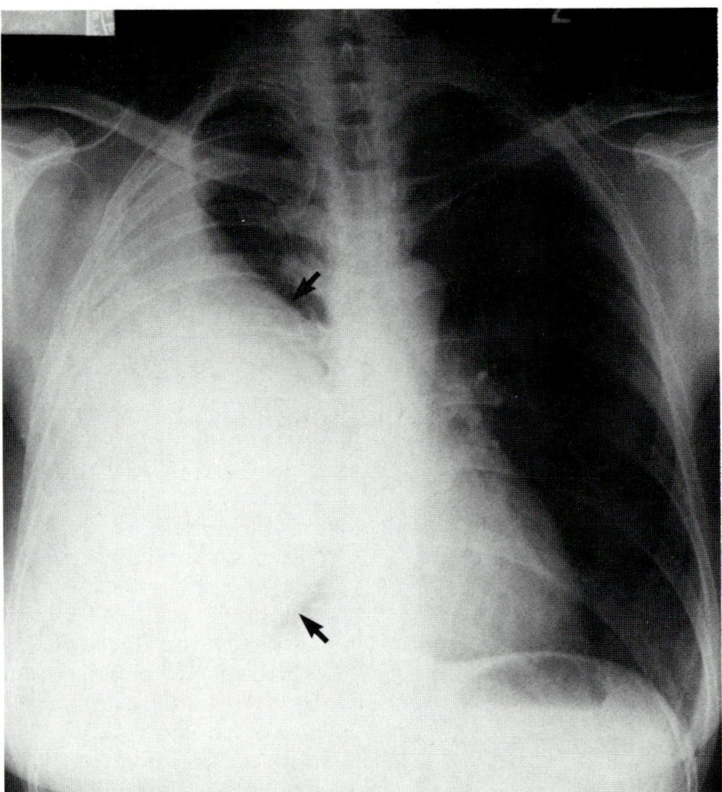

Figure 4.8. Encysted pleural effusion, lying against lateral chest wall: large D-shaped homogeneous opacity with well-defined, smooth medial margin (arrowed)

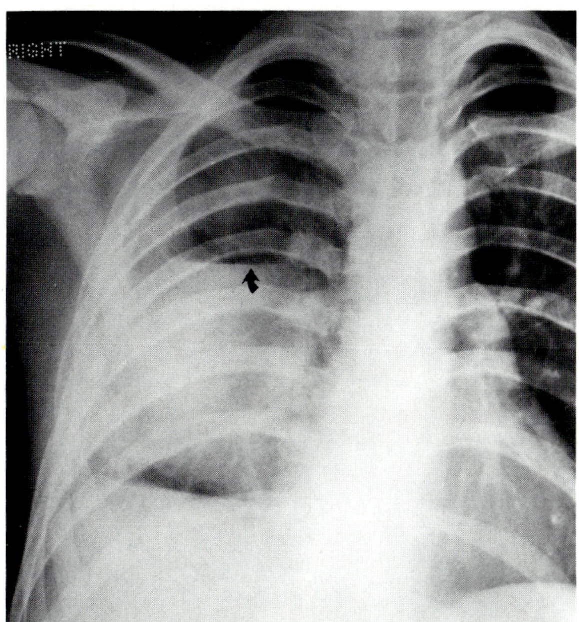

Figure 4.9. Encysted hydropneumothorax on right side: horizontal fluid level seen in upper part of opacity (arrow); ill-defined lower margin of effusion just above diaphragm

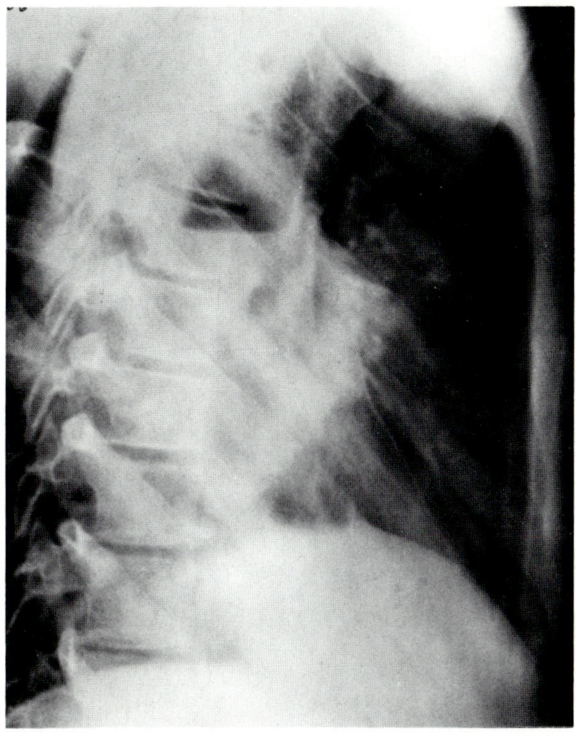

Figure 4.10. Same patient as in *Figure 4.9* (right lateral view). The fluid level is seen posteriorly overlapping the body of the 7th thoracic vertebra, and the homogeneous shadow below has a fairly well-defined convex anterior margin. The thin white line further anteriorly is the interlobar fissure

view it will be seen to lie against the posterior wall of the thorax and to have a well-defined anterior border, usually with an anterior convex curvature (*Figures 4.9 and 4.10*). Sometimes the encysted effusion lies in the interlobar fissure, in which case the lateral view gives a characteristic elliptical homogeneous shadow in the line of the fissure (*Figures 4.11 and 4.12*).

Empyema

When an empyema is suspected clinically, PA and lateral chest films should be taken to show the position of the fluid. The X-ray appearances are the same as those of a serous pleural effusion, either simple or encysted. Occasionally a fluid level is seen (*Figures 4.9 and 4.10*); this appearance may indicate that a bubble of air was introduced at a previous aspiration, or that the organism is of a gas-forming type, or that a bronchopleural fistula is present.

It is sometimes useful to localize the lower limit of an empyema cavity before drainage. This is easily done by introducing a few millilitres of iodized oil into the empyema. When the patient sits up, the radio-opaque oil descends to the bottom of the cavity, the level of which can then be defined in relation to the ribs in further PA and lateral view radiographs.

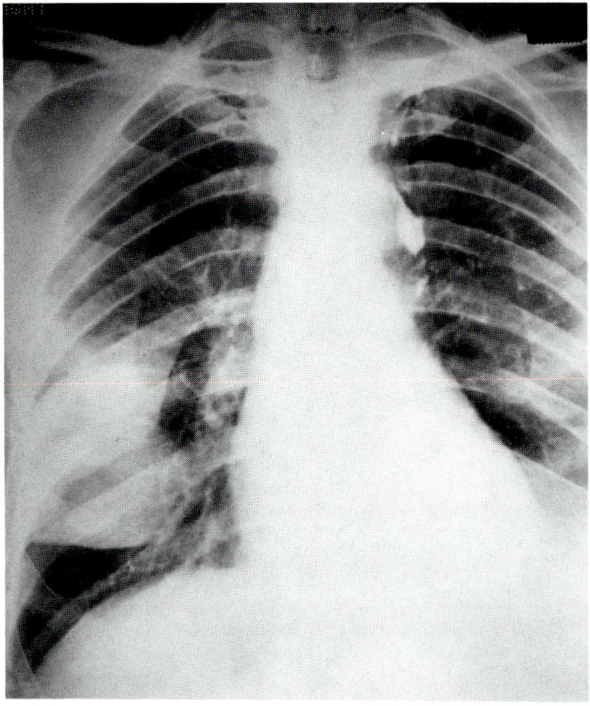

Figure 4.11. Interlobar pleural effusion on the right side; homogeneous shadow between the 4th and 6th ribs anteriorly

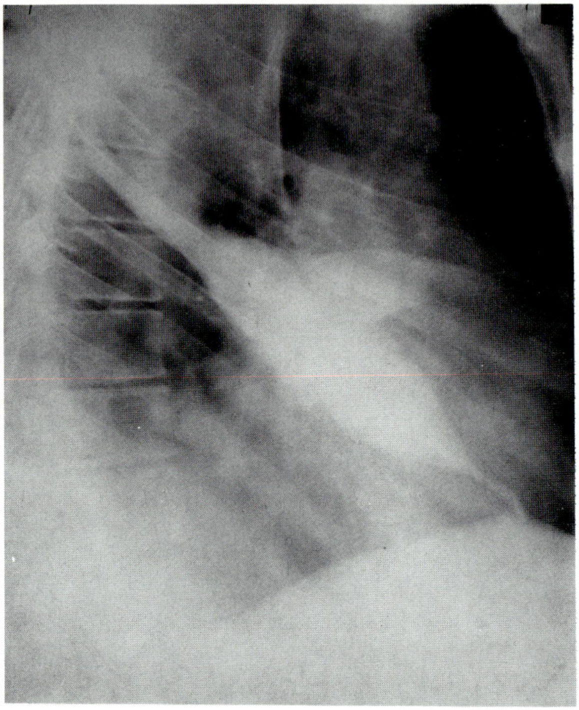

Figure 4.12. Same patient (right lateral view). The elliptical shadow of the fluid in the oblique fissure extends from the 5th thoracic vertebra to meet the diaphragm 4 cm behind the sternum. There is also an anterior extension of fluid into the horizontal fissure

Plain radiographs will be required shortly after initial drainage to confirm that no undrained pockets of fluid remain.

Sinograms for demonstrating size and position of an empyema cavity

Later, if for any reason drainage is unsatisfactory, contrast medium can be injected down the drainage tube and radiographs taken; the size and shape of the residual cavity and its relation to the tube will thus be seen (*Figures 4.13 and 4.14*). The presence and site of a bronchopleural fistula may also be demonstrated by the same method.

Success in this examination depends on attention to detail. A suitable intermediate connection should be fitted between the syringe and the drainage tube. The patient should be positioned so that gravity aids the flow of oil into the cavity. After the injection the syringe and intermediate piece should be disconnected and a spigot placed in the tube to prevent an escape of the opaque medium on to

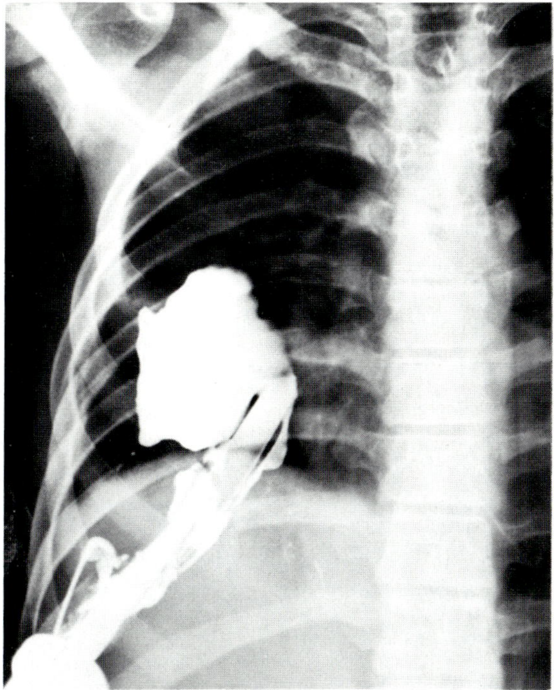

Figure 4.13. Drained empyema; sinogram showing the drainage tube and cavity filled with opaque oil. Same patient as in *Figure 4.9*, 2 weeks later

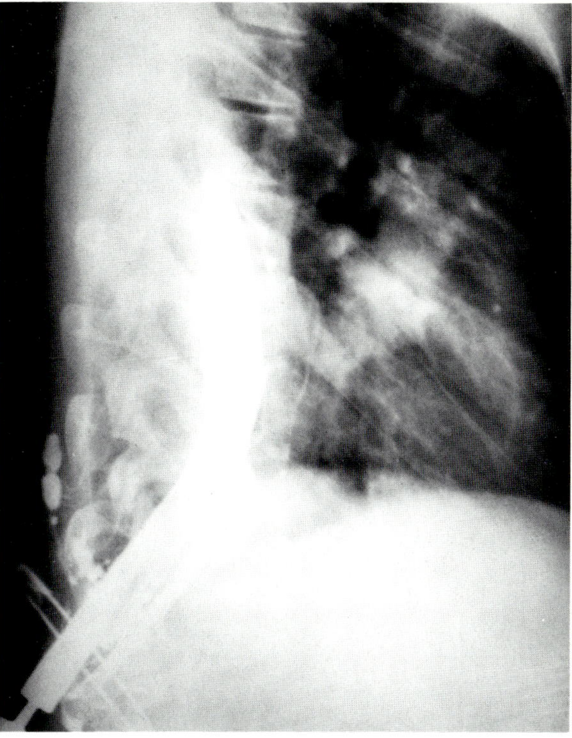

Figure 4.14. Lateral view sinogram of the same patient as in *Figure 4.13*, again showing the position and size of the residual cavity and its relation to the drainage tube

the surrounding skin; light packing should be placed round the tube at its point of entry into the body for the same purpose (this should not be placed round the tube *during* the injection, because of the danger of an air or oil embolus). Radiographs should then be taken with the patient standing to show the relationship of the end of the tube to the bottom of the cavity, and prone or supine if it is necessary to outline the whole cavity—PA (or AP) and the appropriate lateral view are obtained.

Hydropneumothorax

The indications for initial radiography in a hydropneumothorax are much the same as in a simple effusion, and the timing of further X-ray examinations depends on the clinical condition and physical signs. A traumatic haemopneumothorax needs early radiological investigation and further radiographs within a day or so to ensure that drainage is satisfactory and the lung is re-expanding well.

A chest film with the patient standing or sitting shows the upper limit of the fluid ending abruptly with a well-defined horizontal margin (*Figure 4.15*).

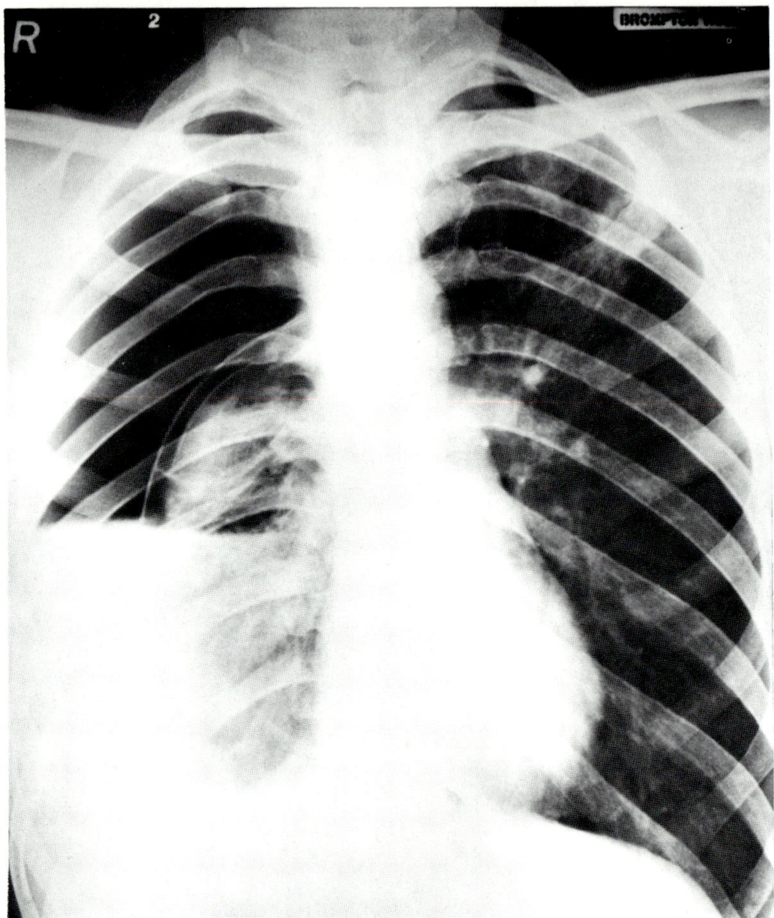

Figure 4.15. Hydropneumothorax on the right side (PA view, patient standing). The transradiant pleural air space, the horizontal fluid level and the edge of the collapsed right lung can be seen

Pneumothorax

Indications for radiology

A large traumatic or a spontaneous pneumothorax presents no difficulties of diagnosis on clinical examination, but radiographs are required to show the degree of relaxation of the underlying lung. If the pneumothorax is small the physical signs are less marked or absent and radiographs will then be necessary for diagnosis.

X-ray appearances

A large pneumothorax with much lung relaxation can be clearly seen in the radiograph (*Figure 4.15*). The pleural air space is hypertransradiant and therefore black, and there is an absence of lung vessel shadows. A well-defined white line marks the site of the visceral pleura covering the relaxed lung. The lung itself may appear grey in colour if it is still partly aerated, or white if it is completely airless (and therefore relatively radio-opaque) as a result of the external pressure or of an associated bronchial obstruction. If the collapse is complete the lung occupies a very small area in the hilar region.

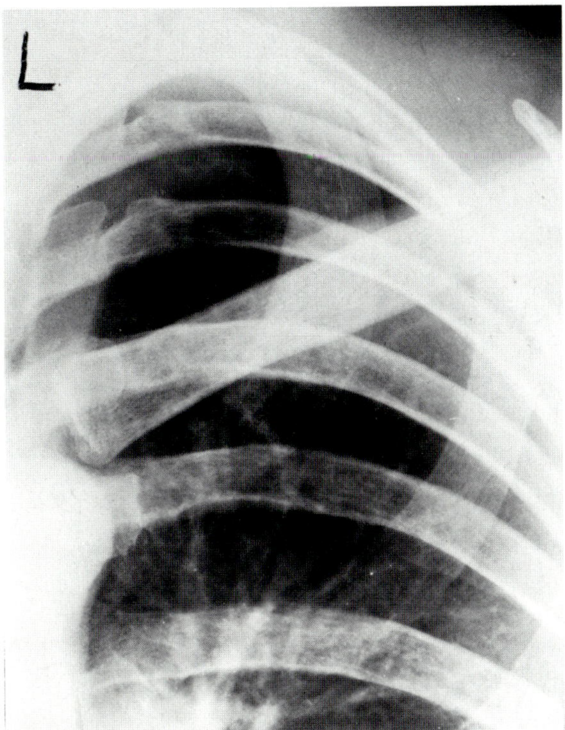

Figure 4.16. Spontaneous pneumothorax; standard inspiration radiograph. The pneumothorax is difficult to see

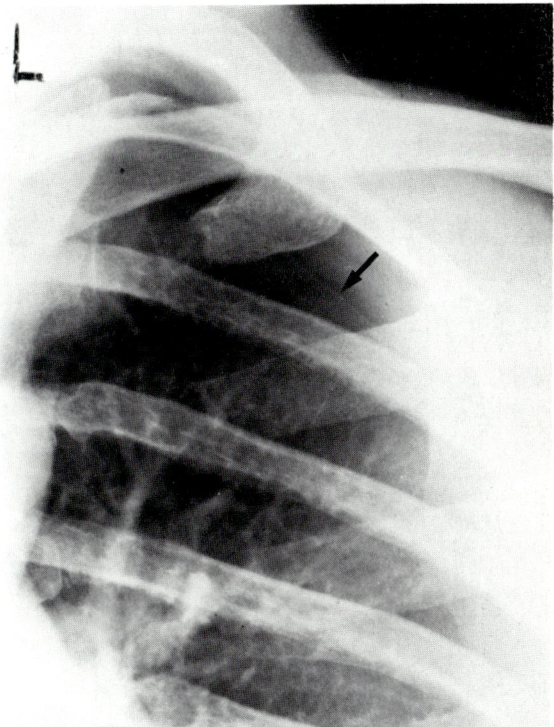

Figure 4.17. Same patient as in *Figure 4.16.* Radiograph on expiration. White line of the visceral pleura over the relaxed lung (arrow) confirms the pneumothorax. There are no pulmonary vessel shadows lateral to the line

A very small pneumothorax may be almost invisible in the routine PA film but may be better seen in one taken during full expiration (*Figures 4.16 and 4.17*).

Tension pneumothorax

It is essential to recognize a tension pneumothorax, since this requires urgent decompression by pleural intubation. The condition is produced by a checkvalve action of a defect in the visceral pleura or injury to the chest wall, allowing air to be drawn into the pleural cavity on inspiration but preventing its escape on expiration. The inspiratory chest film will show a large pneumothorax displacing the collapsed lung and mediastinal structures from their normal positions to the contralateral side of the thorax, and flattening or even inversion of the diaphragm on the affected side (*Figure 4.18*). The condition requires to be diagnosed on an inspiratory film, since some

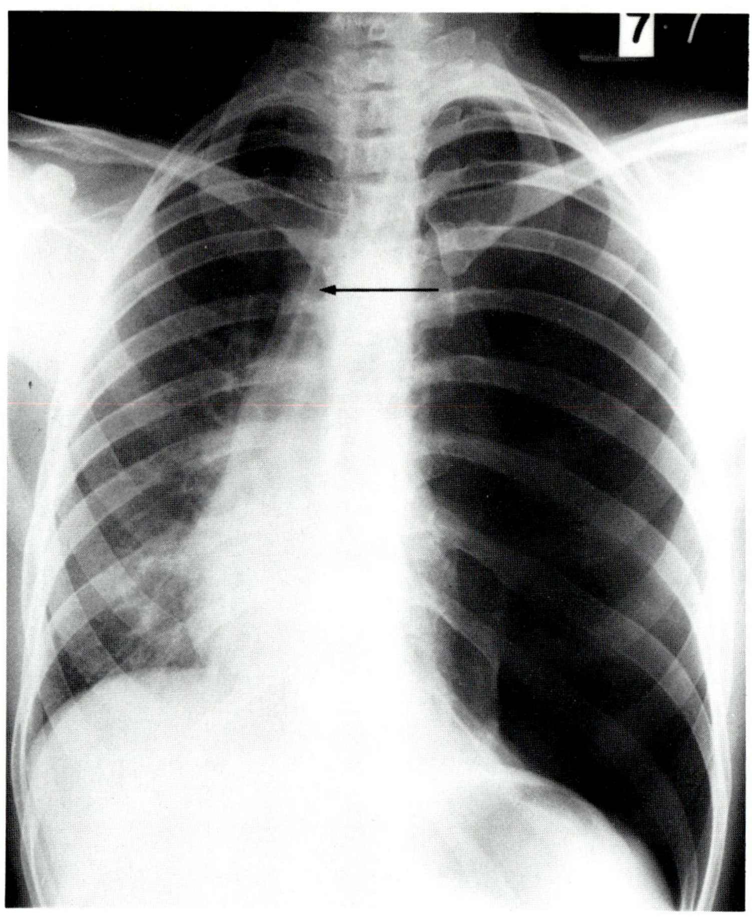

Figure 4.18. Tension pneumothorax on left side. The elevated pressure in the air-filled left pleural space has caused displacement of the heart and trachea (arrow) to the right, depression of the left diaphragm and collapse of the left lung

mediastinal displacement will take place on expiration in the presence of a pneumothorax which is not under tension.

Re-expansion of spontaneous pneumothorax

The patient is usually managed conservatively when the pneumothorax has caused collapse of 20 per cent or less of the lung on the affected side, and, provided that the pleural defect has sealed spontaneously, repeat chest films at fortnightly intervals will show full re-expansion of the lung within a month. It is usual to evacuate the air in the pleural space with an indwelling catheter and water-seal drain when more than 20 per cent of the lung has collapsed. In this case a radiograph should be taken at 24 hours to show whether the lung has completely re-expanded. If re-expansion is good and no air is bubbling from the end of the tube into the water-seal jar the catheter can be withdrawn, and a further radiograph should then be taken 24 hours later to show whether the re-expansion has been maintained.

In most cases of spontaneous pneumothorax the radiograph is otherwise normal, or may show no more than a small apical bulla.

In a few there may be gross emphysema of both lungs, with or without large bullae. Generally a large bulla is more oval in shape than a loculated pneumothorax. Rarely, underlying tuberculosis or a neoplasm may be seen in the re-expanded lung.

Consolidation of the lung

A large shadow occupying the normal position of a lobe, and without evidence of appreciable tracheal or fissure displacement indicating shrinkage, is likely to be caused by consolidation of the lobe. One characteristic radiographic feature of consolidation that is quite often seen is the presence of air-filled, branching bronchi (air bronchogram; *Figure 4.19*). The bronchi are normally invisible on a

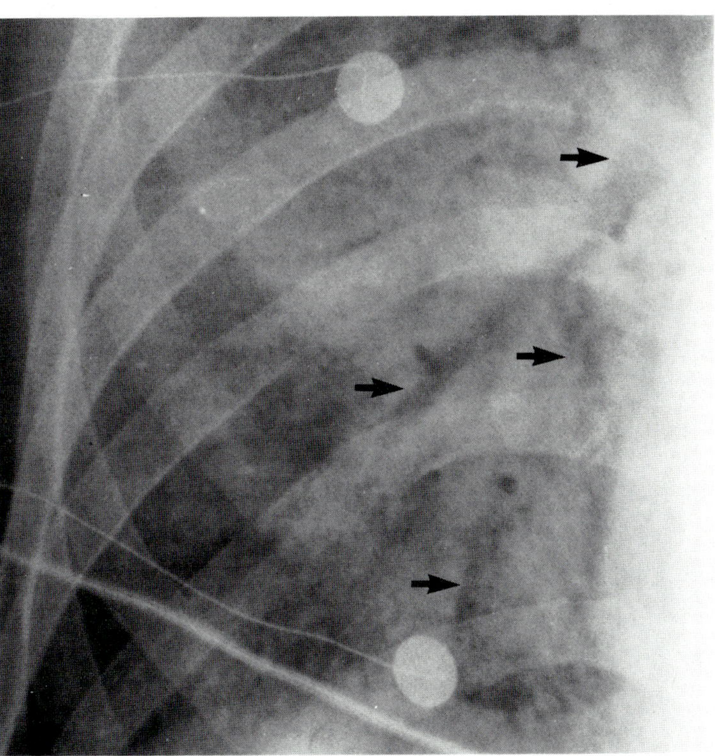

Figure 4.19. Air bronchogram. Branching, air-filled bronchi are visible (arrows), contrasted against opaque lung. This air bronchogram indicates the presence of consolidation

chest X-ray but become visible when the patent lumina are contrasted against the opaque shadows of fluid-filled alveoli in the surrounding lung.

The diaphragm and lateral boundaries of the mediastinum are visible on a normal chest X-ray because they are contrasted against air in the surrounding lungs. Fluid-filled, consolidated lung has the same radiographic density as soft tissue, so that the normal silhouette of the heart border or diaphragm becomes lost when consolidation

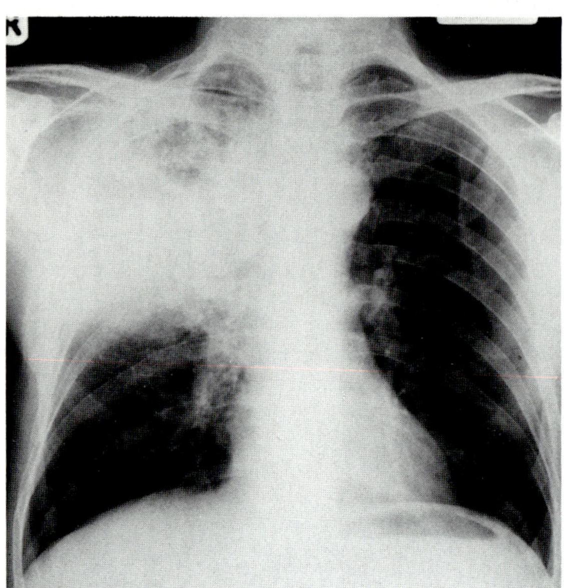

Figure 4.20. Consolidation of right upper lobe. Patchy opacification present in right upper and middle zones. There is no mediastinal displacement

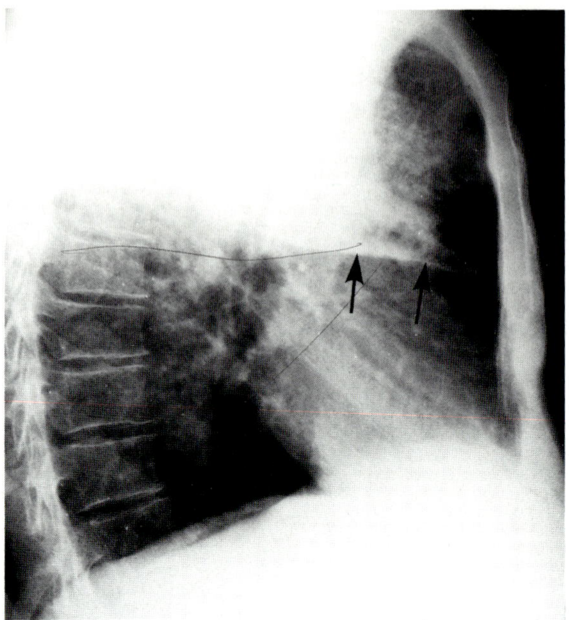

Figure 4.21 Same patient as in *Figure 4.20* (right lateral view). The consolidation is limited inferiorly by the horizontal fissure (arrows), the position of which is normal. Posterior demarcation of the consolidation by the upper portion of the oblique fissure is not clearly defined in this case. Bacterial lobar pneumonia

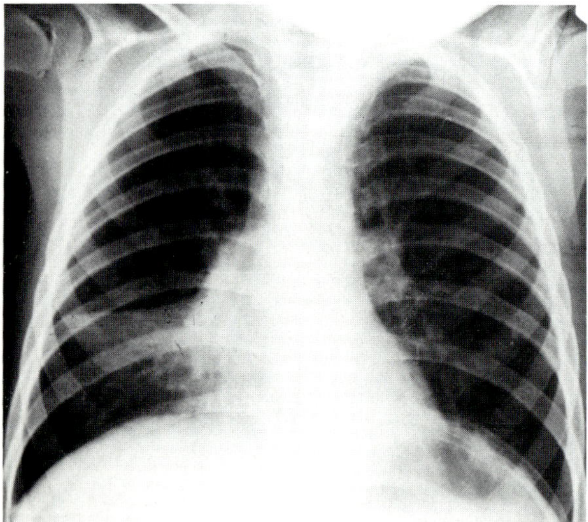

Figure 4.22. Consolidation of middle lobe. Triangular opacity in right lower zone, bordered superiorly by the horizontal fissure. Loss of the outline of the right heart border indicates that the consolidation lies in the anterior portion of the lung adjacent to the heart (silhouette sign)

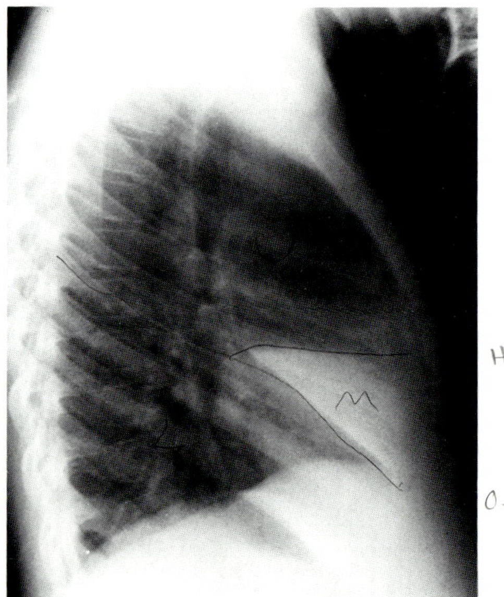

Figure 4.23. Same patient as in *Figure 4.22* (right lateral view). The middle lobe consolidation produces a triangular opacity lying between the horizontal fissure and lower end of the oblique fissure. Both fissures are in normal positions. Simple lobar pneumonia

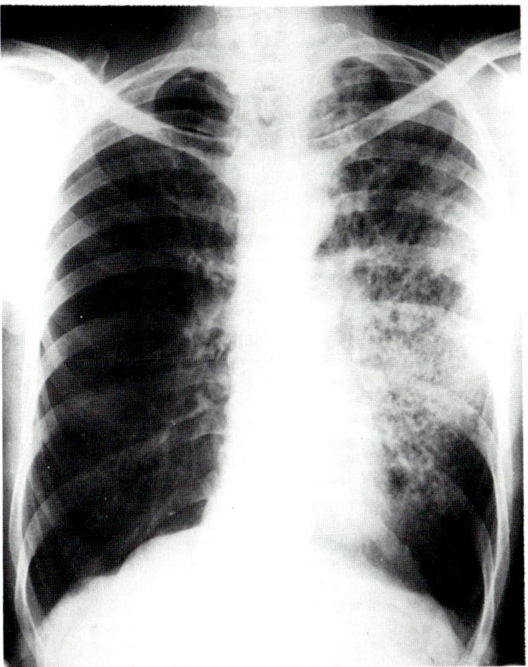

Figure 4.24. Consolidation of left upper lobe. Patchy opacification present in left lung, sparing the lung base. No mediastinal displacement. Left heart border largely obscured, indicating that part of the consolidation involves lung adjacent to it (silhouette sign)

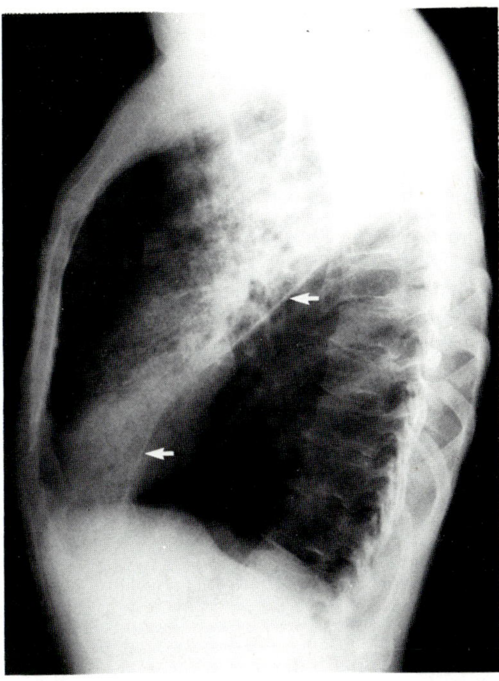

Figure 4.25. Same patient as in *Figure 4.24* (left lateral view). The consolidation is seen to lie entirely in front of the white line of the interlobar fissure (arrows). The fissure is in the normal position, running from the junction of the 4th and 5th dorsal vertebral bodies posteriorly to meet the diaphragm about 4 cm behind the sternum. Simple lobar pneumonia

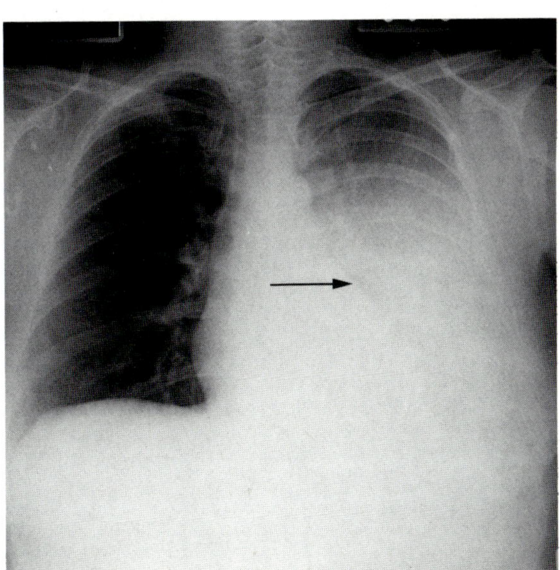

Figure 4.26. Consolidation of left lower lobe. Opacification of lower two-thirds of left lung. No mediastinal displacement. Left heart border visible (arrow)

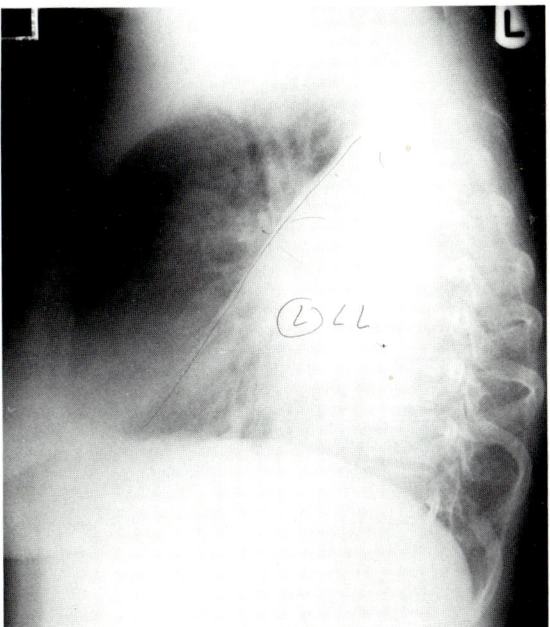

Figure 4.27. Same patient as in *Figure 4.26* (left lateral view). The consolidation lies posteriorly, limited anteriorly by the straight, sharp edge of the fissure. (There is relative sparing of the anterior segment of the lower lobe in this case.) Right lower lobe consolidation would produce a similar shadow on the right side

develops in adjacent lung. Application of this principle, the silhouette sign, is useful in assessing from the PA chest film the lobe involved in consolidation (*Figures 4.22–4.25*).

It is important for the clinician to be familiar with the appearances of consolidation of the lobes of the lungs, and these are shown in *Figures 4.20–4.27*. The appearances can be largely inferred from a knowledge of the surface markings of the lobes as used in physical examination of the patient.

Consolidation is often patchy and non-lobar in distribution and can be due to a great variety of causes, in all of which air in the alveoli is replaced by fluid or cells. Possible causes include infective and aspiration pneumonia, pulmonary oedema from cardiac failure, haemorrhage into the lungs, pulmonary infarction, and malignant infiltration of the alveoli (by alveolar-cell carcinoma of the lung, for example). The radiographic appearances of these conditions may be indistinguishable from each other, with ill-defined shadowing that may contain an air bronchogram, but sometimes the cause can be strongly suggested by the distribution of the shadowing or the presence of associated features. Patchy consolidation associated with areas of cavitation in the upper thirds of the lungs, for example, is likely to be due to pulmonary tuberculosis.

Value of radiology in infective consolidation (pneumonia)

A common cause of consolidation is a bacterial or viral infection. An early radiograph is of value, even when the condition is obvious clinically, in order to define the extent of the pneumonia.

If the patient makes good clinical progress he should have chest films repeated at intervals of 2 or 3 weeks until radiographic resolution is complete. This commonly takes about 6 weeks but may be longer. The importance of following up the patient until full resolution has occurred is that an episode of pneumonia may be the first manifestation of partial bronchial obstruction by a proximal bronchial carcinoma, and in this situation pneumonia may show very protracted clearing, may fail to clear completely or may recur. In these situations, or if there is any appreciable loss of volume associated with a lobar or segmental pneumonia, the patient should be investigated further by bronchoscopy.

Slow initial clinical improvement or return of fever may be due to development of a lung abscess, serous effusion or empyema, in which case more frequent radiographic examination will be required.

Lung abscess

It is rare nowadays for a lung abscess to present with acute fever and foul sputum, so that the diagnosis tends to be made on the X-ray appearances in a patient with a chest infection that is slow to resolve. Serial radiographs are useful to observe the progress of resolution under treatment.

X-ray appearances

The X-ray appearances of a lung abscess are variable but they can be divided into four main types:

1. A well-defined oval or spherical opacity, usually some 2–5 cm in size (*Figure 4.28*). A central cavity with a fluid level is often present at an early stage.

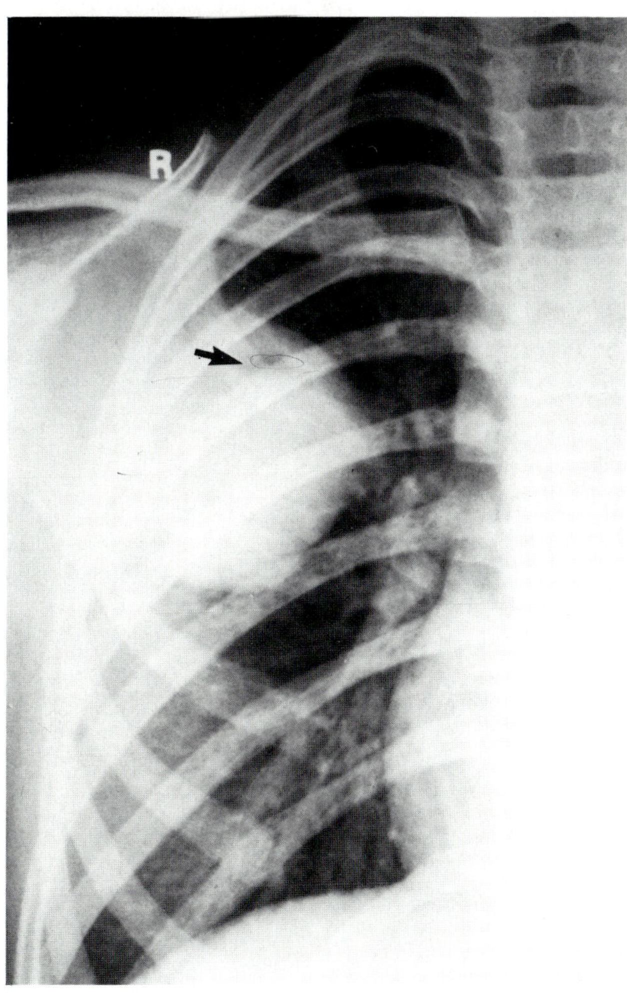

Figure 4.28. Lung abscess. Circumscribed spherical opacity 4 cm diameter in the right mid-zone. A small quantity of air is present within the upper part of the abscess (arrow)

2. A fairly large cavity, with or without a fluid level, round which there is an area of diffuse consolidation, poorly demarcated from the normal lung except where it extends to an interlobar fissure (*Figure 4.29*).
3. An area of diffuse clouding, with multiple small cavities within it, often occupying most of a lobe. This appearance is seen in suppurative pneumonia.

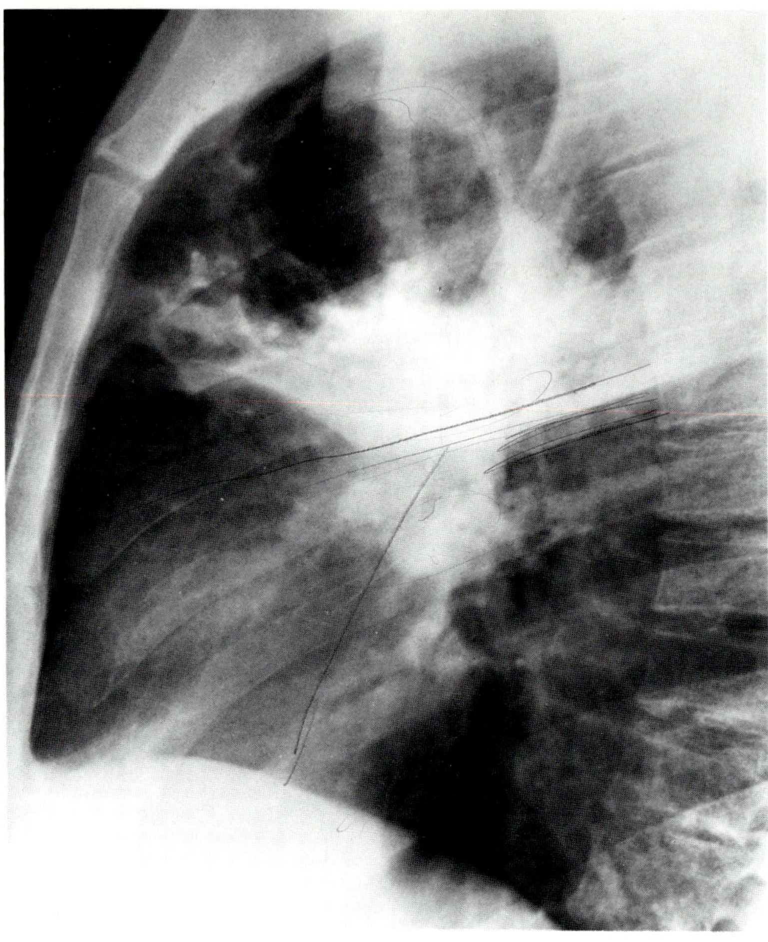

Figure 4.29. Lung abscess; lateral view. A large cavity with a smaller one below. Much surrounding consolidation, limited inferiorly by the interlobar fissures

4. Multiple well-defined oval or spherical opacities, 1–3 cm in size, with central cavitation and fluid levels, due to staphylococcal embolic lesions.

In types 2 and 3 it is sometimes impossible to see an abscess cavity on the routine radiographs, although this can be clearly demonstrated by tomography.

Differential diagnosis

If the clinical and radiological findings are carefully correlated the diagnosis is usually not difficult, although there is often some doubt about the underlying cause and later about the completeness of resolution.

An encysted hydro- or pyopneumothorax may be virtually indistinguishable from a lung abscess on radiographs.

An infected lung cyst or hydatid cyst containing a fluid level will produce similar X-ray appearances.

The well-defined type of lung abscess (type 1 above) is commonly thick walled, the wall thickness being over 5 mm. Several conditions cause similar radiographic appearances, the commonest of these being cavitating pulmonary infarcts and cavitating primary or secondary carcinomas (usually of squamous-cell type). A tuberculous cavity can also present similar appearances but is more commonly thinner walled.

Atelectasis of the lung or of a lobe

Occlusion of a lobar bronchus results in atelectasis (or collapse) of that lobe. The occlusion may be from an intraluminal object such as an inhaled foreign body or mucous plug; from a mural tumour or inflammatory mass; or from pressure on the bronchus from without by hilar lymph glands.

Lobar atelectasis may also be seen without any present evidence of stenosis of the lobar bronchus. It can be the result of a previous transient occlusion such as may ensue from the pressure from enlarged tuberculous glands: these may regress so that the stenosis is relieved, but the lobe may remain small and shrunken if irreversible multiple peripheral bronchial occlusions have occurred, usually consequent on a superadded infection. Similar bronchial occlusions may follow a chronic pneumonia without there having been stenosis of the lobar bronchus at any time.

Pathologically, other changes apart from simple collapse of the lobe are almost invariably present. At the very least there is an outpouring of fluid exudate into the alveoli, and usually there are varying amounts of cellular exudate, so that a combination of consolidation and collapse is found. In addition the bronchi are dilated and full of retained secretions.

X-ray appearances

If a whole lung is collapsed there will be a homogeneous shadow on the affected side, with the heart and trachea displaced towards that side and the diaphragm raised (*see Figure 4.5*). If only a lobe is atelectatic due to bronchial obstruction two characteristic changes will be seen. The first of these is the homogeneous shadow of the collapsed lobe itself, which will occupy much less space than when it is aerated, and the second is the effect of the collapsed lobe on the remainder of the lung and on the mediastinum and diaphragm. Thus lobar collapse will produce some degree of hilar displacement (elevation in upper lobe collapse, descent in lower lobe collapse), increased transradiancy of the remainder of the lung due to compensatory overexpansion of the unaffected lobe or lobes, and some diaphragmatic elevation and mediastinal displacement towards the affected side. These changes may not all be present. For example, in collapse of the smallest lobe, the middle lobe, only the opacity of the collapsed lobe itself is seen, while in upper lobe collapse there may be no appreciable diaphragmatic elevation. Some of these changes

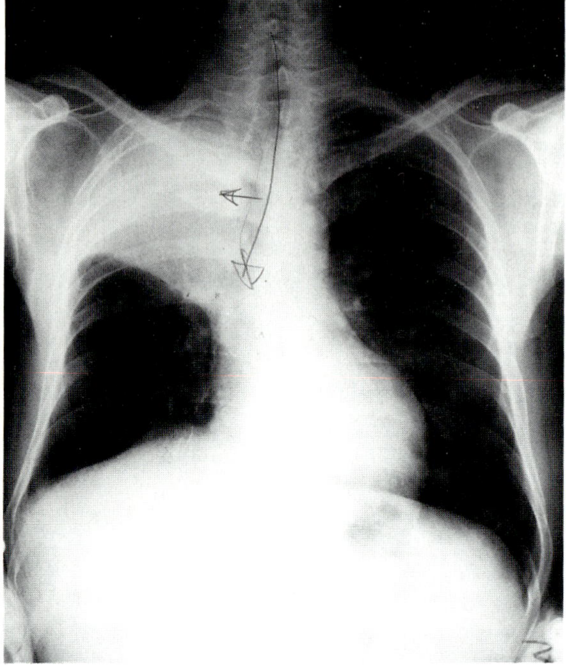

Figure 4.30. Atelectasis of right upper lobe (moderate). Opacity of homogeneous density in upper half of right hemithorax. The horizontal fissure, which forms the inferior border of the opacity, is rotated upwards from the horizontal position, and the trachea is displaced to the right, indicating the effects of lobar shrinkage

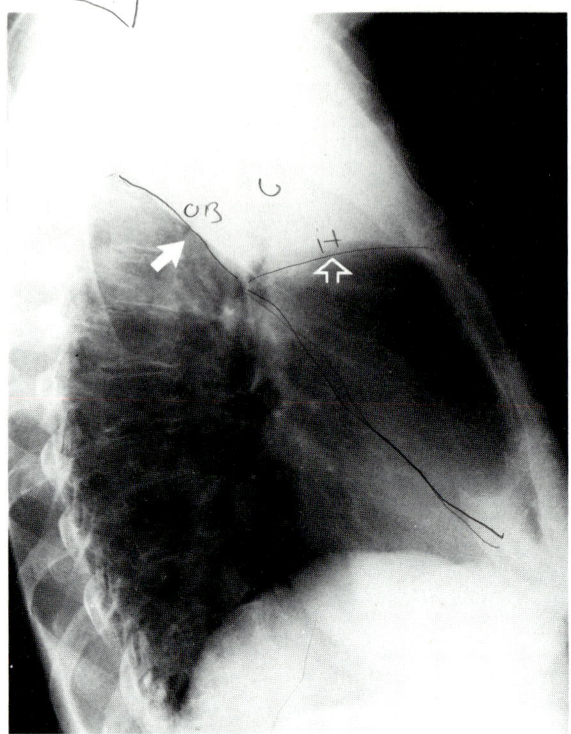

Figure 4.31. Atelectasis of right upper lobe (moderate); right lateral view. The horizontal fissure is displaced and bowed upwards (open arrow) and the oblique fissure is displaced forwards (solid arrow) from the normal positions (cf. *Figure 4.21*); carcinoma in right upper lobe bronchus

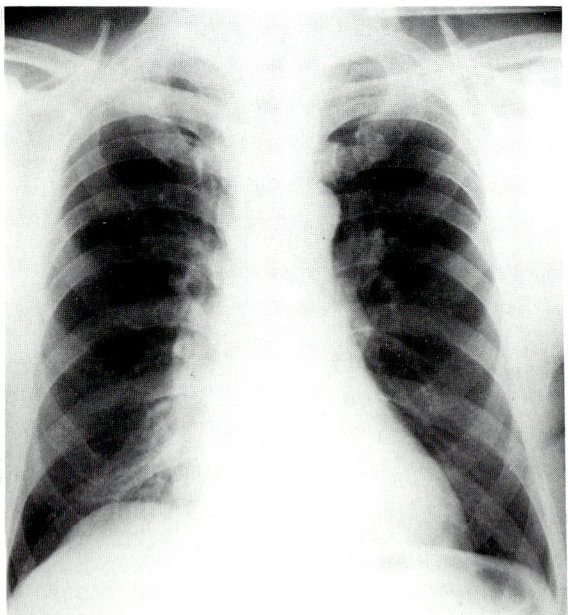

Figure 4.32. Atelectasis of middle lobe. The outline of the right heart border is lost, indicating disease in lung lying adjacent to the heart (silhouette sign)

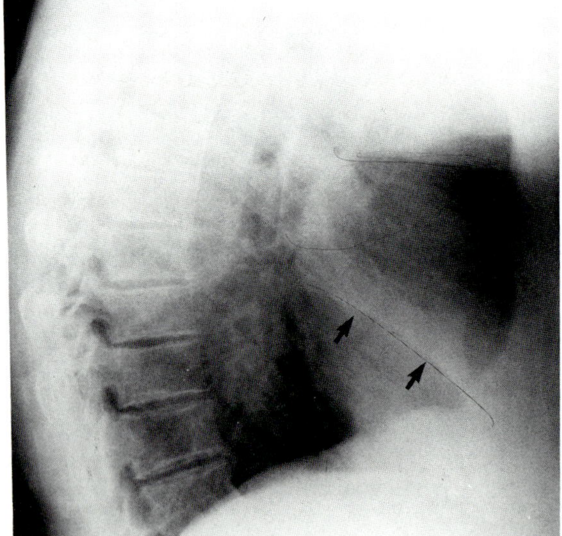

Figure 4.33. Same patient as in *Figure 4.32* (right lateral view). Homogeneous opacity overlying the heart shadow, bordered inferiorly by the oblique fissure which is displaced and bowed upwards (arrows), indicating shrinkage of the middle lobe

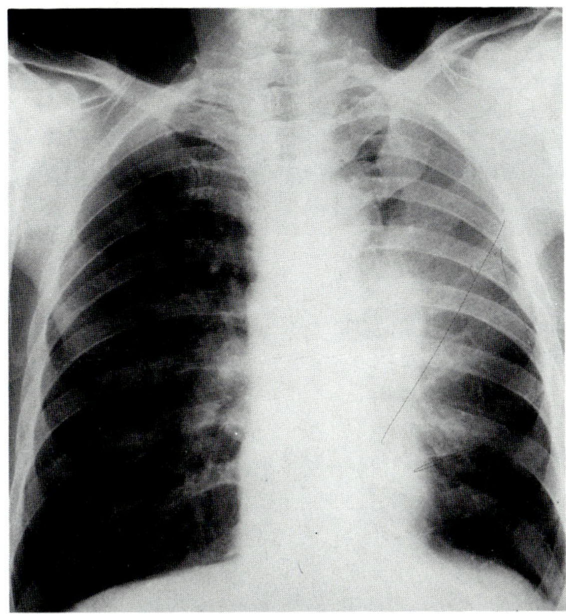

Figure 4.34. Atelectasis of left upper lobe. Opacity of homogeneous density occupying medial portion of upper two-thirds of left lung. The left diaphragm is slightly raised (higher than the right)

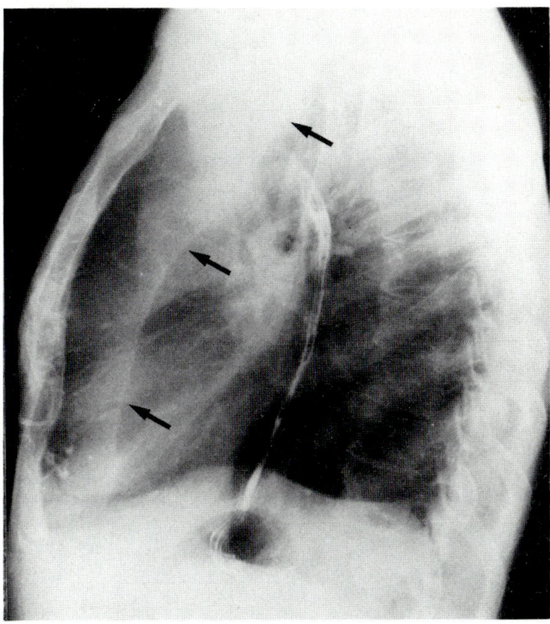

Figure 4.35. Same patient as in *Figure 4.34* (left lateral view). The opacity is bordered posteriorly by the oblique fissure which is displaced forwards from its normal position (arrows), indicating shrinkage of the upper lobe (cf. *Figure 4.25*); carcinoma in the left upper lobe bronchus

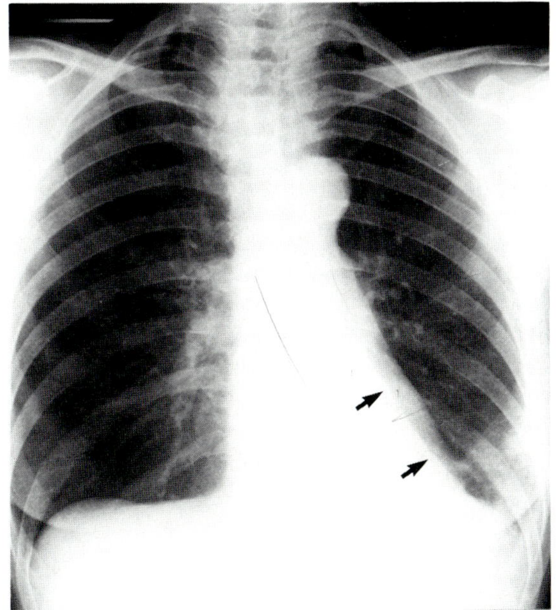

Figure 4.36. Atelectasis of left lower lobe. There is a triangular opacity behind the heart, bounded laterally by the straight edge of the displaced oblique fissure (arrows) running more or less in line with the left heart border. The heart is slightly displaced to the left. Similar changes occur on the right side in right lower lobe atelectasis

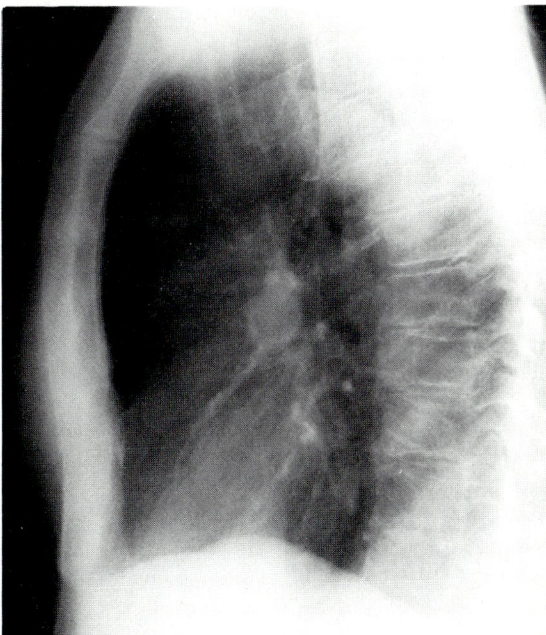

Figure 4.37. Same patient as in *Figure 4.36* (left lateral view). Normally the lower dorsal vertebrae are more transradiant than the upper, and in this case they are of similar density. This is due to the collapsed lower lobe overlying the lower dorsal vertebrae and contributing to the shadow

may be present, however, and they should be looked for as they are useful in substantiating the diagnosis.

It is important to recognize the patterns of collapse of the different lobes of the lung, and these are illustrated in *Figures 4.30* to *4.37*.

The importance of recognizing lobar collapse and distinguishing this from lobar consolidation is that collapse implies the probability of an underlying bronchial obstruction. In a middle-aged or elderly adult this is most commonly due to an underlying bronchial carcinoma, while in a child it may be due to an inhaled foreign body such as a peanut. Bronchoscopy is therefore a mandatory investigation when unexplained lobar collapse is shown on the radiograph.

Pulmonary tuberculosis

The primary infection

The primary lesion, or first infection with tuberculosis, is usually either symptom free or associated with very minor symptoms, so that it generally passes undetected both clinically and radiologically. Sometimes, however, in the case of people who are under careful clinical observation because of contact with the disease, the period during which the Mantoux reaction changes from negative to positive is demonstrated, and the onset of infection thus indicated. At this point there may or may not be visible radiological changes, depending on the size and site of the lesion.

Age of onset

In countries with a high incidence of tuberculosis the primary infection usually occurs in childhood. With improvements in the control of the disease and in living conditions, primary infection may not occur until adult life. Thus a large proportion of adults who did not receive BCG at school may be found to have a negative Mantoux reaction.

X-ray appearances

When visible, the shadow of a parenchymal primary lesion varies in size from a small area of clouding some 2–5 mm wide to an area of consolidation occupying most of a lobe (the smaller lesion is the more common). The shadow has an ill-defined edge and may be present in any part of the lungs. This primary lesion is usually accompanied by visible enlargement of the hilar glands draining the infected area (*Figure 4.38*). When the primary lesion is close to the hilum the two shadows may merge, giving a dumb-bell appearance. The association of a tuberculous pulmonary lesion with enlarged hilar glands is described as the 'primary complex'. A caseous lesion

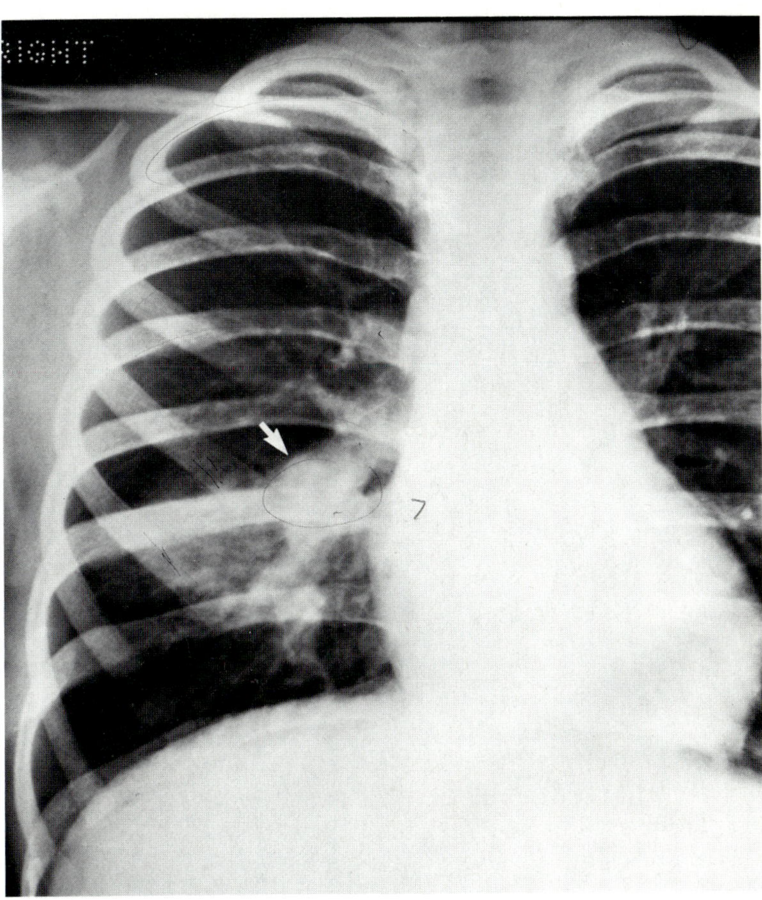

Figure 4.38. Pulmonary tuberculosis: primary lesion in a child aged 4 years; area of diffuse pulmonary shadowing between the anterior ends of the 4th and 5th ribs; associated enlargement of hilar gland (arrow)

may rupture into the pleural space to produce a pleural effusion. This is most common in adolescents and young adults, in whom a pleural effusion may be the presenting feature.

Differential diagnosis

If the change in the Mantoux reaction has passed undetected it will be necessary to distinguish the X-ray shadow of the primary tuberculous complex from the similar pulmonary shadows and associated hilar gland enlargement occasionally seen in measles, whooping cough and other pneumonias. The diagnosis of the latter conditions will usually be obvious clinically or on laboratory investigation. If not, rapid resolution of the lesion—say in 3 weeks—shown by serial X-ray observation will tend to exclude a tuberculous origin.

Resolution of the primary complex

With modern chemotherapy resolution is the rule, but even if the lesion passes undetected and therefore untreated a primary complex tends to resolve, often with some calcification in the lung focus and draining hilar glands.

Progressive primary lesions

Occasionally the primary complex progresses instead of resolving, the opacity increasing in size and finally breaking down with the formation of cavities.

Early secondary or post-primary lesions

An early secondary lesion, like the primary infection, is usually symptomless and without physical signs and may be detected accidentally from a chest radiograph taken during a survey of tuberculosis contacts or for some unrelated purpose. Occasionally it is accompanied or preceded by mild constitutional disturbances, such as loss of appetite or weight, or by a catarrhal 'cold' which does not resolve rapidly.

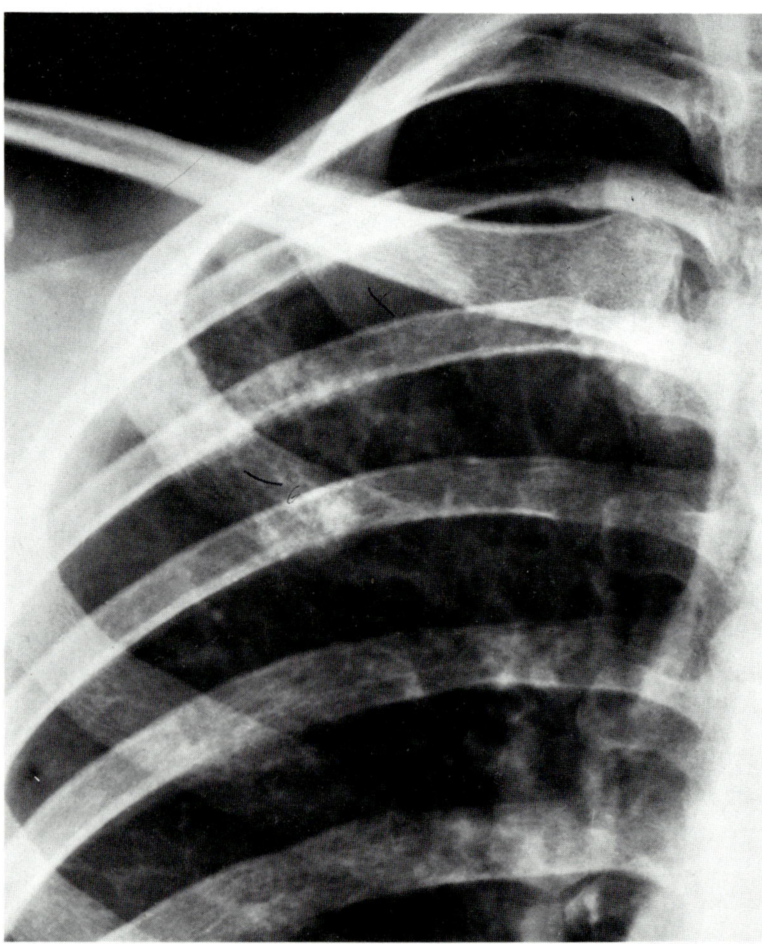

Figure 4.39. Pulmonary tuberculosis: early secondary lesion in a 19-year-old woman. Small area of mottled shadowing in the right first interspace. Contact case; no symptoms

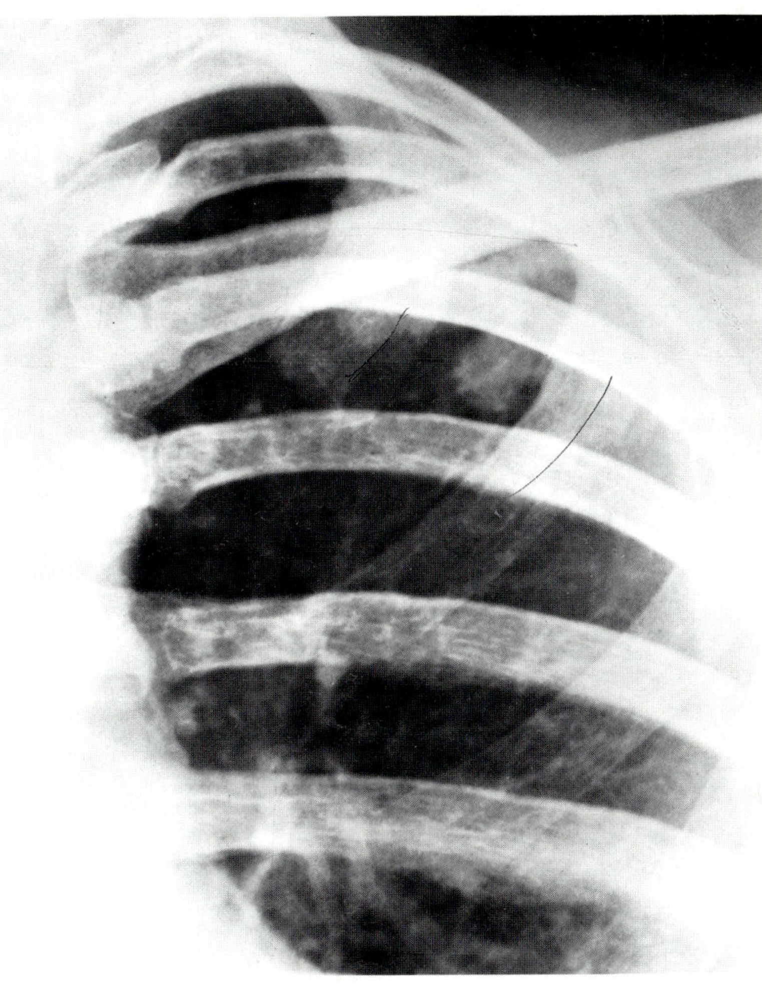

Figure 4.40. Pulmonary tuberculosis: early secondary lesion in a 20-year-old woman. 2 cm round focus in the left first interspace. Contact case

X-ray appearances

Two types of early secondary lesion are seen on the radiograph:
1. A small group of rather low-density mottled opacities, varying in size from 3 to 5 mm (*Figure 4.39*).
2. A homogeneous shadow about 2 cm in size, which may be round and well-defined or more or less rectangular with a rather ill-defined edge (*Figure 4.40*).

Most of these early lesions are in the apical or posterior segments of the upper lobe, or apical segment of the lower lobe, and seen on the radiograph in the upper or middle zones. The lesions may, however, occur anywhere in the lung, and the possibility of post-primary tuberculosis should not be dismissed if the infiltration is in an atypical site. There is no enlargement of the hilar glands in secondary lesions in Caucasians, although this can sometimes occur in Negro or Asian patients.

Established pulmonary tuberculosis

X-ray appearances

If the early secondary lesions progress so that the disease process is well established in the lungs, the radiographs will show more extensive shadows than the small round focus or small area of mottling of an early secondary lesion. Several small areas of clouding or an extensive area of mottling may be seen, often accompanied by ring shadows indicating the presence of cavities

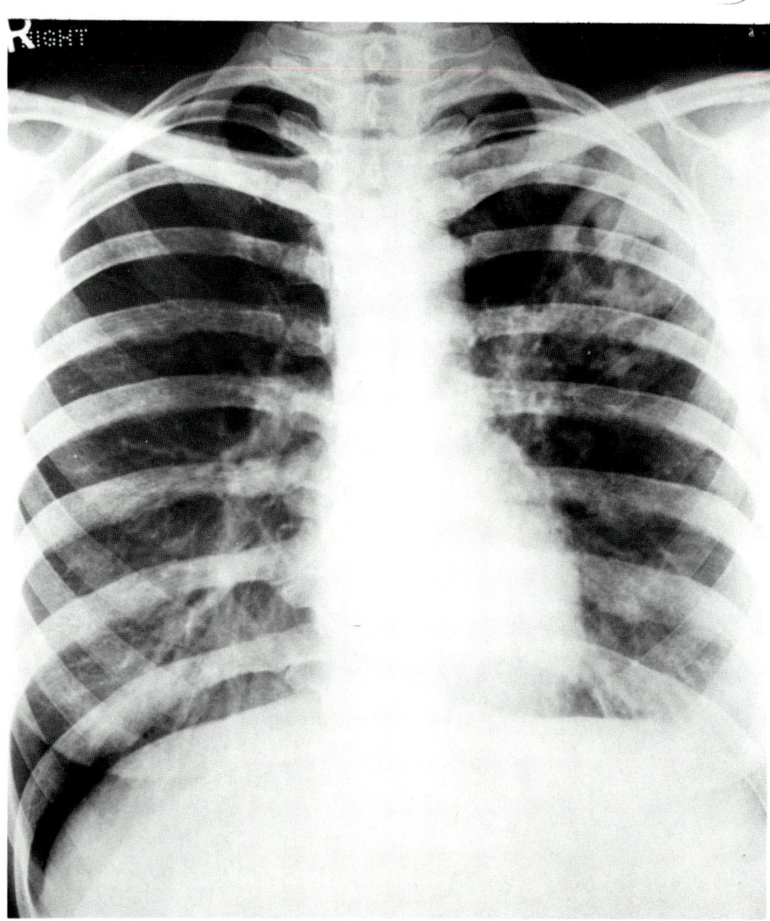

Figure 4.41. Established pulmonary tuberculosis; cavity and mottled shadowing above and lateral to the left hilum

(*Figure 4.41*). Linear shadows, suggesting older fibrotic healing lesions or indrawn pleura, and calcifications are often present concurrently with the mottled shadows of the more recent foci.

Tuberculous cavities

These appear in the radiograph as ring shadows with transradiant centres. They vary in size from a few millimetres to several centimetres. The wall of the cavity is sometimes thin and well-defined, and areas of mottling are usually present in the neighbouring lung (*Figure 4.41*). At other times the cavitation is seen as an irregular translucency in an area of tuberculous pneumonia (*Figure 4.42*).

A fluid level in a tuberculous cavity is relatively uncommon but is occasionally found, so that the presence or absence of a fluid level is of no value in differentiating a tuberculous cavity from a pyogenic lung abscess.

Many tuberculous cavities are invisible in the plain radiographs but can be clearly seen on tomograms (*Figure 4.42*). A cavity appears on a tomogram as a transradiant area surrounded by an opaque

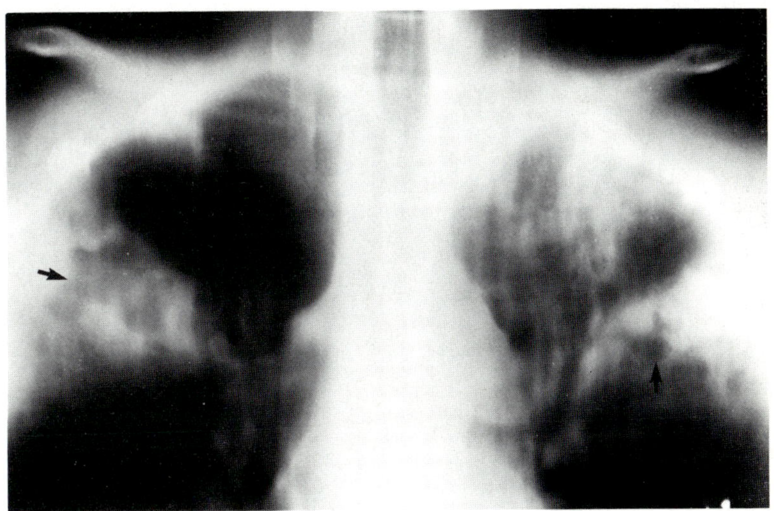

Figure 4.42. Established tuberculosis; tomogram showing cavities (arrows) in areas of tuberculous pneumonia

wall. Some cavities show extremely clearly, and there is no doubt as to the diagnosis; others present considerable difficulties of interpretation, especially if there are many other shadows nearby, the danger being that the shadows of neighbouring structures may be mistaken for the wall of a cavity. After careful study of the tomograms, however, it will usually be possible to tell with certainty whether a cavity is present.

Healing lesions

After chemotherapy many or all of the shadows may disappear and the lungs appear normal. In many cases little residual shadowing is seen but there is evidence of lobar shrinkage. This is indicated by tracheal displacement and/or elevation of the horizontal fissure and hilum. The shrinkage is primarily due to lung destruction. Residual line shadows may represent scars, locally indrawn pleura, or the walls of abnormal bronchi. Calcifications are common. The degree of lung shrinkage with residual cavitation and bronchiectasis may be extreme (*Figure 4.43*).

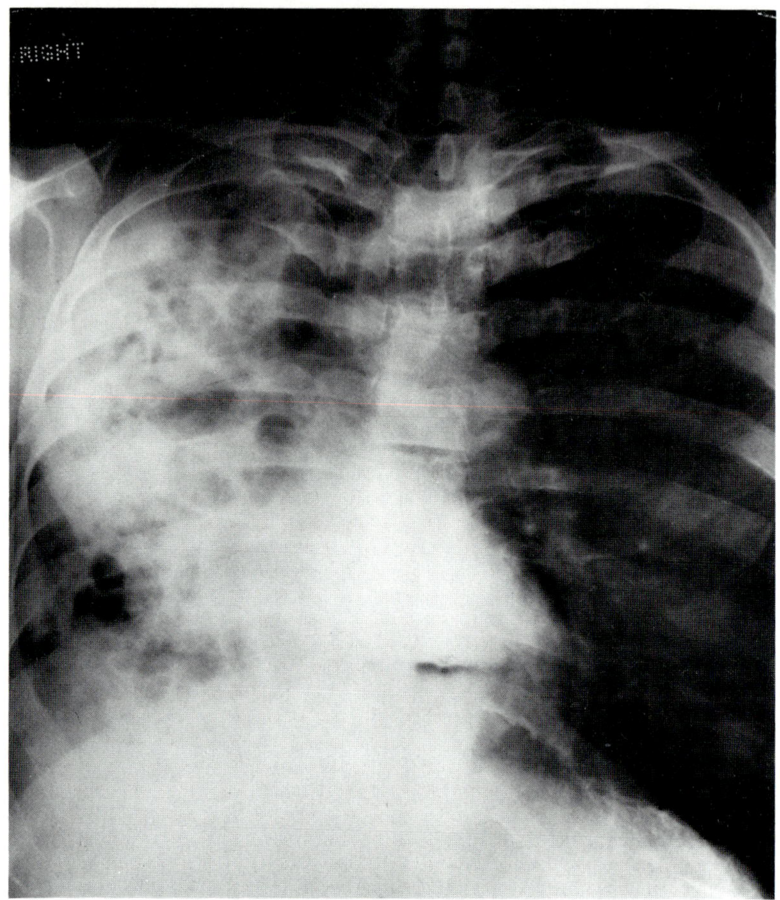

Figure 4.43. Gross destruction of the right lung by tuberculosis. Opacity caused by fibrosis and consolidation; spherical transradiant areas indicate cavitation and bronchiectasis; heart and trachea displaced to the right due to lung destruction. Tubercle bacilli were present in the sputum

The place of radiology

In diagnosis

Obviously, the finding of tubercle bacilli in the sputum, on laryngeal swabs or after gastric lavage is the only definitive evidence for diagnosis. An X-ray examination may nevertheless draw the clinician's attention to the presence of tuberculosis in patients who have no symptoms and no sputum, or only mild symptoms. There may even be sputum in which no bacilli are found at the first examination; in such cases, the positive X-ray findings suggest the need for a more careful and persistent search for the bacilli, which often proves fruitful.

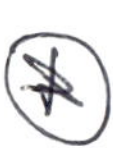

The X-ray appearances alone are not sufficient evidence for a diagnosis of pulmonary tuberculosis, since the shadow of almost any tuberculous lesion can be mimicked by that of some non-tuberculous lesion. It is therefore most important to substantiate the diagnosis from the sputum bacteriology. When, however, sputum smears and culture are negative, typical chest X-ray changes and a strongly positive tuberculin test provide almost certain evidence of activity.

Radiographs usually show with clarity the extent and distribution of the lesions—in fact, they are the only means of achieving this during life—so that they are essential even when the diagnosis can be made on the clinical and bacteriological findings.

In assessing activity

It is not possible to assess the degree of activity of a tuberculous lesion from an isolated radiograph. The presence of cavities is usually associated with tubercle bacilli in the sputum; while calcified and streaky or linear opacities, in the absence of any low-density shadow, usually denote quiescent or even healed lesions. A patient showing much mottling and cavitation may nevertheless be well stabilized in relation to the infection and remain symptom free for long periods; whereas another, showing rather fibrotic linear opacities, may have active and spreading disease. The activity of the lesion is best judged from a careful correlation of the clinical findings with those of serial radiographs at suitable intervals. Calcified hilar glands are of no clinical significance except to show that the patient has had a primary infection and has overcome it; they have no prognostic significance should he develop secondary lesions.

In controlling treatment

Once chemotherapy has been started, no further radiographs need be taken for 3 months unless there is some specific clinical indication. In a recent acute lesion resolution may be well advanced by then, but in well-established disease clearing may not be apparent for 6 months or a year, and considerable residual shadowing may persist indefinitely.

Aspergilloma

Sometimes one or more lung cavities become progressively filled with a growth of aspergillus, which forms a fungal ball. This most commonly occurs in healed tuberculous cavities, so that the aspergilloma is usually seen in the upper lobes; but the cavities in cystic bronchiectasis, lung abscesses and neoplasia can also be involved. An aspergilloma has a characteristic radiological appearance, the fungal ball being separated from the wall of the cavity by a thin crescent of air (*Figure 4.44*). Tomography may be required to define the typical appearance clearly. Occasionally, blood clot or a carcinoma arising within a cavity can give a similar appearance. An aspergilloma can be distinguished, however, as this is commonly freely mobile within the cavity (as can be shown by repeat radiographs with the patient in different positions), and the serum

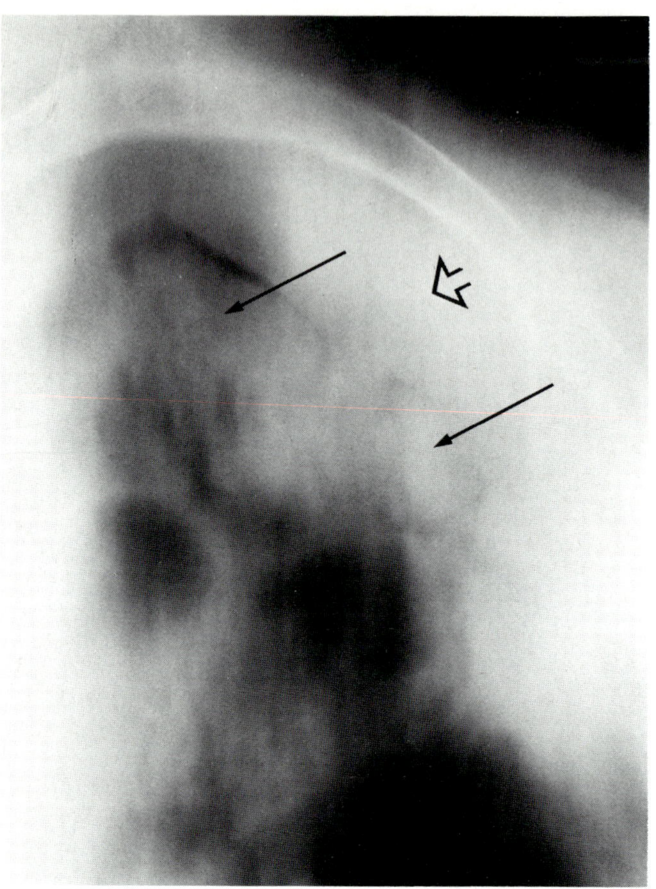

Figure 4.44. Aspergilloma. Fungus balls (long arrows) occupy two healed tuberculous cavities in the left upper lobe. Characteristic crescents of air separate the fungal balls from the walls of the cavities. Greatly thickened overlying pleura (open arrow)

precipitins for aspergillus will be positive. Adjacent pleural thickening commonly accompanies the development of an aspergilloma.

The condition may give rise to no symptoms or it may be suggested by episodes of haemoptysis developing in a patient with previous tuberculosis. The haemoptyses are occasionally severe.

Multiple small nodular shadows

When multiple small nodular shadows are seen in the lungs and there are no immediate clinical clues to indicate their cause, a careful study of the size, clarity of outline, distribution and any associated shadows will often be rewarding.

Miliary tuberculosis

This may present with the classic features of fever, choroidal tubercles, splenomegaly, characteristic chest X-ray changes, and a positive tuberculin test. However, the manifestations may be minimal and non-specific, the patient exhibiting only fever and anaemia.

The characteristic radiographic appearance is of small, very discrete shadows, many of which look as if they could be picked out with tweezers (*Figure 4.45*). These shadows vary in size, from 1 to 4 mm, from patient to patient but are fairly equal in size in any one case. The distribution is even and all zones are affected, including the apices. There may be other evidence of pulmonary tuberculosis

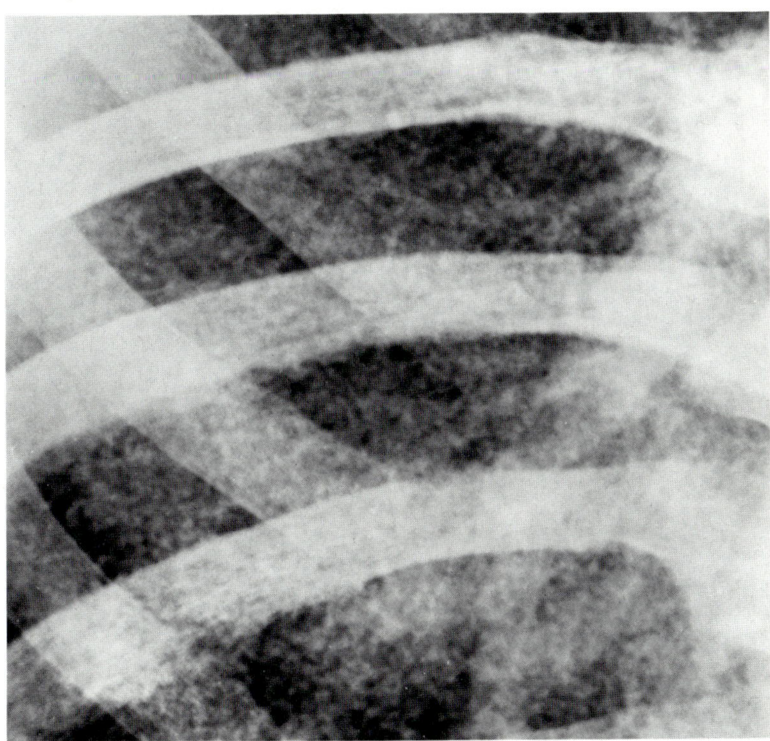

Figure 4.45. Miliary tuberculosis in a man aged 22, who had suffered 4 weeks' fever and malaise

such as a cavity, or the hilar glands may be enlarged. Very few conditions give shadows really like those of miliary tuberculosis. In coal workers there is a mid-zone predominance and the nodular shadows are less even in size and less discrete; in sarcoidosis the nodular shadows tend to be larger and less discrete; in secondary carcinoma deposits they are fewer and larger. The lesions of miliary tuberculosis usually show radiographic clearing after 3 or 4 months of treatment. Resolution is sometimes more protracted, and occasionally the lesions calcify.

In the cryptic form of miliary tuberculosis, in which the patient presents with the non-specific manifestations of pyrexia and anaemia, difficulty in diagnosis may be increased by the fact that the lesions are too small to be seen on the radiograph. The possibility of this important condition should therefore not be discounted by the finding of a normal X-ray. The typical radiographic appearance may be seen in the undiagnosed case on a follow-up film taken after an interval of several weeks.

Sarcoidosis

In pulmonary sarcoidosis the nodular shadows are as a rule larger, less well defined, fewer and less evenly distributed than in miliary tuberculosis, and the symptoms are less marked. Hilar gland enlargement usually precedes the nodular shadowing, may coexist with it for a time (*Figure 4.46*) and generally disappears before the

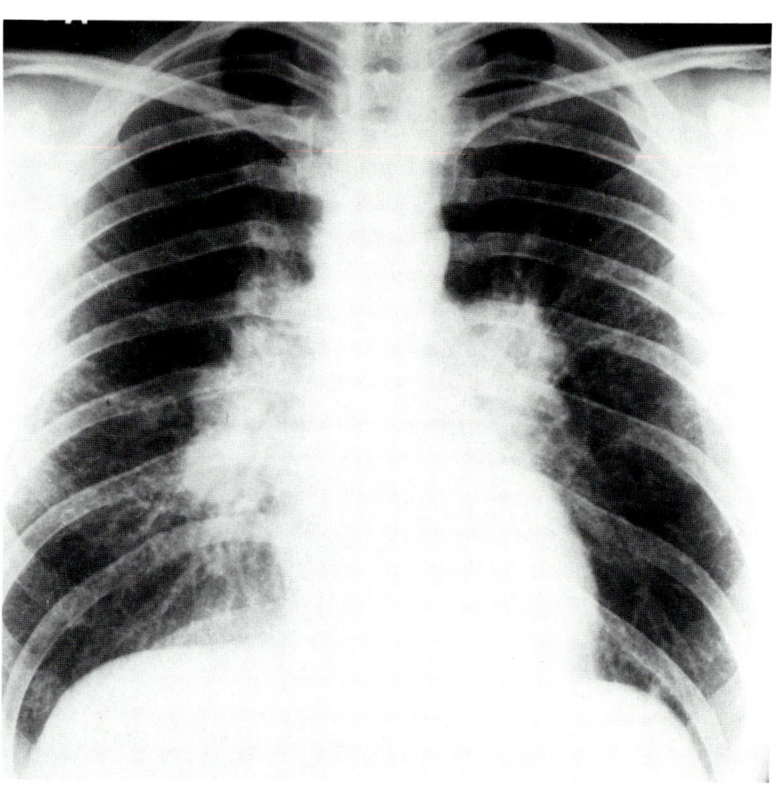

Figure 4.46. Sarcoidosis: hilar gland enlargement and parenchymal infiltrates. Rounded, well-defined shadows produced by enlarged glands at the hila. 2–4 mm diameter nodular infiltrate in middle zones

lung shadowing also resolves. Occasionally, instead of spontaneous resolution taking place the lung shadowing becomes more confluent as extensive pulmonary fibrosis develops. This serious outcome can be averted to a large extent with corticosteroid therapy. Differentiation will need to be made from tuberculosis in a patient presenting with diffuse pulmonary lesions, and from primary tuberculosis or lymphoma where there is hilar adenopathy alone. This may be impossible on clinical grounds, although in general a patient with sarcoidosis will be less constitutionally upset. Confirmation of a negative tuberculin test may be all that is required to infer a diagnosis of sarcoidosis in a young woman presenting with erythema nodosum and bilateral hilar lymphadenopathy. In less clear-cut cases the Kveim test or demonstration of sarcoid granulomas in tissue obtained by lymph node biopsy, transbronchial lung biopsy or biopsy of other organs will establish the diagnosis.

In most patients with sarcoidosis, hilar gland enlargement (with or without accompanying mediastinal gland enlargement) is the sole radiographic finding, and pulmonary parenchymal nodulation does not occur at any stage of the disease. The extent of glandular enlargement tends to be similar on the two sides (*Figure 4.46*), although occasionally one hilum shows much greater enlargement than the other.

Occupational pulmonary diseases

Sometimes a person working in an industry such as coal mining is sent for a radiograph to see if the nature of the work is having any ill effects on the lungs; in other instances abnormal shadows are found in a radiograph and it is only with great difficulty that these can be related to an industrial process. Such was the case in persons living adjacent to a factory using beryllium, and in a woman who merely dusted the clothing of her sister who worked in an asbestos factory.

The common radiological finding is that of small nodular shadows.

Coal wo.

The nodular shadows start predominantly in the mid-zones but may spread to all zones. The size varies from pinpoint to 2 or 3 mm in

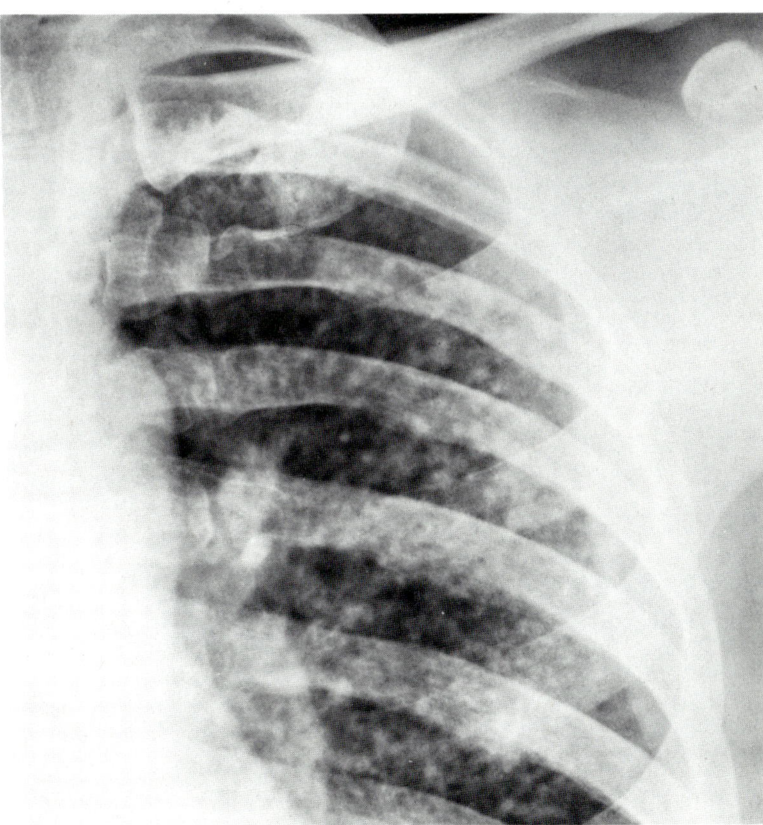

Figure 4.47. Pneumoconiosis. Mottled shadows 1–3 mm in diameter, some dense and sharp, others poorly demarcated. The changes were widespread in both lungs. Man aged 33, a coal miner in South Wales for 15 years, with little disability

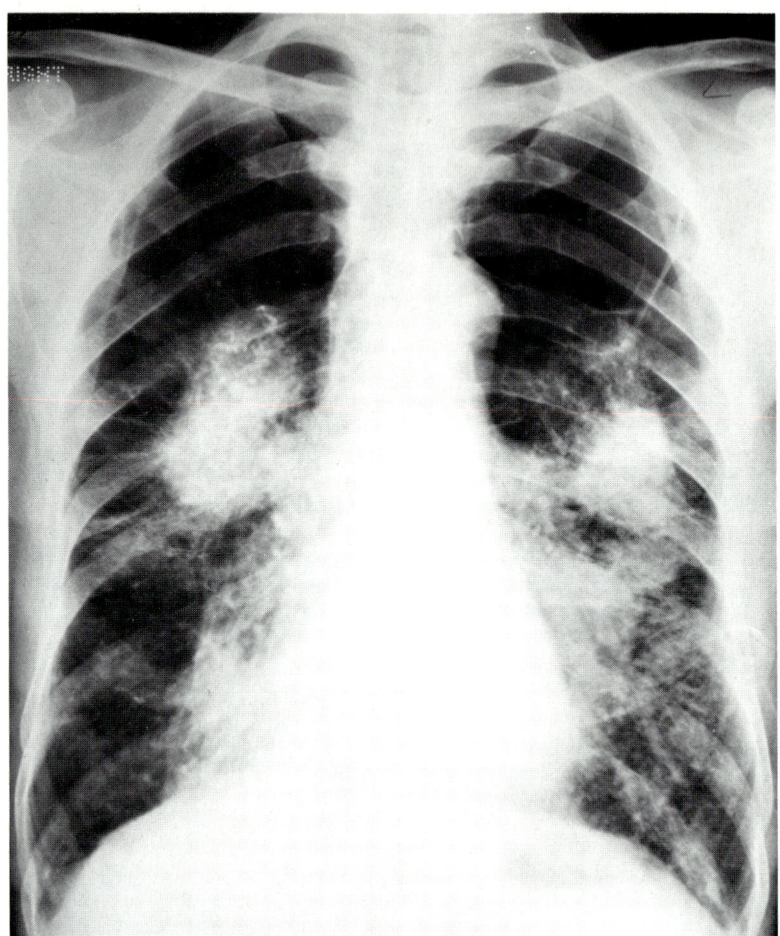

Figure 4.48. Pneumoconiosis with pulmonary massive fibrosis. Gross emphysema of upper lung fields. Massive confluent shadows in mid-zones. Line shadows and nodules. Man aged 47, a coal miner for 23 years. Severe dyspnoea for the past 6 years

diameter, and the outline of the nodules is usually ill-defined (*Figure 4.47*). Short basal horizontal line shadows above the costophrenic recesses are seen in some cases. A few miners progress from this state of simple pneumoconiosis to develop complicated pneumoconiosis, manifest radiologically by the formation in the lungs of large masses which are composed of dense fibrous tissue (pulmonary massive fibrosis). These masses tend to be situated in the upper or middle zones and are often bilateral (*Figure 4.48*). The lungs distal to the masses become grossly emphysematous, and the patients usually suffer from severe dyspnoea.

Silicosis

Not to be confused with the simple nodulation of coal workers is the rather better-defined, coarser, 2.5 mm diameter nodulation occurring among workers who coincidentally mine silica, as in the Rand gold mines and some iron mines, or among those exposed to silica dust, as in some sand blasting. As in coal workers' pneumoconiosis, areas of progressive massive fibrosis with severe disability may develop later.

Iron workers

Haematite miners, and other workers exposed to iron dust such as spot welders, inhale the iron particles which, because of their high atomic weight, give the lungs a snowstorm appearance. Many are without symptoms unless the iron ore is mixed with silica, when they may develop fibrotic lesions from this, leading to dyspnoea. Similar dense shadows may be seen in barium and tin workers.

Asbestos workers

Anyone working with asbestos is at risk, including boiler scalers, pipe laggers, and even demolition workers. The radiological changes may be very insignificant at first and consist of no more than a ground-glass haze with a few nodular shadows in the lower half of the lungs. Later, in addition to the nodules, there may be a fine reticular appearance (*Figure 4.49*). The appearances are the same as those of fibrosing alveolitis due to other causes, and apart from the presence of an excess of asbestos fibres and asbestos bodies the pathology is the same.

In some cases only these lung shadows can be seen, while in others localized, flat lesions are also visible arising from the pleura. These pleural plaques may be of soft-tissue density or calcified (*Figure 4.50*).

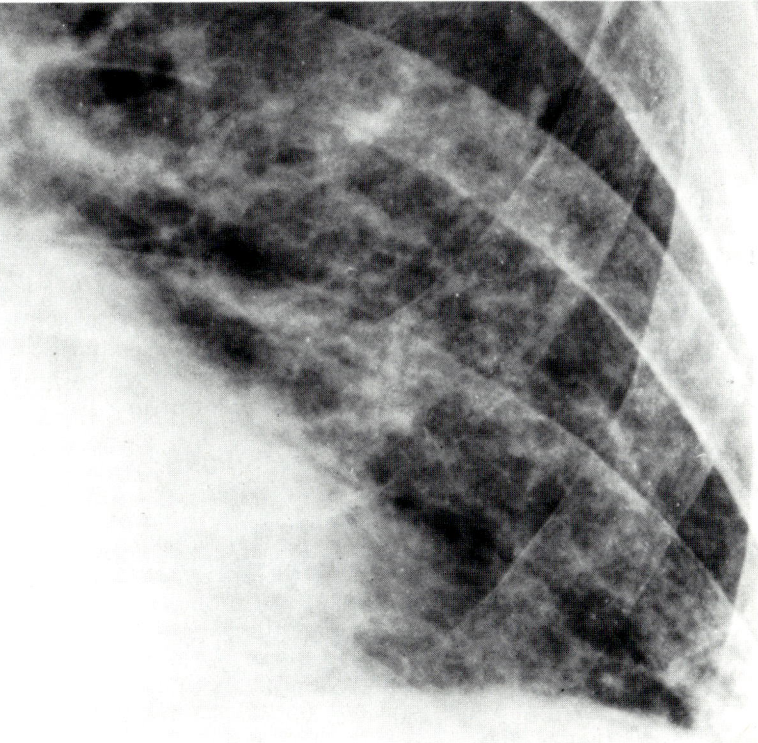

Figure 4.49. Asbestosis in a man aged 69, a former asbestos-factory worker: short line shadows and fine reticular pattern; recent dyspnoea; post-mortem showed asbestos bodies and fine fibrosis

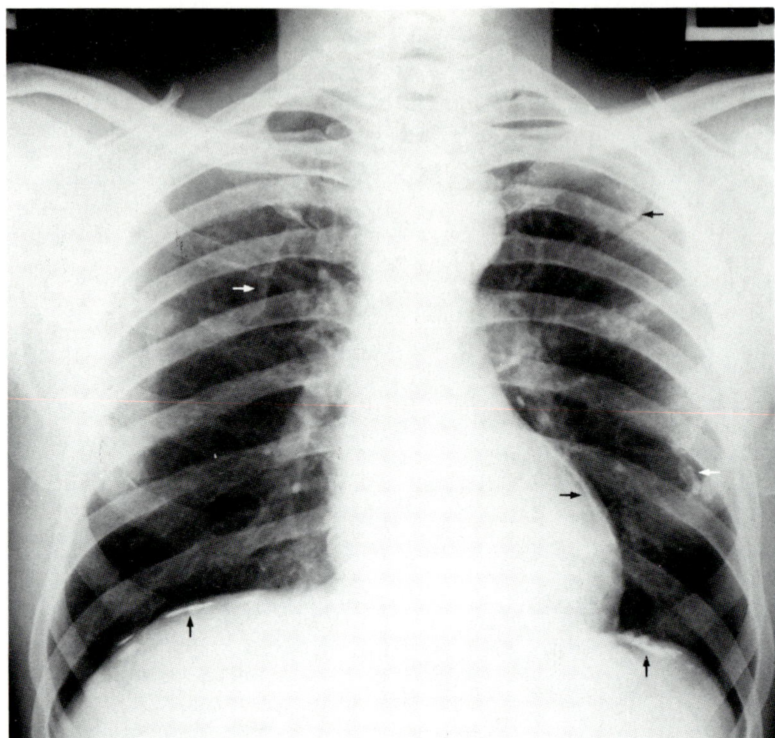

Figure 4.50. Calcified pleural plaques in asbestos worker. Calcified plaques are present in the pleura overlying the diaphragm and mediastinum and beneath the thoracic cage (several arrowed)

The findings of shadows like fibrosing alveolitis together with pleural shadows will strongly suggest this condition, since pleural shadows do not occur in fibrosing alveolitis from other causes. In other patients only pleural shadows can be seen. The pleural changes are typically bilateral, and the plaques arise from the diaphragmatic pleura as well as from the pleura underlying the chest wall. Pleural calcification from a previous haemothorax or tuberculous empyema is unilateral except in rare instances in which both sides of the chest have been involved, and the calcification rarely involves the diaphragmatic pleura in these conditions.

Patients with pleural plaques are usually asymptomatic, while those with lung changes may develop severe dyspnoea and respiratory failure. A few patients exposed to asbestos develop a malignant mesothelioma of the pleura, characterized radiologically by lobulated masses arising from the pleura and a pleural effusion. The incidence of mesothelioma arising from the peritoneum and of bronchial carcinoma is also increased in asbestos workers.

Acute extrinsic allergic alveolitis

The antigens of several inhaled organic dusts set up an allergic response at alveolar level. A common cause is *Thermopolyspora polyspora* found in mouldy hay and causing farmer's lung; another is the proteins in bird droppings, particulary of pigeons and budgerigars, causing bird fancier's lung. Mushroom and malt workers and workers in many other industries can also be affected. Exposure to a large amount of antigens such as in cleaning out a pigeon loft, or a barn with mouldy hay, may lead to acute dyspnoea and fever, and ill-defined nodular shadows may be seen in the lungs. These may take months to resolve, and if contact is continued may cause fibrosing alveolitis.

Haemosiderosis

In about 10 per cent of patients suffering from severe mitral stenosis nodular shadows are seen in the lungs, predominantly in the mid-zones, due to deposits of haemosiderin.

Much rarer is the condition of idiopathic haemosiderosis in children or in young adults, who present with repeated haemoptyses and fine lung nodulation, also due to haemosiderin deposits. The condition appears to be due to an immune reaction on the alveolar wall which becomes damaged, and red cells then leak out from the alveolar capillaries. Histologically the iron particles from the disintegrated red cells are mainly in macrophages in the interalveolar spaces and are in small conglomerations, and the radiographic shadow is a composite one produced by a number of such foci superimposed. The prognosis is variable, and some patients die of associated immune-complex glomerular basement membrane lesions.

Fibrosing alveolitis

This condition when acute is also known as the Hamman–Rich syndrome, and when chronic as diffuse idiopathic interstitial pulmonary fibrosis. It presents with dyspnoea, clubbing and a low gas transfer factor (TCO). It may occur in any age group from young adulthood to old age. In the early stage there are pinpoint nodular shadows and a ground-glass haze; later, larger shadows may be seen, and finally 5 mm ring shadows with walls the thickness of a hair and with transradiant centres giving the lung a honeycomb appearance. The diaphragms are often high due to loss of lung volume. The changes first develop in the lower zones in idiopathic fibrosing alveolitis, but in the more advanced stages the disease may also involve the middle zones. The pulmonary fibrosis that may develop in rheumatoid arthritis or scleroderma or from asbestos exposure has a similar appearance and distribution (*see Figure 4.49*). The fibrosis occurring in bird fancier's lung tends to involve predominantly the upper halves of the lungs. The ring shadows sometimes seen in the lungs in histiocytosis X are often widely distributed and larger in size (1–3 cm diameter).

Secondary malignant deposits

Blood-borne metastases to the lung can cause widely distributed small nodular shadows resembling the appearances of miliary

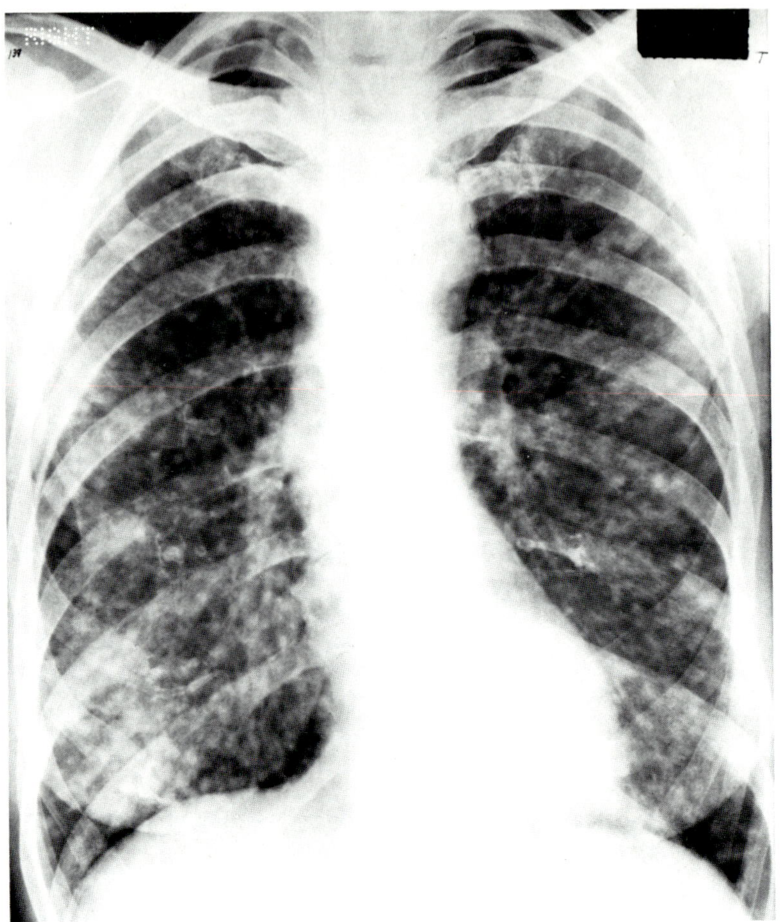

Figure 4.51. Miliary carcinomatosis: shadows 3–5 mm in size, scattered throughout the lungs; secondary deposits from primary carcinoma of the stomach

tuberculosis. Often, however, the nodules of secondary deposits are larger (some measuring 1 cm or so in diameter; *see Figure 4.51*) and less numerous than are typically seen in miliary tuberculosis.

Involvement of the lymphatics of the lung by malignant disease can produce visible lymphatic A lines (1–2.5 cm long lines of the width of a hair situated midway between the hilum and lung periphery, pointing in the direction of the hilum; *see Figure 4.73*) and lymphatic B lines (1–3 cm long lines running horizontally above the costophrenic angles at the extreme periphery of the lung; *see Figure 4.74*). These can be seen either when the lymphatics are invaded by malignant cells or obstructed by malignant tumour in the mediastinum. Similar appearances occur in pulmonary oedema. Enlargement of the heart usually points to the latter condition as the cause, although the pericardium may be invaded by malignant tumour causing a pericardial effusion and hence an enlarged cardiac shadow. Furthermore, pulmonary oedema can be present without cardiac enlargement after an acute myocardial infarction or overhydration with intravenous fluids. Malignant infiltration can usually be distinguished from pulmonary oedema on clinical grounds, but in cases of doubt it is worth repeating the chest X-ray after diuretic therapy, when clearing would indicate a cardiac cause.

Nodular shadowing in the lung may coexist with lymphatic shadowing in disseminated malignant disease.

Miscellaneous

Fine nodular shadowing in the lungs may be seen in pulmonary oedema, histoplasmosis and occasionally in viral pneumonia. 3–5 mm very radio-opaque (dense), well-defined circular shadows are present in the lower half of the lungs in some cases of mitral stenosis and represent small intrapulmonary bone nodules. Calcified pulmonary nodules of similar size are sometimes found 3 years or more after severe chicken-pox with intrapulmonary involvement. Tiny dense opacities can represent residues of contrast media in the lungs after bronchography.

Bronchiectasis and bronchography

Patients with bronchiectasis may present with haemoptysis without other symptoms or signs, or with persistent cough and foul sputum. A history of pneumonia complicating measles or whooping cough or other contagious diseases in childhood, or of tuberculosis, is often present. The incidence of and morbidity from bronchiectasis have declined considerably since the advent of antibiotic treatment.

Repeated haemoptyses are fairly common in this condition since there is often dilatation of the bronchial arterial system, and rupture of one of these vessels, perhaps by inflammatory ulceration, gives rise to copious arterial bleeding.

Most patients with bronchiectasis will have an abnormal chest X-ray, with features suggesting the presence of the condition. Bronchography, however, is required for absolute confirmation of this diagnosis and to establish the extent and distribution of the disease within the lungs.

Chest X-ray appearances

One of the more obvious changes that may be observed on a chest film is atelectasis of a lobe, due to obstruction of the peripheral bronchi. The degree of atelectasis of an affected lobe is highly variable, ranging from slight volume loss to complete collapse. Parallel line shadows representing the walls of a dilated bronchus, lying 5–8 mm apart and separated from each other by an area of transradiancy, may be seen when the bronchus is free of secretions. When much secretion is present a band-like shadow about 8 mm wide, often with a rounded end (gloved finger shadow), may be visible.

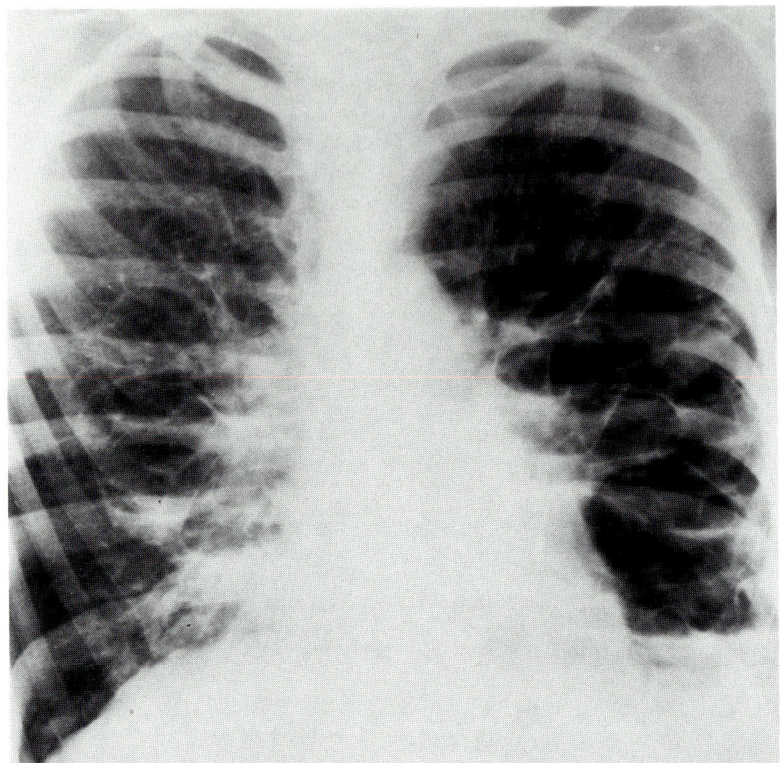

Figure 4.52. Cystic bronchiectasis: multiple ring shadows with walls of hair-line width, representing grossly dilated bronchi, are shown in both lungs; several of the cystic bronchi contain small quantities of fluid

Hairline ring shadows 1–2 cm in diameter will suggest cystic bronchiectasis (*Figure 4.52*). If some secretion is also present a half-moon shadow will be seen in the lower half, the straight upper margin representing the fluid level.

Bronchography

Confirmation of a diagnosis of bronchiectasis and assessment of its extent and anatomical location provide the main indications for bronchography. The technique involves opacifying the airways with oily iodine-containing contrast media. This is achieved by injecting the contrast medium either through a catheter passed transnasally and positioned with its tip lying in the lower trachea, or through a needle or fine catheter passed percutaneously through the cricothyroid membrane into the larynx. The procedure can be performed under local anaesthesia of the upper airways, or after general anaesthesia. The examination carries a small but nevertheless well-recognized risk of reaction to the contrast agent. Serious reactions include bronchospasm, anaphylaxis and even death. For this reason the examination should be undertaken only if it is thought that the information that it would provide would make a positive contribution to the management of the patient. Bronchography should not be performed, for example, to show the extent of the disease in a patient with known bronchiectasis unless surgical resection of affected segments is being considered. The examination is contraindicated in patients with respiratory failure and should be undertaken in asthmatics only if it is thought that the value of the information so obtained would outweigh the above-average risk in these patients.

In a patient with normal lungs the walls of the bronchi are seen to be parallel, and regular branching of the bronchi occurs, the bronchi becoming progressively smaller as the lung periphery is approached (*Figure 4.53*). Normally the alveoli do not fill with the oily contrast

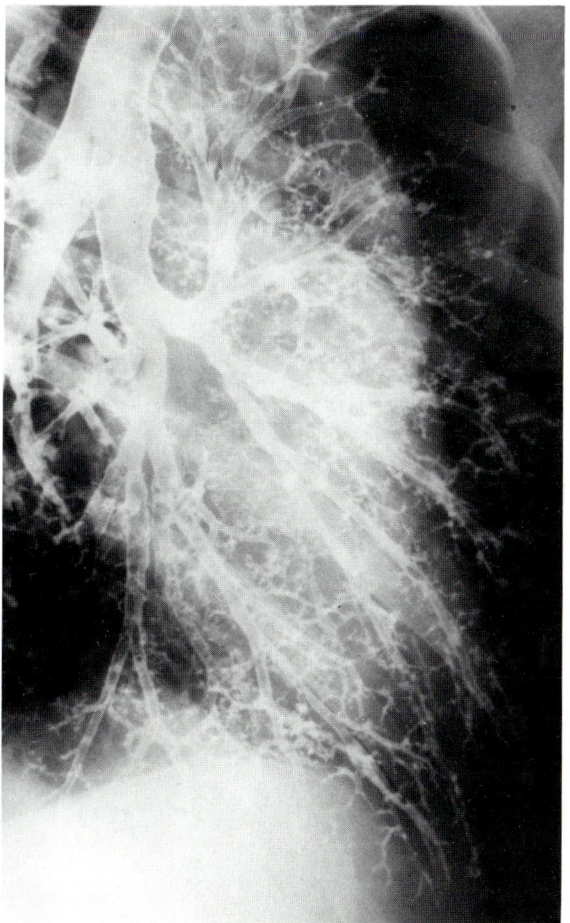

Figure 4.53. Normal bronchogram. Oblique view of left lung. The bronchi show regular branching and progressive reduction of size to the lung periphery

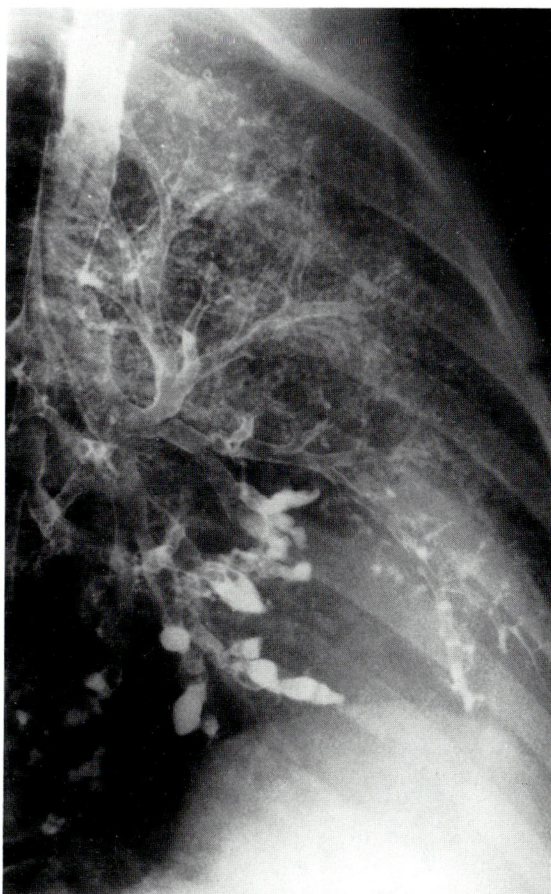

Figure 4.54. Varicose bronchiectasis. Bronchogram; oblique view of left lung. Irregular dilatation of bronchial branches of inferior segment of lingula and basal segments of lower lobe. The bronchi terminate in tapered or squared endings and there is absence of peripheral bronchial filling in affected segments

medium and there is a shallow non-opacified band of lung immediately below the pleura. In bronchiectasis, bronchi of one or more segments of the lung are dilated, and filling of only the proximal four or so bronchial divisions takes place due to the bronchi being occluded distally. The dilated bronchi may have parallel walls so that they are cylindrical in appearance, or the walls may show local areas of concentric widening interspersed with constrictions so that the appearance resembles that of varicose veins (varicose bronchiectasis, *Figure 4.54*), or the contrast may outline 1–2 cm diameter balloon-like expansions of the bronchi (cystic bronchiectasis). Two or all three of these morphological types of bronchiectasis may be present in the same patient, and the type bears little relationship to the severity of symptoms or prognosis.

It is important to remember that reversible bronchial dilatation occurs in pneumonia. If there is a possibility of bronchiectasis predisposing to an episode of pneumonia a bronchogram should be deferred for 3 or 4 months after the acute episode to avoid confusion in interpreting any bronchial dilatation that may be present.

Bronchography used to be used extensively in the investigation of pulmonary shadows of unestablished nature and in patients with undiagnosed haemoptysis or cough. Nowadays the greater availability of sputum cytology examination and of techniques of bronchial washing, fibreoptic bronchoscopy combined with transbronchial biopsy, and percutaneous needle aspiration biopsy of peripheral lesions have led to a very substantial diminution in the role of bronchography. It is clearly infinitely preferable to view a bronchial abnormality directly through a bronchoscope and to obtain material for histological or cytological examination, resulting in a definitive diagnosis, than simply to outline the surface of a lesion where this projects into or obstructs a bronchus. Establishing a diagnosis of bronchiectasis or showing the extent of the disease provide virtually the sole indications for bronchography at the present time. It is tempting to use the technique to investigate a patient with haemoptysis or with malignant cells in the sputum who has a normal chest X-ray and normal bronchoscopy findings. The yield from bronchography in these situations in the absence of any localizing features (e.g. visible bleeding from one of the bronchi on bronchoscopy) is, however, negligible.

Asthma, chronic bronchitis and emphysema

Asthma

Bronchial asthma is a condition characterized by recurrent generalized airways obstruction which is reversible, either naturally or after the administration of certain drugs (e.g. adrenalin or corticosteroids). The reversibility may be obvious clinically, or detected only by observing an improvement in the forced expiratory volume in one second, or in the peak flow rate. The most important clinical manifestations are periodic attacks of wheezing and dyspnoea. In some patients external allergens such as those of pollen, the house-dust mite or animal dander can be incriminated in provoking the attack (extrinsic asthma) while in others no such cause can be found (intrinsic asthma).

Radiology plays little part in the diagnosis of this condition which is usually obvious clinically. The chest X-ray is normal in most patients with asthma, even during an attack. This is particularly the case in patients with late-onset asthma who develop symptoms for the first time after the age of 30. In these patients the chest X-ray is almost invariably normal, however severe the attack. In 20–30 per cent of children with the condition minor chest X-ray abnormalities can be seen. These rarely occur during a mild attack of short duration but may be present during a severe protracted episode when the diagnosis is clinically obvious. The changes that may occur are evidence of overinflation of the lungs, manifest by unduly low, flattened diaphragms; 'tramline' and ring shadows representing the thickened walls of bronchi; and some hilar enlargement representing proximal pulmonary arterial enlargement from reversible pulmonary artery hypertension. The vessel markings of the lungs themselves are normal in size and distribution in asthma (cf. emphysema).

The main value of the chest X-ray in asthma is to exclude other conditions presenting with wheeze and dyspnoea, such as a centrally situated bronchial neoplasm in an adult patient. The chest X-ray is also of use in excluding complications of asthma such as a pneumothorax.

In a small proportion of patients with asthma a sensitivity reaction may arise to *Aspergillus fumigatus*. This is characterized by mucus plugging of segmental bronchi, the plugs containing aspergillus and numerous eosinophils. The plugs are sometimes seen as band-like or V- or Y-shaped shadows of homogeneous density lying within the dilated branching bronchi. Alternatively, areas of patchy consolidation or atelectasis, commonly in the upper halves of the lungs, may be present. These are usually transitory but recurrent, and repeated episodes may result in bronchiectasis. The condition is suspected from the above radiographic appearances occurring in an asthmatic, and confirmed by demonstrating aspergillus and eosinophils in the sputum, the presence of blood eosinophilia, and an immediate positive skin reaction to the injected antigen. In addition, serum precipitens for *Aspergillus fumigatus* are present in over 50 per cent of cases.

Chronic bronchitis

In uncomplicated chronic bronchitis the plain radiograph is usually normal. This is not surprising because the proximal bronchi are not appreciably thickened macroscopically, only the gland layer being hypertrophied, and there is little evidence of past or present inflammatory changes. In most patients with chronic bronchitis there is no radiological evidence of overinflation of the lungs despite physiological evidence of airways obstruction and air trapping. The diaphragm is at a normal level and is curved.

cases showing radiographic change. These are usually seen just above one or both of the diaphragms. They have been attributed to several possible pathological processes, including areas of localized atelectasis, lung fibrosis, locally indrawn pleura, and thrombosed vessels surrounded by oedema. Horizontal line shadows above the diaphragm are non-specific features of pulmonary thromboembolism, being commonly seen in patients hypoventilating due to severe pain after abdominal surgery or myocardial infarction, and in patients with retained bronchial secretions producing basal atelectasis.

3. Pleural effusion. This is a common non-specific manifestation of pulmonary embolism.
4. Transradiancy of a lobe or lung. This is produced by cessation of perfusion and therefore reduction of size of the peripheral pulmonary vessels after occlusion of a lobar or main pulmonary artery. This change may be seen in a patient developing severe dyspnoea of acute onset several days after abdominal surgery or major trauma.
5. Enlargement of a proximal pulmonary artery. This is produced by mechanical stuffing of a pulmonary artery by thrombus, and this change is most readily appreciated when earlier films of the patient are available for comparison.
6. Changes of cor pulmonale with enlargement of both hila due to pulmonary artery hypertension.

In summary, the disadvantages of the chest radiograph in the diagnosis of pulmonary thromboembolism are that many pulmonary emboli produce no radiographic change, and when changes do occur these are non-specific and usually do not develop for 24 hours or more after the acute episode.

Isotope lung scanning

The perfusion lung scan is the most commonly performed investigation in pulmonary thromboembolism. The radiopharmaceutical is prepared by binding a radioactive substance, usually technetium-99m, to particles—commonly albumin aggregates—of 15–35 μm diameter. This is injected intravenously, and after passage through the right side of the heart enters the pulmonary vessels. The lung capillaries trap particles larger than 7–8 μm diameter, so that these injected particles produce in effect multiple tiny pulmonary emboli. If the pulmonary vascularity is normal gamma-camera images of the lungs show even distribution of the particles throughout both lungs. If one or more of the pulmonary arteries is obstructed by clot the lung scan shows defects corresponding with the regions that are not being perfused (*Figure 4.58*). Typically, these defects are multiple and some are roughly hemispherical, with their bases lying on the pleura and with convex, smooth, inner margins facing the hila. These must correspond with areas of chest X-ray normality, since consolidation in the lung, bullae, etc., will be associated with areas of defective perfusion.

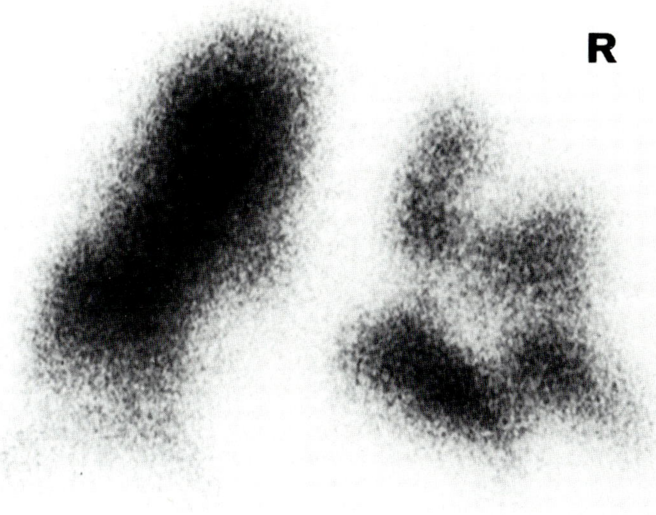

Figure 4.58. Multiple pulmonary emboli. (Perfusion lung scan: posterior projection; gamma-camera recording.) Large perfusion defects ('white' areas representing deficient perfusion distribution) in right lung

Perfusion defects, however, can occur in patients with asthma, chronic bronchitis or emphysema without radiographic abnormality. It is important, therefore, to establish whether the patient has clinical or simple laboratory evidence of airways obstruction at the time of the examination. If this is present a ventilation scan, involving the inhalation of radioactive gas, may be carried out to establish whether the perfusion abnormalities correspond with areas of ventilation abnormality (obstructive airways disease) or are unassociated with any significant ventilation abnormality (pulmonary thromboembolism).

The advantages of the perfusion lung scan are that it is abnormal immediately after the clinical episode of embolism, is simple and safe and involves no discomfort to the patient, and is highly sensitive. A negative perfusion lung scan will exclude the possibility of pulmonary thromboembolism demonstrable by any other means.

Pulmonary angiography

The technique has been mentioned on page 187. The radiographic findings are entirely specific and diagnostic when the contrast outlines the characteristic filling defects of clot within an artery (*Figure 4.59*), or when abrupt cut-off of a vessel is seen, indicating occlusion. The disadvantages are that the investigation is highly specialized, and—as with all angiographic procedures—associated with a certain morbidity. Cardiac arrhythmias commonly occur as the catheter is advanced through the right ventricle, and ECG monitoring is required. The specific changes of pulmonary embolism will be overlooked in small vessels.

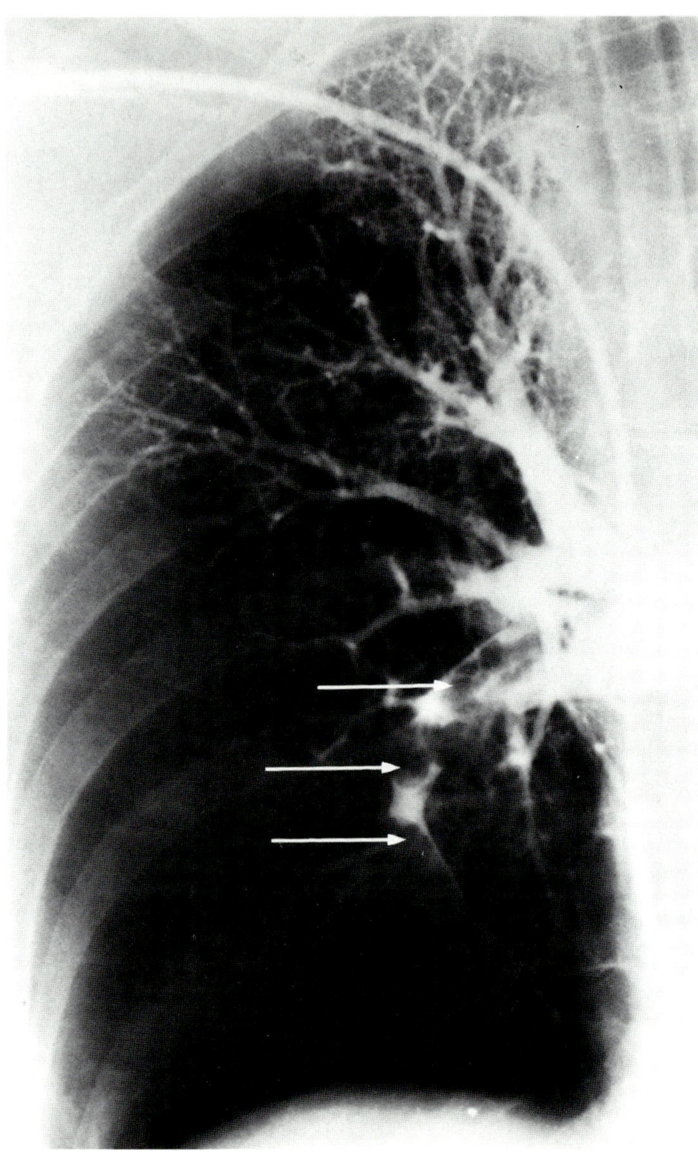

Figure 4.59. Pulmonary thromboembolism; pulmonary arteriogram: absent perfusion of lower lobe of right lung due to thrombus producing large filling defects (arrowed) within the lower lobe artery; normal perfusion of upper lobe

Comparison of scanning and angiography in pulmonary embolism

As mentioned, a technically satisfactory negative perfusion lung scan excludes the possibility of pulmonary thromboembolism demonstrable by angiography or other means. A positive perfusion scan may be produced by causes other than pulmonary thromboembolism, most commonly obstructive airways disease. The incidence of false-positive scans is not exactly established. Patients with positive scans which are not clearly due to thromboembolism can if necessary be investigated further with ventilation scans or pulmonary angiography.

Pulmonary angiography is less sensitive than perfusion lung scanning but can show unequivocal changes of clot within the large and medium-sized pulmonary arteries. Pulmonary angiography, however, is a complex procedure with a recognized morbidity. While the frequency of use of angiography in the diagnosis of pulmonary thromboembolism varies considerably from centre to centre, one absolute indication is to demonstrate the position and extent of clot within the pulmonary vasculature in patients who are being considered for emergency thrombectomy.

Intrathoracic neoplasms

Carcinoma of the lung

Indications for radiology

Whenever a bronchial carcinoma is suspected a full X-ray examination of the chest should be carried out. The clinical evidence of this

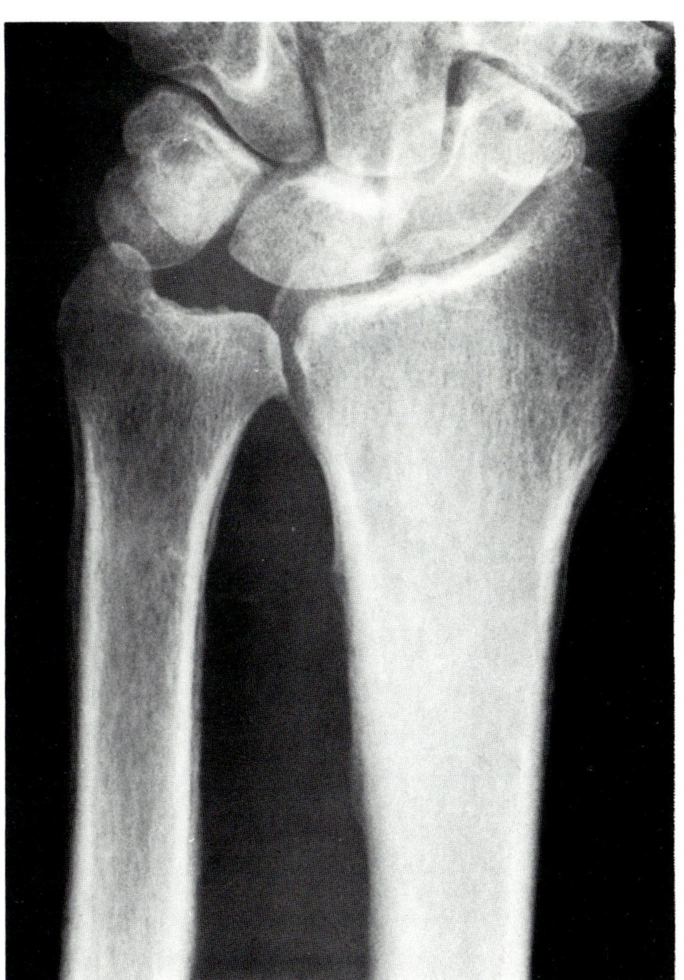

Figure 4.60. Hypertrophic pulmonary osteoarthropathy: periosteal reaction on distal radial and ulnar shafts; similar changes were present in opposite wrist and on both distal tibiae and fibulae; bronchial carcinoma

Sometimes both lung fields are riddled with small deposits, when the condition is termed miliary carcinomatosis (*see Figure 4.51*). These appearances and the appearances of lymphatic carcinomatosis have been described on pages 221–222.

Usually the correlation of X-ray appearances and clinical findings leaves no doubt as to the diagnosis, but while the deposits are still very small they may be invisible or be mistaken for old inflammatory lesions. A further radiograph in one or two months' time will show an increase in size which may confirm the diagnosis.

Malignant deposits in the mediastinal glands may produce lobulated widening of the mediastinal shadow and may be radiologically indistinguishable from non-neoplastic causes of glandular enlargement.

Secondary deposits may occur in the ribs, when their presence will be indicated by areas of erosion or, in the case of sclerotic deposits from prostatic and certain other tumours (*see* page 87), by areas of increased density.

Elevation of the right diaphragm may be evidence of deposits in the liver if no other cause is found, but such a radiological finding is insufficient in itself to be of value.

Mediastinal masses

Mediastinal masses are often asymptomatic, but when due to malignant disease may produce constitutional upset, respiratory difficulties from tracheal compression or invasion, or swelling of the face from superior vena caval obstruction.

Mediastinal lesions may widen the mediastinal shadow on both sides (*Figure 4.67*) or may be confined to one side only. When both sides are involved, as in *Figure 4.67*, there can be no doubt as to the mediastinal origin of the abnormality, but in unilateral lesions it is sometimes impossible to establish from the chest film whether a mass is situated in the mediastinum or medially within the lung (and in fact a medially situated bronchial carcinoma may invade the mediastinum by direct spread to involve both lung and mediastinum). Compared with pulmonary tumours, however, mediastinal masses typically have very smooth margins abutting on lung, since irregularities of their surfaces are 'ironed out' by the overlying layers of parietal and visceral pleura (*Figure 4.69*). Furthermore, it may be obvious from the visible portion of a rounded shadow that the bulk of the mass is too medially situated to lie in lung.

The diagnostic possibilities of a mediastinal mass depend on whether the mass is situated anteriorly, centrally or posteriorly within the mediastinum, different groups of conditions characteristically occupying these different sites. As a general rule, therefore, a lateral film is required for full assessment of a mediastinal mass. Only very occasionally is a mediastinal opacity sufficiently well characterized on a PA film to obviate the need for a lateral radiograph.

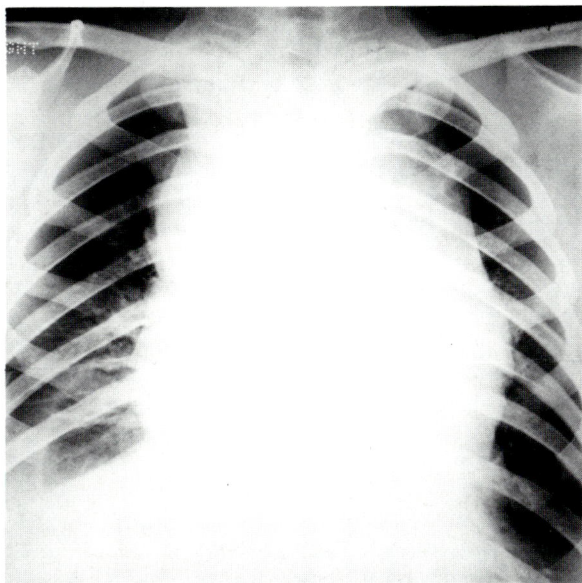

Figure 4.67. Anterior mediastinal lymphoma: massive, lobulated, well-defined tumour involving both sides of mediastinum

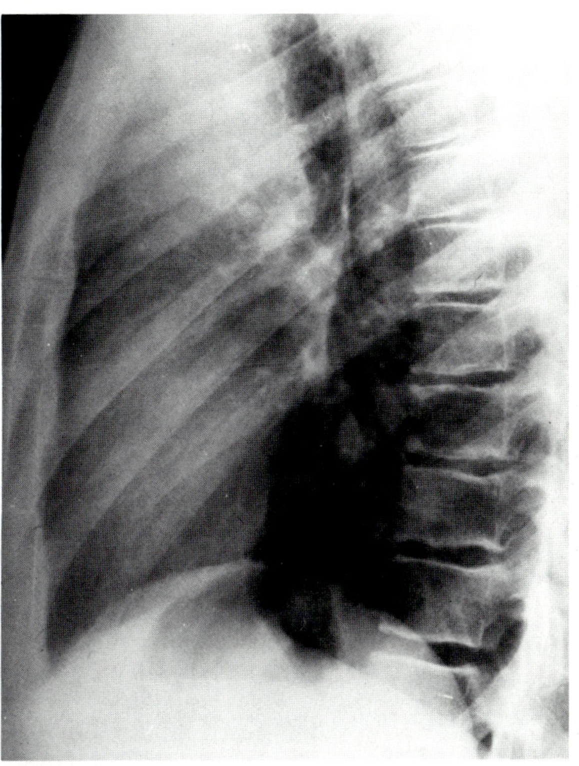

Figure 4.68. Lymphoma (lateral view). The PA view was similar to *Figure 4.67*. There is loss of the normal retrosternal transradiancy above the heart, which indicates that the tumour is situated anteriorly

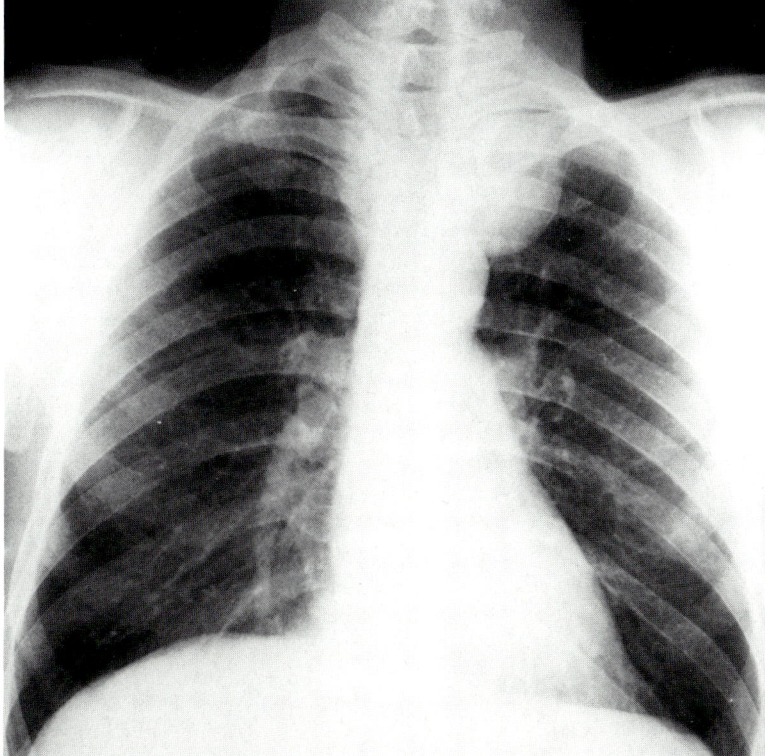

Figure 4.69. Posterior mediastinal neurofibroma. Homogeneous opacity with completely smooth, rounded lateral margin abutting on lung and blending medially with the mediastinal shadow. The posterior position was confirmed on the lateral view

Anterior mediastinal shadows

These refer to masses situated behind the sternum and in front of the heart and great vessels arising from the heart. Enlarged glands in any part of the mediastinum typically produce a lobulated border to the widened mediastinum, and gross bilateral lobulated mediastinal widening involving the anterior or anterior and middle mediastinal compartments is commonly seen in thoracic lymphomas (*see Figure 4.67*). The retrosternal position is confirmed on the lateral view by loss of the normal retrosternal transradiancy (cf. *Figure 4.68* with *Figure 4.6*). With a large retrosternal mass this region will appear relatively white in comparison with the blacker retrocardiac area. Tuberculosis and metastases also cause enlargement of anterior mediastinal glands, although generally to a lesser degree than may be found in lymphoma.

Retrosternal goitres may widen the upper mediastinum anteriorly, although 20 per cent descend into the thorax between the trachea and oesophagus. Commonly these are calcified and produce tracheal displacement. An associated goitre in the neck may be palpable.

Thymic and dermoid tumours and cysts are usually situated adjacent to the upper border of the heart. These may be of homogeneous soft-tissue density or may contain calcium. Calcification is also commonly seen in the walls of aortic aneurysms. A diagnosis of a thymic tumour will be suggested in a patient suffering from myaesthenia gravis with an anterior mediastinal mass.

Pericardial fat pads produce low-density triangular shadows at the cardiophrenic angles, and pleuropericardial cysts give rise to rounded opacities of soft-tissue density at these sites and, less commonly, at other sites adjacent to the pericardium.

Middle mediastinal shadows

The lateral view may show that the retrosternal transradiancy is clear and that the shadow shown on the anterior view lies at the level of the trachea. Middle mediastinal opacities are most commonly due to paratracheal gland enlargement (*see Figure 4.64*), which may be unilateral or bilateral. Involvement of several glands produces a lobulated border to the mediastinum, as already described. When glands are suspected, it is important to ascertain whether the hilar glands are also enlarged and whether the lungs show abnormality. Although very considerable overlap of disease patterns occurs, and dogmatic rules cannot be applied, the following are useful working principles:

1. Unilateral paratracheal or hilar gland enlargement is likely to be due to disease in the corresponding lung—e.g. primary tuberculosis in a child or young adult (*see Figure 4.38*), or bronchial carcinoma in a middle-aged or elderly patient (*see Figure 4.64*).
2. Bilateral hilar gland enlargement without enlargement of mediastinal glands is likely to be due to sarcoidosis, particularly if the patient is well (*see Figure 4.46*).

3. Bilateral paratracheal and anterior mediastinal gland enlargement without hilar gland enlargement is likely to be due to lymphoma (*see Figures 4.67* and *4.68*).
4. Both sarcoidosis and lymphoma can produce bilateral hilar and paratracheal gland enlargement, with or without associated lung infiltrates. Differentiating features are that a patient with sarcoidosis with these manifestations usually has fairly mild constitutional upset, whereas a patient with lymphoma is ill: and sarcoidosis very rarely involves anterior mediastinal lymph glands, which are commonly enlarged in lymphoma.

Other causes of middle mediastinal masses are bronchogenic cysts and aneurysms of the arch of the aorta. These produce localized, well-defined mediastinal swellings.

Posterior mediastinal shadows

These represent shadows lying behind the heart and great vessels arising from and entering the heart. The commonest tumours producing localized swellings in this region are those derived from neural tissue (*Figure 4.69*). These may be associated with vertebral or rib anomalies, e.g. separation or erosion of the ribs by an interposed tumour.

Aneurysms of the descending aorta (*see Figures 4.82 and 4.83*) and lesions of the oesophagus, e.g. achalasia (*see Figures 4.90 and 4.91*) produce widening of the mediastinum posteriorly. Aortography provides definitive evaluation of aortic lesions in the thorax.

The heart and aorta

Posteroanterior and lateral chest radiographs should be taken whenever a cardiac condition is diagnosed or suspected. From this the size, shape and position of the heart can be seen, as can the aorta and the proximal and peripheral pulmonary vessels. This information may be of value either at the time or for comparison with other radiographs at a later date. Oblique views are contributory in special situations but are rarely performed routinely. Only an anteroposterior view may be feasible in patients presenting with acute cardiac disease such as myocardial infarction.

Heart size, shape and position

Heart size

The maximum transverse diameter of the heart, representing the horizontal distance between the extreme edges of the heart borders, is a useful measurement. Gross enlargement is usually obvious, and any heart with a transverse diameter exceeding 15.5 cm on a PA film is probably diseased unless the person is very tall, heavy and in an occupation involving much physical effort. It is often stated that the transverse diameter of the heart should not exceed half the maximum internal transverse diameter of the thorax, and the two measurements are usually expressed as a ratio (the cardiothoracic ratio). Use of this ratio is of less value than an absolute measurement of cardiac diameter, since in many normal individuals diameters of, for example, 14 cm and 23 cm are found, giving a ratio of 60 per cent.

The only reliable way of detecting early cardiac enlargement is by comparison with a pre-existing radiograph. Certain conditions must be fulfilled. The radiographs that are being compared must be PA views, taken with the patient upright, in deep inspiration, at a tube-to-film distance of 2 m (6 ft). An AP view at 1.2 m (4 ft) on partial expiration may show a transverse diameter 3 cm larger than one taken immediately afterwards in the standard manner.

Finally, it has been shown that in normal persons radiographed from time to time the average difference in the cardiac transverse diameter at different dates is 0.5 cm, but can vary by 1.0 to 1.5 cm. In only 2 per cent of healthy individuals is the difference 2 cm or more, so that in the presence of cardiac disease any enlargement greater than 1.5 cm is usually significant. The systole–diastole difference is usually less than 0.5 cm; but if the patient strains to hold the breath in this may raise the intrathoracic pressure, restrict the systemic venous return and produce a temporary reduction in heart size.

The shadow of a pericardial effusion may be indistinguishable from that of an enlarged heart on the plain radiograph, and the two may coexist.

The more common causes of enlargement of the heart shadow are:
1. Ischaemic heart disease.
2. Systemic hypertension.
3. Rheumatic heart disease.
4. Left-to-right shunts and other congenital heart disorders.
5. Pulmonary arterial hypertension.
6. The cardiomyopathies.
7. Pericardial effusion.

These conditions are discussed in the following sections.

Cardiac shape (*see Figures 4.2 and 4.6*)

On the PA film the right atrium forms the normal, slightly convex right heart border. Above this and the hilar shadow the right mediastinal border is often vertical, formed by the lateral wall of the superior vena cava. In older people the unfolded aorta may give a convex margin to the mediastinum on the right side at the level of and just above and below the hilum. This can usually be seen to be continuous with the shadow of the aortic arch.

On the left side the aortic knuckle produces a shadow just below the sternal end of the clavicle, and the left wall of the descending aorta is seen running downwards in continuity with this, almost vertically in young adults and often showing considerable unfolding and tortuosity in the elderly. The main pulmonary artery causes a slight convexity below the aortic knuckle at the level of the left hilum. The wall of the left ventricle forms the left heart border. The left atrial appendage may contribute to the upper part of the left cardiac border but this produces a separate convex shadow only when the atrium is enlarged.

The right ventricle lies immediately behind the sternum and lower left costal cartilages and forms the anterior border of the heart shadow seen on the lateral film. The upper two-thirds of the posterior border of the heart is formed by the left atrium, which lies immediately in front of the oesophagus. The lower third is repre-sented by the left ventricle.

Position of the heart

Normally between two-thirds and three-quarters of the diameter of the heart lies to the left of the midline. Alteration in the position of the heart is most commonly produced by disease of the lung or pleura: the heart is displaced to the side of a collapsed lobe or lung and away from a large pleural effusion (*see Figures 4.5 and 4.3, respectively*). The heart is often considerably displaced to the left in patients with pectus excavatum. A mirror image of the normal heart shadow will be seen in a patient with dextrocardia, the left ventricle forming the right heart border. There may be associated mirror transposition of the abdominal organs in this condition, in which case the air bubble of the gastric fundus will be visible beneath the right diaphragm and the homogeneous shadow of the liver beneath the left.

Cardiac chamber enlargement

Hypertrophy of a cardiac chamber does not produce detectable abnormality of the cardiac silhouette: recognition of chamber enlargement requires the chamber to be dilated. The left atrium is unique in producing specific radiographic features indicating dilatation. While there are signs ascribed to enlargement of the other chambers, these are less reliable and should be interpreted in the clinical context in each case.

Left atrial enlargement

The features of enlargement, as commonly seen in mitral regurgitation, are:

1. The presence of a double shadow to the right heart border, the left atrium producing a second convex shadow that does not extend down as far as the diaphragm (*Figure 4.70*). This can

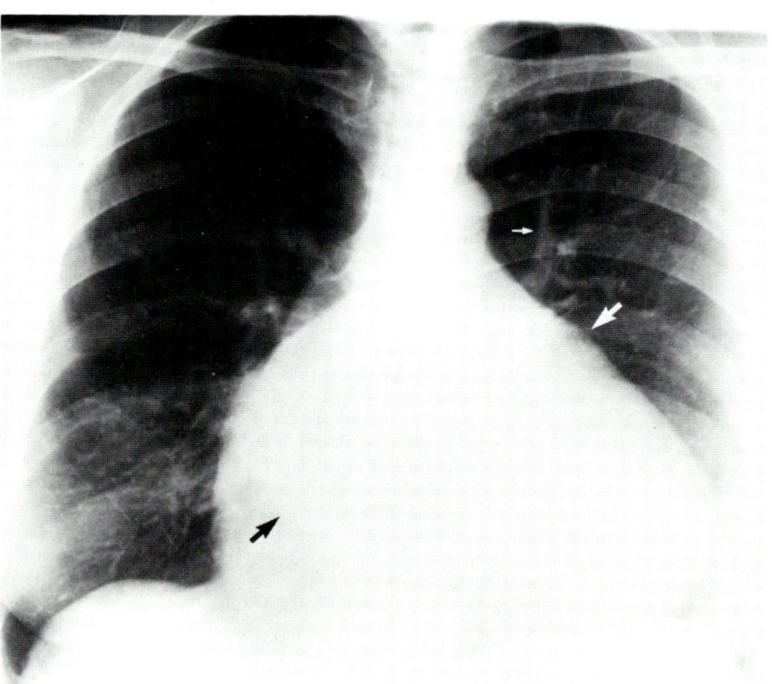

Figure 4.70. Mitral valve disease (mixed stenosis and incompetence). PA film showing enlarged heart, edge of enlarged left atrium (black arrow), enlarged left atrial appendage (large white arrow), and enlarged upper lobe vein (small white arrow)

usually be distinguished from the shadow of an unfolded ascending aorta, as the latter can be traced upwards to show its continuity with the shadow of the aortic knuckle.

2. The left atrial appendage produces a convex bulge on the left heart border just below the hilum (*Figure 4.70*).

3. The left main bronchus is elevated and the angle between the right and left main bronchi increased.

4. The barium-filled oesophagus is pushed backwards by the enlarged atrium lying immediately in front of it. The oesophagus may also be displaced to the right, or occasionally to the left.

Enlargement of other chambers

Enlargement of the right atrium may produce a larger than normal extension of the heart shadow to the right of the midline and an almost horizontal upper right heart border, but these signs require cautious interpretation. Enlargement of the right ventricle produces anticlockwise rotation of the heart about its vertical axis, so that the apex may lie several centimetres above the diaphragm. Conversely, the heart rotates in a clockwise direction about its vertical axis with left ventricular enlargement, so that the apex may descend below the level of the upper margin of the diaphragm.

It is worth re-emphasizing that while these features may be present, they are neither specific nor highly reliable. As will be seen in the following sections, plain film signs of changes in the pulmonary circulation often provide far more valuable evidence of abnormal cardiac flow or pressures than do changes in the heart shape. Furthermore, electrocardiography and echocardiography provide far more accurate assessment of hypertrophy or dilatation of the left and right ventricles than can be obtained from plain films.

Other investigative techniques

Fluoroscopy

Fluoroscopy is useful in the investigation of abnormal cardiac contraction and in the detection and localization of cardiac calcification. A patient with protracted cardiac failure after a myocardial infarction may be found on fluoroscopy to have no contraction of an area of the left ventricle, or to have a ventricular aneurysm. In this latter situation the diseased portion of the ventricular wall expands during ventricular systole (paradoxical pulsation) while the healthy part contracts normally.

It may not be possible to establish from plain films whether an area of calcification represents calcification in one of the valves of the heart or calcification in the lumen (in thrombus), in the wall of a cardiac chamber, or in the pericardium or coronary arteries. This can often be resolved by fluoroscopy. One particular difficulty is in distinguishing on plain films between aortic valve and mitral valve calcification. On fluoroscopy the up-and-down movement of the aortic valve can be differentiated readily from the characteristic side-to-side elliptical movement of the mitral valve.

Angiocardiography

A catheter can be positioned with its tip in any of the cardiac chambers for the injection of contrast medium. The right side of the heart and the pulmonary artery are catheterized from an arm vein or the femoral vein, and the left cardiac chambers from the femoral, brachial or axillary artery. Alternatively, a catheter can be passed across the interatrial septum at the level of the foramen ovale to enter the left atrium from the right atrium (Brockenborough technique). Correct positioning of the catheter tip is established by fluoroscopy.

Angiocardiography provides detailed information of cardiac anatomy and function. The technique is indispensable in investigating the anatomy of complex congenital heart disease. It is also of the utmost value in the accurate determination of the severity of acquired valve disease, such as the relative contributions of stenosis and incompetence in a patient with disease of the mitral valve. Cineangiography of the left ventricle shows the anatomical site of an area of absent contraction or paradoxical movement of the wall, and also furnishes information about the function of the ventricle. This function is commonly expressed in terms of the ejection fraction, which is the proportion of the ventricular content ejected in systole. This can be assessed reasonably accurately by direct inspection of the cine-recording of the opacified chamber. Angiocardiography is conveniently carried out at the same examination as cardiac catheterization performed for the measurement of chamber pressures and blood oxygen concentrations.

Coronary arteriography provides the only means of determining the exact site and extent of disease of the coronary arteries and is essential in patients who are being considered for coronary artery surgery. The procedure is combined with left ventriculography so that the extent of associated impairment of left ventricular function can be assessed.

Echocardiography

Echocardiography (ultrasound examination of the heart) has acquired an important role as a non-invasive means of investigating cardiac disorders. Echocardiography is complementary to the clinical examination and other results of investigation, and the findings require to be considered in the context of the full clinical picture.

The transducer is held directly over the right ventricle of the heart in an intercostal space to the left of the lower sternum. The direction of the ultrasound beam for examination of the mitral valve is shown in *Figure 4.71*. With only minor movements of the probe echoes can be obtained from the anterior and posterior mitral valve cusps, from the walls of the ventricles and left atrium, and from the anterior and posterior walls of the root of the aorta. The echoes are usually viewed as a time–position display on the cathode ray oscilloscope, and permanent recordings can be made as shown in *Figure 4.72*.

Alternatively, real-time echocardiography can be performed.

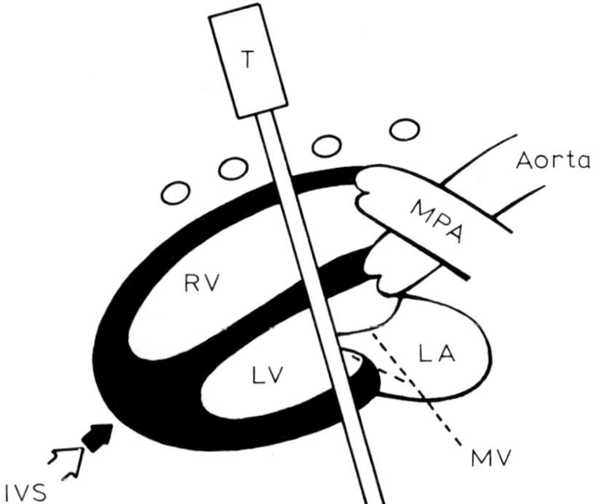

Figure 4.71. Echocardiography. Diagram of longitudinal section of heart to show path of ultrasound beam (two parallel lines) for scan of mitral valve cusps illustrated in *Figure 4.72*. IVS, interventricular septum; LA, left atrium; LV, left ventricle; MPA, main pulmonary artery; MV, mitral valve; RV, right ventricle; T, transducer on anterior chest wall

This provides a two-dimensional image of the heart and is similar in principle to real-time scanning of other regions of the body (*see* page 11). Information can be obtained from the display about the movements of the mitral valve cusps, and sometimes vegetations can be seen on the cusps themselves. A left atrial myxoma can be diagnosed and its size determined by this technique. Since echoes are returned from the walls of the ventricles, including the interventricular septum, thickening of the walls of one or both ventricles due to hypertrophy or dilatation of the ventricular chambers can be demonstrated. As has already been mentioned, chest X-ray evidence of ventricular enlargement is imprecise, and ultrasound provides an accurate, alternative, non-invasive method of assessment. Since the ultrasound beam can be directed at the aortic root, the distance between the echoes from the anterior and posterior

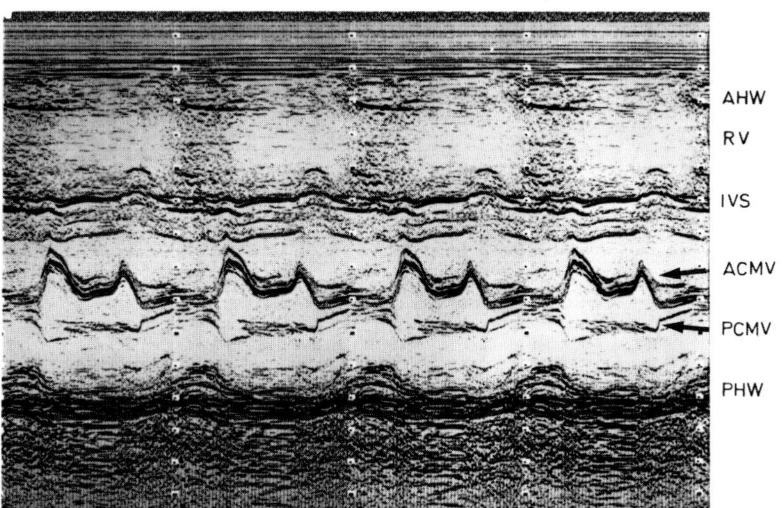

Figure 4.72. Mitral valve echocardiogram, with transducer in position shown in *Figure 4.71*. Slightly thickened but normally opening valve cusps. AHW, anterior heart wall; RV, right ventricular cavity; IVS, interventricular septum; ACMV and PCMV, anterior and posterior mitral valve cusps; PHW, posterior heart wall

walls can be used to detect aneurysmal dilatation of the root of the aorta, and a dissection extending proximally to the root can also be diagnosed.

Ultrasound is an extremely sensitive technique for detecting pericardial effusions. In most cases only small quantities of fluid need to be present in the pericardial cavity for the diagnosis to be made.

Pulmonary oedema

Pulmonary oedema is an extremely common radiographic finding, due in the great majority of cases to ischaemic heart disease causing left ventricular failure and much less frequently to other conditions, e.g. mitral valve disease. In failure of the left side of the heart the upper zone veins dilate and there is some vasoconstriction of the lower zone arteries and veins, so that the upper zone vessels are seen to be larger than those of the lower zones on the chest X-ray. The probable mechanism for this is as follows. The pulmonary venous pressure is elevated in left heart failure. The additional effect of hydrostatic pressure causes the pressure in the lower zones to be greater than that in the upper zones in the erect patient. A critical pressure is reached, whereby the venous pressure at the lung bases exceeds the osmotic pressure and some perivascular oedema starts to form. This causes local hypoxia which in turn produces reactive vasoconstriction with diversion of blood to the upper zones.

Pulmonary oedema is at first interstitial, in the perivascular space, and this may be seen radiologically when there is no clinical evidence of pulmonary oedema. More severe oedema results in fluid accumulating in the alveolar air spaces. The earliest changes of interstitial oedema are blurring of the normally distinct hilar shadows and vessels to the lower zones. The right basal artery (the artery to the lower lobe) is usually clearly seen on a radiograph, and blurring of this on a good quality PA radiograph may indicate early oedema (*Figure 4.73*). This is sometimes most readily appreciated by comparing the current radiograph with the patient's previous examinations. Lymphatic A and B lines are common, distinctive findings in interstitial pulmonary oedema. As previously described, lymphatic A lines are 1–2.5 cm long and the width of a hair, situated midway between the hilum and lung periphery, pointing in the direction of the hilum (*Figure 4.73*). Lymphatic B lines are lines of similar width, 1–3 cm long, running horizontally above the costophrenic angles at the extreme periphery of the lung (*Figure 4.74*).

Alveolar oedema is manifest by the development of frank consolidation (replacement of air in the alveoli by fluid). The diagnosis of pulmonary oedema as the cause of pulmonary opacification is strongly suggested when the shadowing occupies a symmetrical mid-zone distribution, resembling the silhouette of a butterfly or bat's wings (*Figure 4.75*). A more patchy and less characteristic middle and lower zone distribution is more often seen, however.

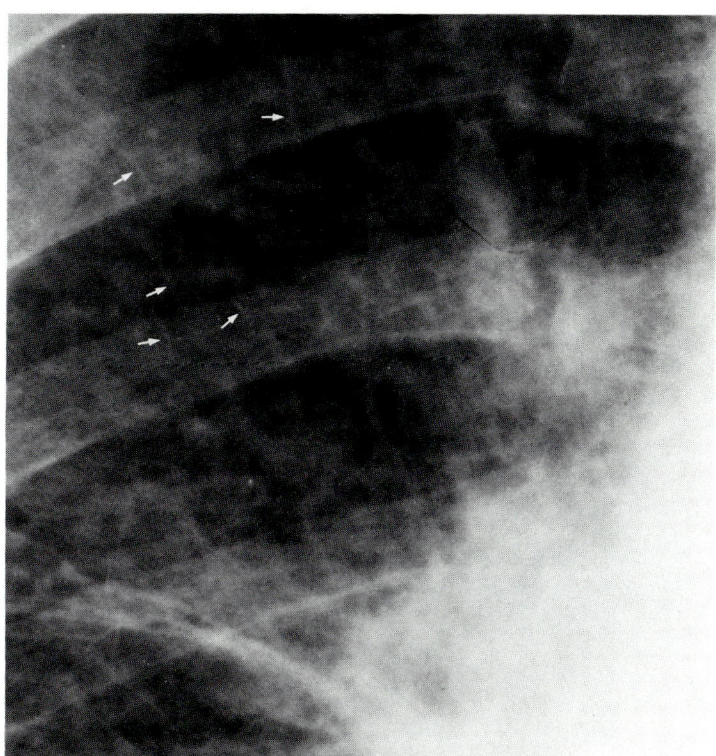

Figure 4.73. Pulmonary oedema: lymphatic A lines (arrows) and blurred hilar shadows; myocardial infarction

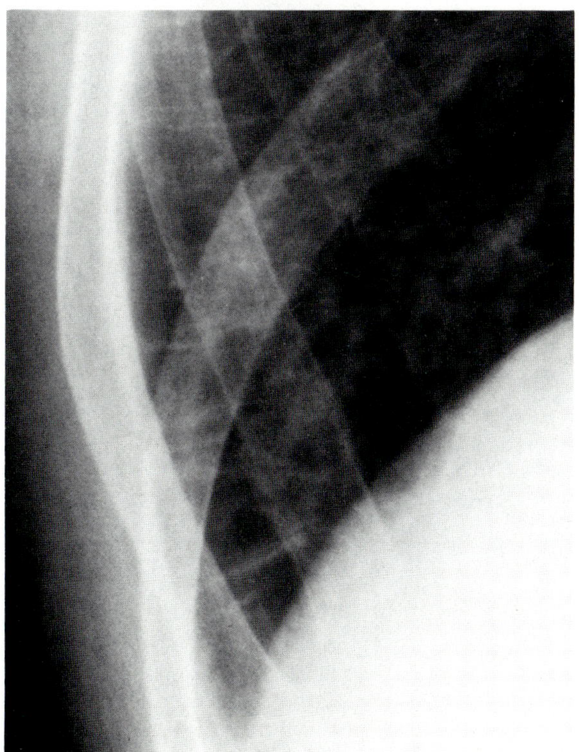

Figure 4.74. Pulmonary oedema; lymphatic B lines (horizontal line shadows above costophrenic angle); mitral stenosis

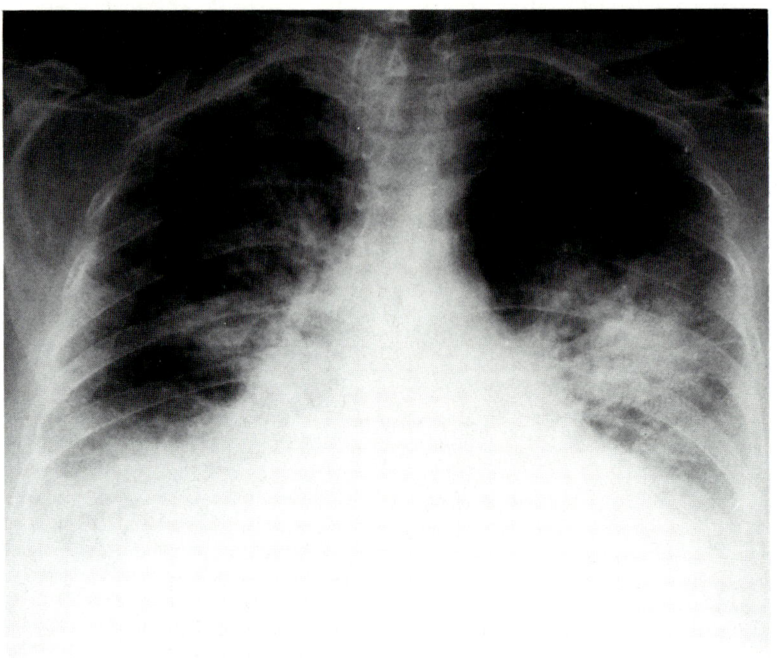

Figure 4.75. Pulmonary oedema: bilateral perihilar (bat's wings) and basal consolidation; small pleural effusions also present; ischaemic heart disease

Sometimes the consolidation is virtually unilateral, developing on the dependent side when the patient has been lying on his side for a period of time.

A right-sided pleural effusion or bilateral pleural effusions are common signs of cardiac failure. It is unusual for a patient to develop an effusion from this cause solely or predominantly on the left side, and when this is found another cause for the effusion—such as pulmonary embolism or infection—should be considered. However, a predominantly left-sided effusion will occur in cardiac failure when the right pleural space has been largely obliterated by previous pleural disease.

Differential diagnosis

Consolidation due to pulmonary oedema is not diagnostic in appearance, and the main differential diagnosis is from infective pneumonia. Features favouring a diagnosis of pulmonary oedema due to heart failure are enlargement of the heart and upper zone vessels on the PA film and prominent changes of interstitial oedema (blurred hilar and basal artery shadows and lymphatic lines). A patient with pulmonary oedema may, however, have a normal sized heart, this being seen, for example, shortly after an acute myocardial infarction or when a patient without heart disease has been overhydrated with intravenous fluids. Conversely, it is common for elderly patients with enlarged hearts from ischaemic heart disease to be admitted to hospital with pneumonia. Assessment of the cause of consolidation must therefore be considered in the clinical context, and quite frequently a patient will have both pulmonary oedema and pneumonia. The response of pulmonary oedema to diuretics is often rapid, and complete or very substantial clearing of the lungs in 24–48 hours favours oedema rather than infection.

The commonest causes of lymphatic A and B lines are pulmonary oedema and malignant disease, the lines in the latter condition being due either to a combination of lymphatic obstruction and oedema in the surrounding tissues, or to frank malignant invasion. Differentiation between an episode of heart failure and diffuse carcinomatosis is usually obvious on clinical grounds. Radiologically, an enlarged heart will favour pulmonary oedema, although the heart shadow may be enlarged due to malignant invasion of the pericardium in diffuse tumour spread. Pleural effusions are common in both conditions. Lobulated glands widening the mediastinum are sometimes seen, substantiating a diagnosis of diffuse malignant disease.

Ischaemic heart disease

Chest films should be taken on patients admitted to hospital after an acute myocardial infarction. These will assess the extent of clinically detected pulmonary oedema or may show the presence of pulmonary oedema before it is clinically apparent. Chest films will also show whether pleural effusions are present. The films are taken as AP views on acutely ill patients and, as already mentioned, an accurate assessment of cardiac size cannot be obtained from these. Nevertheless, the serial films obtained may suggest that the heart shadow is enlarging, and this will serve to alert the physician to the possible development of a pericardial effusion or cardiac dilatation.

Development of a left ventricular aneurysm is one cause of protracted cardiac failure after myocardial infarction. This is sometimes manifest on plain films as a distinct localized bulge of the left heart border (*Figure 4.76*). Fluoroscopy may confirm the paradoxical movement of this area, the bulge expanding further during contraction of the ventricle in systole. Fluoroscopy provides a quick, simple means of examining for a cardiac aneurysm, but aneurysms are not always detected by this technique and cineventriculography is a more sensitive and precise method of investigating this condition. Radiological detection of a ventricular aneurysm is important since resection of a proven aneurysmal segment may significantly benefit the patient.

Detailed assessment of the severity and positions of stenoses and occlusions of the coronary arteries can be obtained only from coronary arteriography (*see* page 250). This technique is now well established, and in experienced hands carries a very low morbidity. Nevertheless, as with other invasive procedures, this examination is carried out only when it is expected that the results will contribute significantly to management. Only a small percentage of patients with ischaemic heart disease require this investigation, and these

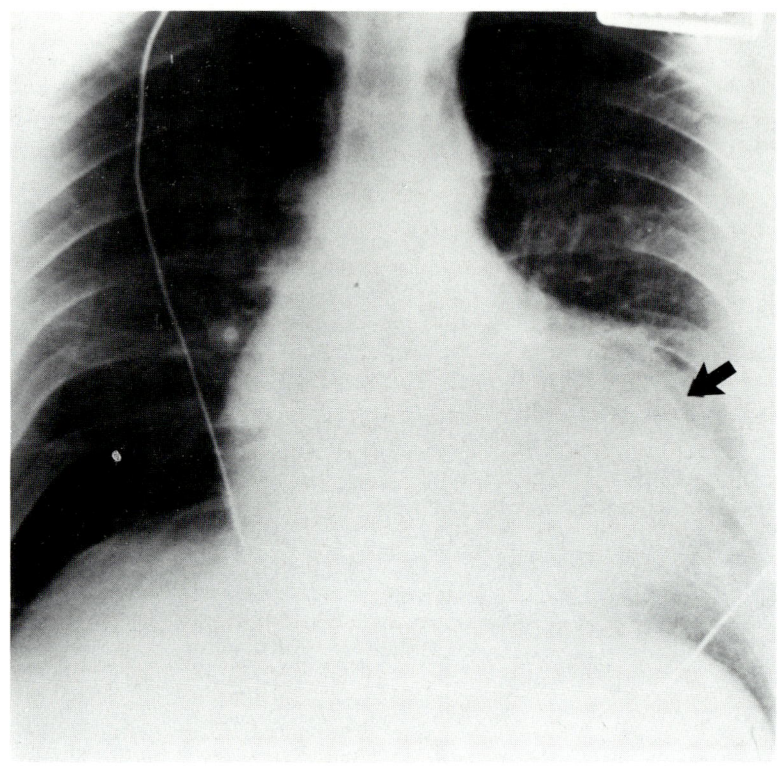

Figure 4.76. Left ventricular aneurysm from previous myocardial infarction: enlarged heart with localized bulge on left heart border (arrow)

include patients with intractable angina, patients in whom the diagnosis of coronary artery disease is not certain, and patients who are being considered for coronary artery surgery.

Rheumatic heart disease

The presence of acquired valve lesions may be manifest on the plain radiographs by features of specific chamber enlargement together with changes in the pulmonary circulation. A diseased valve usually exhibits both stenosis and incompetence, and the relative contribution of each cannot be ascertained from plain films. Furthermore, the appearances of the heart may be complicated by the fact that more than one valve is diseased. In general, gross dilatation of a cardiac chamber immediately proximal to a diseased valve is more likely to be produced by incompetence than by stenosis of that valve. Angiocardiography is necessary for detailed assessment of the severity of disorder of the valve. Valve calcification can be confirmed by fluoroscopy (*see* page 249).

Mitral valve disease

Mitral stenosis

The cardiac transverse diameter is usually within normal limits, but calcification of the mitral valve and moderate enlargement of the left atrium (*see Figure 4.70*) may be seen. Elevation of the pulmonary venous pressure in mitral stenosis leads to diversion of blood to the upper zones of the lungs with visible enlargement on the radiograph of these vessels relative to the lower zone vessels. This feature of pulmonary venous hypertension has already been described in the section on pulmonary oedema.

As in left ventricular failure, pulmonary oedema will develop if the pulmonary venous pressure becomes critically high. Sustained elevation of the venous pressure in mitral stenosis will cause pulmonary arterial hypertension. This will produce enlargement of the main and proximal pulmonary arteries. Severe pulmonary arterial hypertension can lead in turn to right heart failure with dilatation of the right ventricle and atrium.

Mitral incompetence

The plain film appearances can overlap with and mimic those of mitral stenosis, and stenosis and incompetence usually coexist to a variable degree. Gross aneurysmal dilatation of the left atrium may occur in incompetence to an extent that is not found in mitral stenosis, and features of pulmonary hypertension and pulmonary oedema are rarer in incompetence than in stenosis.

The severity of stenosis and regurgitation are evaluated by angiography, the contrast being injected into the left atrium to show the degree of stenosis and into the left ventricle to assess for regurgitation.

Haemosiderosis

Chronic pulmonary venous hypertension due to mitral stenosis can result in capillary dilatation and small haemorrhages. The freed iron tends to collect in the interstitial tissues in clumps, producing fine nodular shadows on the radiograph, mainly in the mid-zones (*see* page 221). The nodules resemble those of miliary tuberculosis in appearance, but the predominant middle zone distribution and the presence of mitral heart disease assist in establishing the true nature of the shadows. The shadows may slowly resolve over a period of several months after successful valve surgery.

Pulmonary ossification

A few 2–5 mm diameter well-defined very dense circular shadows are sometimes seen in the middle and lower zones in patients with mitral stenosis. Histologically these represent small areas of bone formation within the lung.

Aortic valve disease

The chest X-ray may show features compatible with enlargement of the left ventricle, and evidence of dilatation of the ascending aorta.

Both of these changes tend to be more marked in aortic incompetence than in stenosis. Some functional mitral incompetence may occur secondary to the left ventricular failure, but it is rare for the left atrium to be recognizably enlarged. Angiography can be performed to assess the degree of valve disorder, the injections being made into the aorta just above the valve for the evaluation of incompetence and into the left ventricle for the assessment of aortic stenosis.

Tricuspid valve disease

Right atrial enlargement may occur with tricuspid disease, the dilatation being greater in incompetence than in stenosis. Right ventricular enlargement may also be present in incompetence. As already mentioned, plain film evidence of right atrial and ventricular enlargement is insensitive and imprecise. Right heart failure may lead to distension of the superior vena cava, sometimes seen as a straight vertical shadow producing widening of the upper mediastinum on the right side. This is also an insensitive radiological sign, and evidence of right heart failure is far more readily and reliably diagnosed clinically.

Left-to-right shunts

This section refers to the radiographic changes in atrial and ventricular septal defects and in patent ductus arteriosis.

The chest radiograph will be normal when the left-to-right communication is small or of only moderate size. In the presence of large left-to-right shunts the heart is enlarged. There is enlargement also of the main pulmonary artery and generalized enlargement in both lungs of the proximal, medium-sized and small pulmonary artery branches (*Figure 4.77*). The plain radiograph, however, is an insensitive index of shunting, the pulmonary to systemic flow ratio requiring to be at least 3:1 or 4:1 before pulmonary plethora can be recognized.

Later, the resistance in the pulmonary circulation may increase due to the development of arteriolar vasoconstriction in response to the sustained elevation of pulmonary arterial pressure, and the shunt will reverse when the pulmonary pressure exceeds that of the systemic circulation (Eisenmenger syndrome). This change may be evident on the radiograph by the presence of oligaemic instead of plethoric peripheral lung fields, and of further enlargement of the main and proximal pulmonary arteries due to development of severe pulmonary arterial hypertension (*Figure 4.78*). Peripheral pulmonary oligaemia is an insensitive indicator of shunt reversal, this being obvious only when a considerable right-to-left shunt is present.

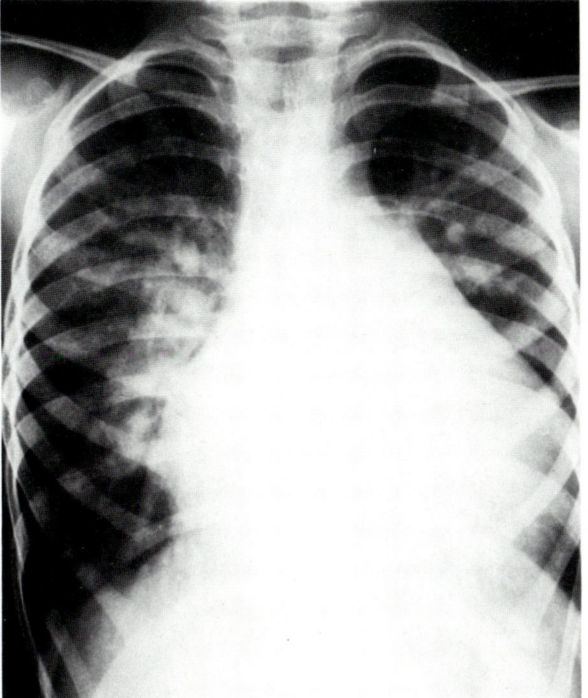

Figure 4.77. Ventricular septal defect with large left-to-right shunt. Enlarged heart and pulmonary plethora (enlarged hilar and peripheral pulmonary vessels)

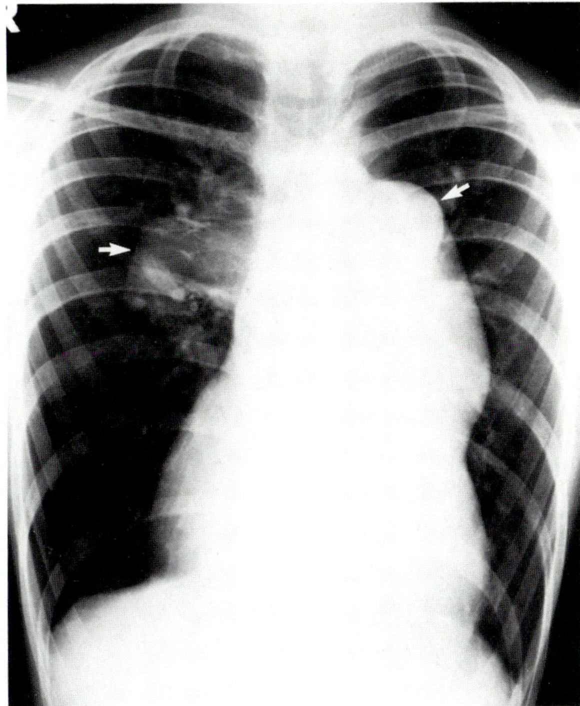

Figure 4.78. Septal defect with reversed (right-to-left) shunt in a 10-year-old girl. The main and proximal pulmonary arteries (arrows) are grossly enlarged from pulmonary arterial hypertension. The lungs are oligaemic

When the characteristic changes of a large left-to-right shunt are usually easily recognized, it is in general difficult to tell the site of the shunt from the radiograph alone. Enlargement of the aortic arch and calcification in the ductus ateriosus may be seen in conjunction with the above features when the shunt is due to a patent ductus. Conversely, in an atrial septal defect some rotation of the aortic arch may occur rendering the aortic knuckle less prominent than usual. A feature sometimes seen in patients with ventricular septal defects is an inequality in the pulmonary pleonaemia, the pulmonary vessels being generally enlarged but particularly so in the right lung, usually in the upper and middle zones. Knowledge of the age of the patient is of some help in diagnosis: radiographic features of a shunt in an elderly person are almost always due to an atrial septal defect.

If further information to that obtained from the clinical, plain chest X-ray and electrocardiographic findings is required cardiac catheter studies and angiocardiography can be performed to assess in detail the shunt and associated pulmonary vascular changes.

Differential diagnosis

Enlargement of the main pulmonary artery (due to pulmonary arterial hypertension) and of the heart are seen in patients with mitral stenosis (*see* page 257). Features distinguishing this condition radiographically from left-to-right shunts are that in mitral stenosis the upper-zone vessels are enlarged but the lower zone vessels are constricted, while in left-to-right shunts the lung fields show generalized pleonaemia. Further, when mitral stenosis has reached a degree of severity to cause radiologically obvious pulmonary arterial hypertension (enlargement of the pulmonary artery) it is common to see some evidence of pulmonary oedema, such as lymphatic B lines above the costophrenic angles. In contrast, heart failure causing pulmonary oedema is less commonly seen in patients with communications between the pulmonary and systemic circulations.

Enlargement of the main pulmonary artery

Several conditions, some of which have already been mentioned, can cause main pulmonary artery enlargement, seen on the plain radiograph as a convex bulge immediately below the shadow of the aortic knuckle. The causes of pulmonary artery enlargement are as follows:

1. Pulmonary stenosis. Post-stenotic dilatation of the main pulmonary trunk and left pulmonary artery occur with stenosis of the pulmonary valve (*Figure 4.79*). This post-stenotic dilatation is due to the effect of the jet of blood on the wall of the artery or to turbulence thereby produced in the immediate post-stenotic region. In contrast, stenosis below the pulmonary valve (infundibular stenosis) is associated with a small main pulmonary artery, seen on the X-ray as a distinct bare area below the aortic knuckle. The pulmonary vascularity is normal unless a right-to-left intracardiac shunt is also present, since the right ventricle maintains a normal cardiac output.

2. Increased pulmonary blood flow. The main, proximal and distal pulmonary vessels are enlarged in large left-to-right shunts (*see* above). Pulmonary artery enlargement is only rarely recognized in high cardiac output states such as thyrotoxicosis.

3. Secondary to pulmonary arteriolar vasoconstriction:
   (a) Vasoconstriction in response to hypoxia gives rise to pulmonary arterial hypertension with enlargement of the main and proximal pulmonary arteries, and sometimes to right heart failure (cor pulmonale). This change is commonly seen during an exacerbation of chronic bronchitis.
   (b) In response to pulmonary venous hypertension, as in sustained left ventricular failure and mitral stenosis.
   (c) Eisenmenger syndrome (*see* page 258).

4. Secondary to organic occlusion or obliteration of the peripheral pulmonary vessels:
   (a) Pulmonary thromboembolism. Multiple small peripheral emboli can cause severe pulmonary arterial hypertension with enlargement of the main and proximal pulmonary arteries, and

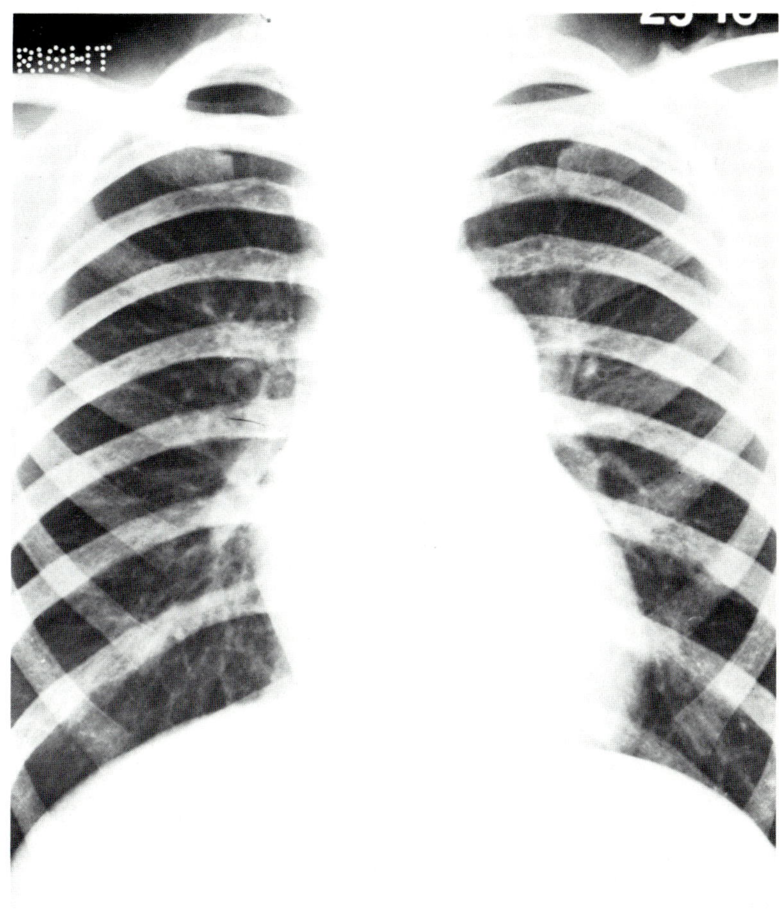

Figure 4.79. Pulmonary valve stenosis in a 7-year-old asymptomatic girl. Pulmonary systolic ejection murmur. Enlarged main pulmonary artery. Normal hilar and pulmonary vessels

right heart failure with enlargement of the heart. Peripheral pulmonary oligaemia may be recognizable on the chest film in this serious condition.

(b) Eisenmenger syndrome, when peripheral vascular obliteration follows vasoconstriction.

(c) Certain collagen diseases, e.g. polyarteritis nodosa, systemic lupus erythematosus.

(d) Diffuse pulmonary fibrosis.

(e) Idiopathic pulmonary hypertension.

5. Idiopathic. A large main pulmonary artery shadow is sometimes seen in the absence of heart or lung disease, particularly in adolescents. Sometimes prominence of the pulmonary artery shadow in this situation is brought about by a scoliosis or by the patient being slightly rotated. At other times no cause is apparent, but before concluding that the finding is of no significance the possibility of a previously undetected pulmonary stenosis with post-stenotic dilatation should be excluded clinically and electrocardiographically.

The cardiomyopathies

The heterogeneous group of conditions classified as the cardiomyopathies are characterized by disorder of the myocardium. These present with congestive cardiac failure (the congestive cardiomyopathies) or with gross hypertrophy of the myocardium of the left ventricular outflow tract causing obstruction to ventricular emptying (hypertrophic obstructive cardiomyopathy). This group of disorders is usually subdivided for purposes of classification into the primary cardiomyopathies, in which disease is confined to the myocardium, and the secondary cardiomyopathies, in which the myocardial disease forms part of a more widespread systemic disorder.

The appearances on the chest X-ray are non-specific. Enlargement of the heart, due to generalized hypertrophy and dilatation of cardiac chambers, is usually present. The heart is sometimes rather globular in shape and usually shows diminished pulsation on fluoroscopy, so that the features may mimic and must be differentiated from a pericardial effusion. In some patients difficulty is experienced both clinically and radiologically in distinguishing congestive cardiomyopathy from ischaemic heart disease. In others, hypertrophic obstructive cardiomyopathy may mimic aortic stenosis (or, since secondary mitral incompetence is common) mitral-valve disease of rheumatic origin.

Echocardiography or angiocardiography can be performed to exclude a pericardial effusion of any appreciable size (*see* page 263). Differentiation from ischaemic heart disease can be made in difficult cases by angiography. In the congestive cardiomyopathies there is generalized impairment of ventricular contraction and the coronary arteries are usually normal, while in ischaemic heart disease absent or paradoxical movement of the ventricular walls is patchy and coronary angiography shows stenoses and occlusions of the coronary arteries.

The pericardium

Pericardial effusion

The causes of pericardial effusion are:

1. Infective: viral (usually Coxsackie), pyogenic or tuberculous.
2. Traumatic: injuries to the thorax or cardiac surgery.
3. Neoplastic: invasion by bronchogenic carcinoma or other malignant tumours.
4. Metabolic uraemia.
5. Connective tissue disorders: rheumatoid arthritis, systemic lupus erythematosus or polyarteritis nodosa.
6. Myocardial infarction.

The presence of a pericardial effusion may be strongly suggested by the chest film and fluoroscopic appearances, but these investigations are insensitive in the absence of a considerable volume of fluid. The chest X-ray features are of enlargement of the cardiac shadow which becomes globular in shape, the two sides being almost symmetrical in appearance (*Figure 4.80*). The shape is seen to alter on films taken with the patient erect and supine due to redistribution

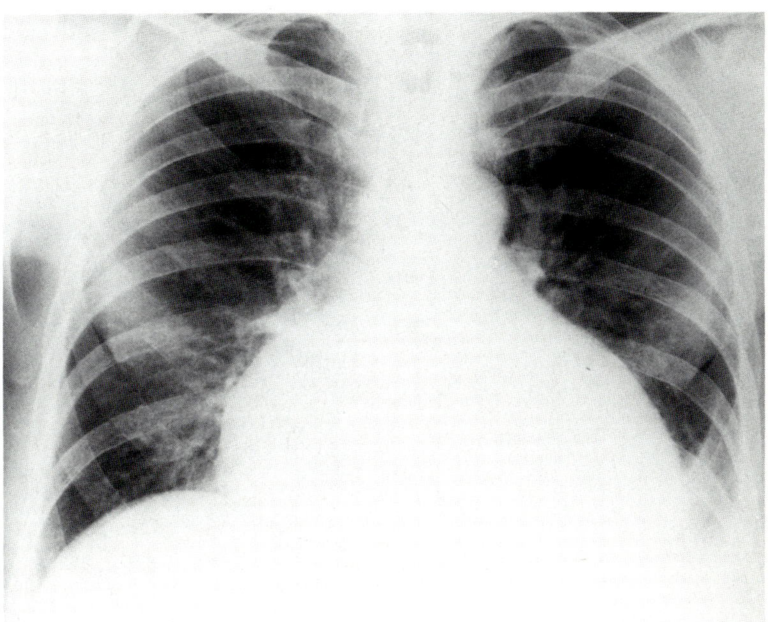

Figure 4.80. Pericardial effusion. Symmetrical, globular enlargement of cardiac silhouette. A small left pleural effusion is also present

of the fluid under the effect of gravity. A useful early sign of the development of a pericardial effusion is sudden increase in the diameter of the heart shadow, a feature that can be detected when a patient has comparable previous chest films available for comparison. Concurrent pleural effusions are present in two-thirds of cases. The characteristic fluoroscopic finding is of markedly reduced cardiac pulsation, but as previously mentioned this may also be seen in the cardiomyopathies.

The definitive investigations for confirmation of a pericardial effusion are echocardiography and contrast opacification of the right atrium and ventricle. Echocardiography is a sensitive, reliable, non-invasive method for the detection of pericardial fluid and is the investigation of choice in centres where this facility is available. The angiographic diagnosis of a pericardial effusion entails the injection of contrast through a venous catheter positioned with its tip in either the superior vena cava or right atrium. The right atrial and right ventricular walls are thin, and in a normal person only a narrow soft-tissue shadow separates these opacified chambers from the translucent lung. In the presence of a pericardial effusion the shadow of soft-tissue density, representing the wall of the cardiac chamber and surrounding pericardial fluid, is abnormally wide. This investigation, although invasive, is simple to perform and can be carried out in a critically ill patient in the ward.

Constrictive pericarditis

Constrictive pericarditis is characterized by gross fibrosis of the pericardium, which restricts diastolic expansion of the ventricles. Tuberculous pericarditis is a well-recognized cause, and less commonly the condition follows suppurative or viral pericarditis. Other rare aetiological factors are haemopericardium, rheumatoid arthritis and irradiation of the chest. Often no obvious cause is found in patients presenting with the condition.

The shadow of the heart may be normal in size, or slightly increased by the overlying thickened pericardium. Calcification of the pericardium is present in 50 per cent of cases. This can be linear

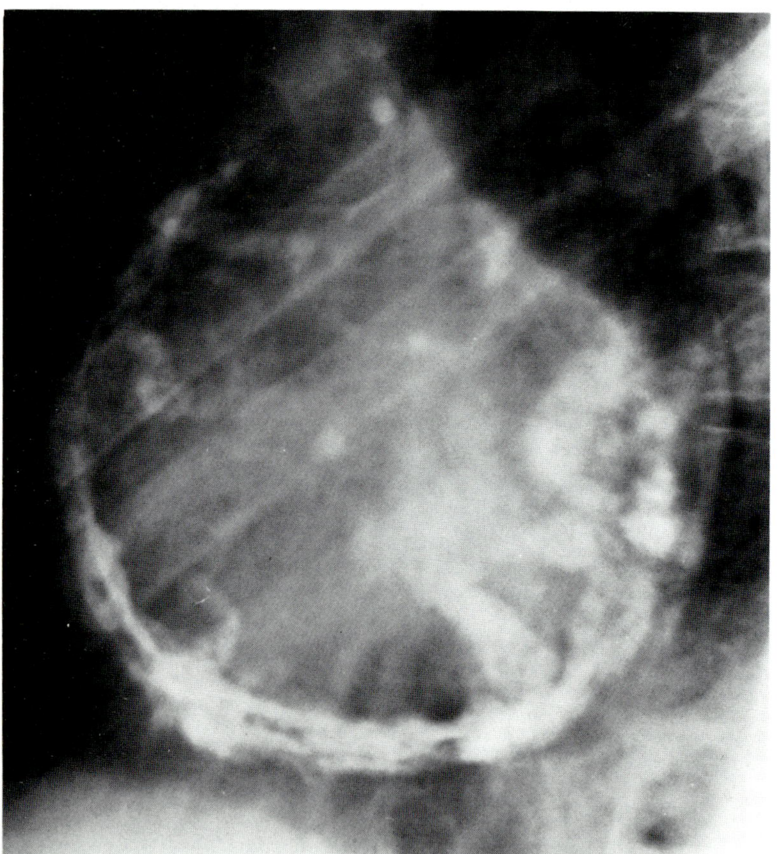

Figure 4.81. Constrictive pericarditis: oblique view of heart showing heavily calcified, thickened pericardium encasing the heart

or take the form of thick plaques. The calcification can be very widespread and obvious, encasing the heart (*Figure 4.81*), or it can be sparse and seen only on lateral or oblique films. Associated pleural effusions are present in 50 per cent of cases.

On fluoroscopy the characteristic finding is gross reduction of the amplitude of cardiac pulsation. Confirmation that calcification seen on the chest X-ray lies within the pericardium can also be obtained by fluoroscopy.

The thoracic aorta

Widening of the aortic arch and tortuosity of the descending aorta are common findings on the PA radiograph in elderly people. These usually represent simple ageing changes without aneurysm formation. Calcification in the aortic wall at any site, but especially in the arch, is often seen in atheromatous degeneration. Calcification in the wall of the ascending aorta also occurs in syphilitic aortitis.

The main radiographic sign of an aneurysm is loss of parallelism of the aortic walls. Only the outer border of the thoracic aorta, abutting on the lung, can be seen on a PA radiograph: the medial wall is invisible. It may therefore be impossible on this view to distinguish between a fusiform aneurysm and simple unfolding. An aneurysm will, however, be very strongly suggested by the presence of a local aortic bulge; by a wide aortic shadow in a young person, particularly after recent trauma (*Figures 4.82* and *4.83*); and if rapid increase in the width of the aortic shadow is evident on serial films. Occasionally an aneurysm simulates a mediastinal neoplasm. Sometimes it presses on a bronchus, causing atelectasis of the lung thus simulating a bronchial neoplasm.

The whole aortic shadow is often clearly visible on a lateral chest film, and lack of parallelism of the walls can frequently be confirmed

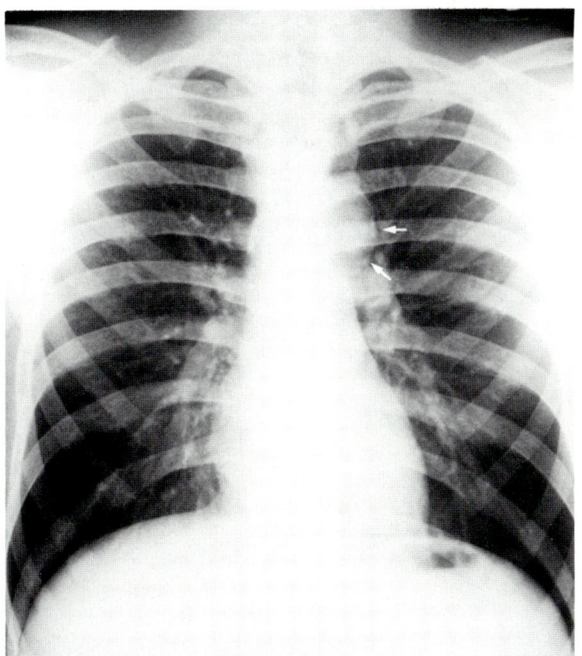

Figure 4.82. Traumatic aneurysm of aorta: calcification (arrows) in wall of enlarged aortic knuckle; male, aged 21, struck chest on steering wheel of car in head-on collision 3 years previously

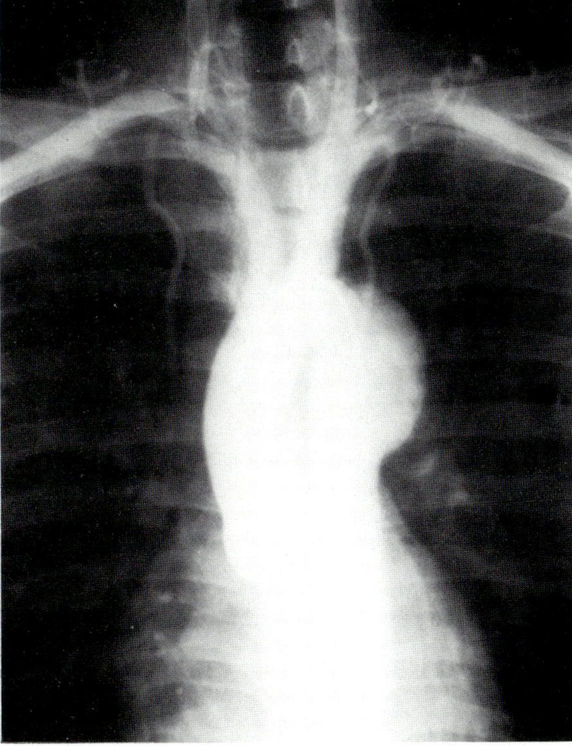

Figure 4.83. Arch aortogram in same patient as in *Figure 4.82*, showing aneurysm of distal part of arch and adjacent proximal descending aorta

on this view. The oesophagus may be seen to be displaced on barium swallow examination.

Aortography is indicated to confirm the diagnosis or provide precise anatomical delineation in situations where this information would influence patient management. Urgent aortography is mandatory when there is any suggestion of aortic injury after blunt chest trauma: if surgical repair of a traumatic aneurysm or rupture can be undertaken in time the prognosis is generally favourable.

A dissecting aneurysm may be present with acute chest pain suggestive of myocardial infarction. The plain radiographs may show a wide mediastinum, or sudden enlargement of the aortic shadow in comparison with a previous radiograph. Extrapleural blood, a pleural effusion or consolidation from bleeding into the lung may be present. An angiogram will be of value, particularly if surgical intervention is contemplated, to confirm the diagnosis. The most common specific angiographic features are compression of the true aortic lumen and opacification of the false lumen.

Coarctation of the aorta may be discovered during routine medical or chest X-ray examination of asymptomatic young adults: at other times patients with this condition present with symptoms of hypertension. The aortic narrowing is usually at the level of the ductus. The characteristic features that may be seen on the PA chest film include widening of the upper mediastinal shadow (due to enlargement of the left subclavian artery), a double aortic knuckle (the lower of the two bulges being produced by post-stenotic dilatation of the proximal descending aorta), and rib notching. Notching is due to pressure erosions of the walls of the intercostal grooves produced by the enlarged, tortuous intercostal arteries. It involves the lower surfaces of the 4th to 8th (sometimes 3rd to 9th) ribs, is usually bilateral and symmetrical, and is most reliably identified on the posterolateral portions of these ribs.

Coarctation is treated surgically, and the exact site and severity of the stenosis and any associated aortic-valve abnormality are assessed preoperatively by aortography.

The oesophagus

Carcinoma of the oesophagus

Dysphagia arising for the first time in a middle-aged or elderly patient is an ominous symptom, often indicating the presence of a carcinoma of the oesophagus or cardia. Weight loss may be a prominent feature.

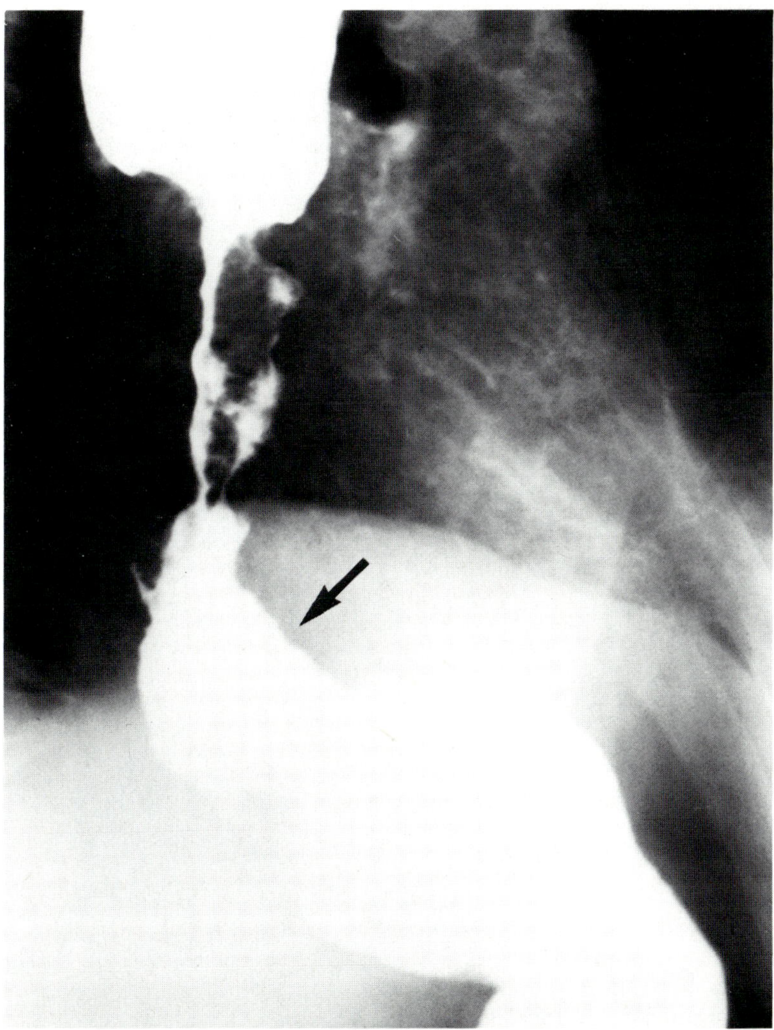

Figure 4.84. Carcinoma of lower oesophagus, cardia and adjacent stomach: highly irregular oesophageal stricture with abrupt 'shouldered' proximal margin; the adjacent stomach is narrowed and has an irregular edge (arrow) due to tumour infiltration

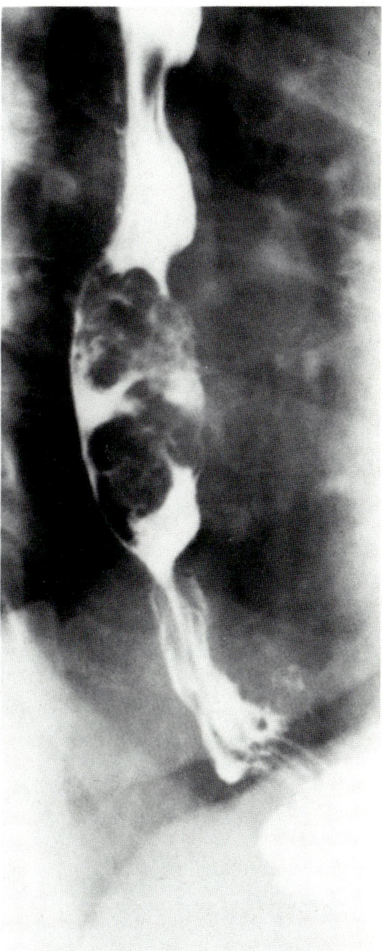

Figure 4.85. Large polypoid lower oesophageal carcinoma. Barium seen tracking in grooves on the tumour surface. Tumour is distending the lumen. Dysphagia for 10 months. An impacted food bolus gives a very similar radiological appearance

Oesophageal carcinoma is unfortunately often advanced by the time of the radiological examination, and the commonest appearance is of a highly irregular stricture with destroyed mucosa, and with abrupt 'shouldered' demarcation between the abnormal and adjacent normal segments (*Figure 4.84*). Less commonly, the tumour shows as an irregular polypoid mass encroaching on the barium-filled oesophageal lumen (*Figure 4.85*).

The level at which the patient feels food sticking is not a reliable pointer to the level of the organic lesion, and it is mandatory that patients with dysphagia have a radiological examination of the stomach as well as of the oesophagus and are prepared for this by fasting in the standard manner for barium meal examination. Unless this is done tumours encroaching on the lower oesophagus from the cardia and adjacent fundus or lesser curve of the stomach can be overlooked or diagnosed with less certainty (*Figure 4.86*).

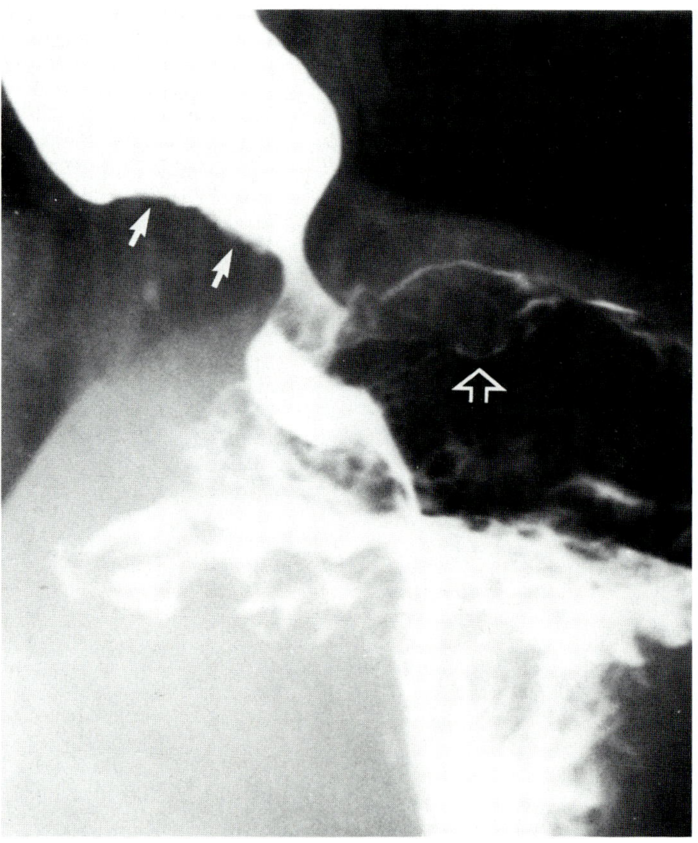

Figure 4.86. Carcinoma of lower oesophagus and adjacent gastric fundus: irregular lower oesophageal margin (small arrows); more certain evidence of tumour is provided by the irregular filling defect in the adjacent gastric fundus (open arrow)

Small oesophageal carcinomas can occasionally be overlooked altogether on barium examination and at other times may be indistinguishable radiologically from benign strictures. It is therefore essential that disproportionate emphasis is not placed on a negative or equivocal barium examination and that oesophagoscopy is carried out as a supplement to the barium study in any patient whose symptoms suggest a possible carcinoma.

Hiatus hernia and benign oesophageal strictures

In a hiatus hernia of sliding type the gastro-oesophageal junction lies above the diaphragm and the cardiac end of the stomach protrudes through the diaphragmatic hiatus into the thorax. The

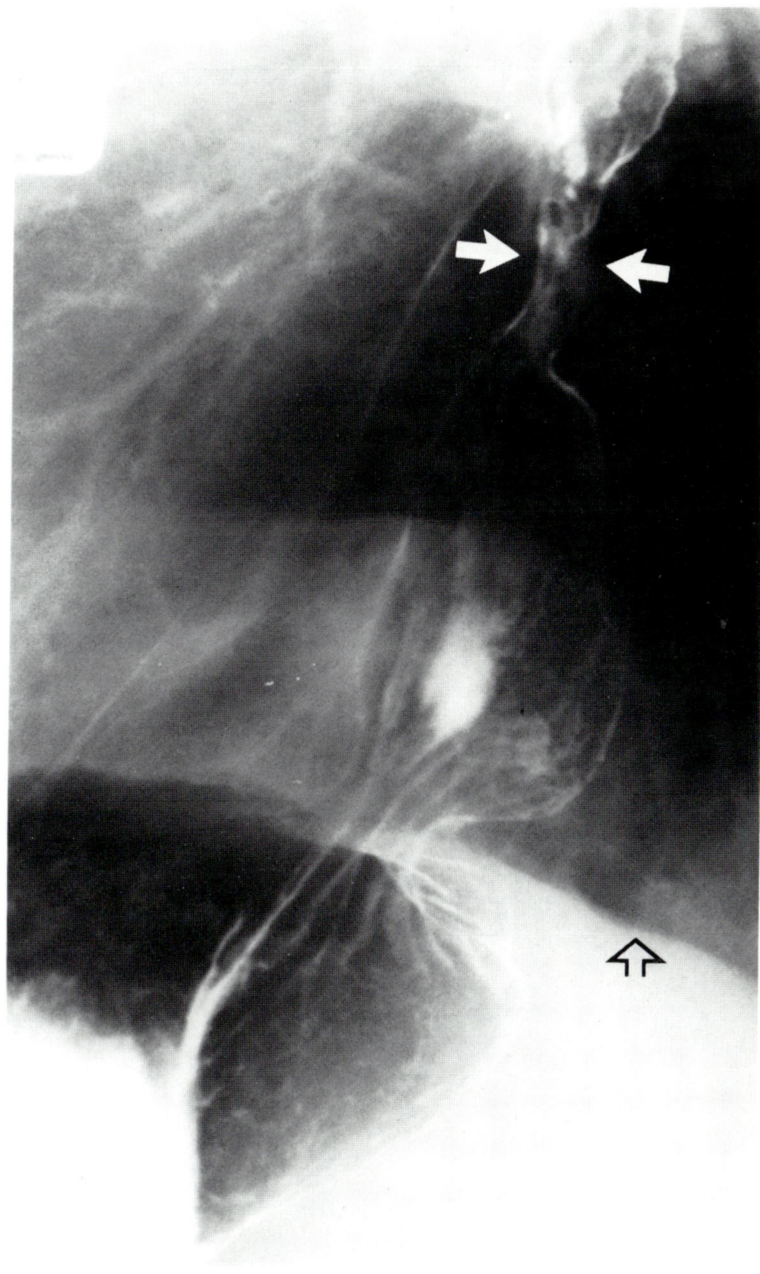

Figure 4.87. Hiatus hernia with benign stricture (white arrows) at gastro-oesophageal junction: the walls of the stricture are smooth, and the upper and lower margins of the stricture show gradual tapering. Diaphragm is indicated by open arrow

presence of part of the stomach within the thorax is obvious on barium examination when the hernia is large; when it is small, recognizable gastric mucosal folds can be seen passing through the hiatus and converging above the diaphragm. The normal angle of entry of the oesophagus into the stomach is lost with this type of hernia, and gastro-oesophageal reflux occurs. This may cause oesophagitis, which in turn may lead to ulceration and stricture formation in the lower oesophagus (*Figure 4.87*). In these circumstances the patient may present with lower retrosternal pain or dysphagia.

A small sliding hiatus hernia with some reflux can be demonstrated quite often in middle-aged or elderly patients examined for

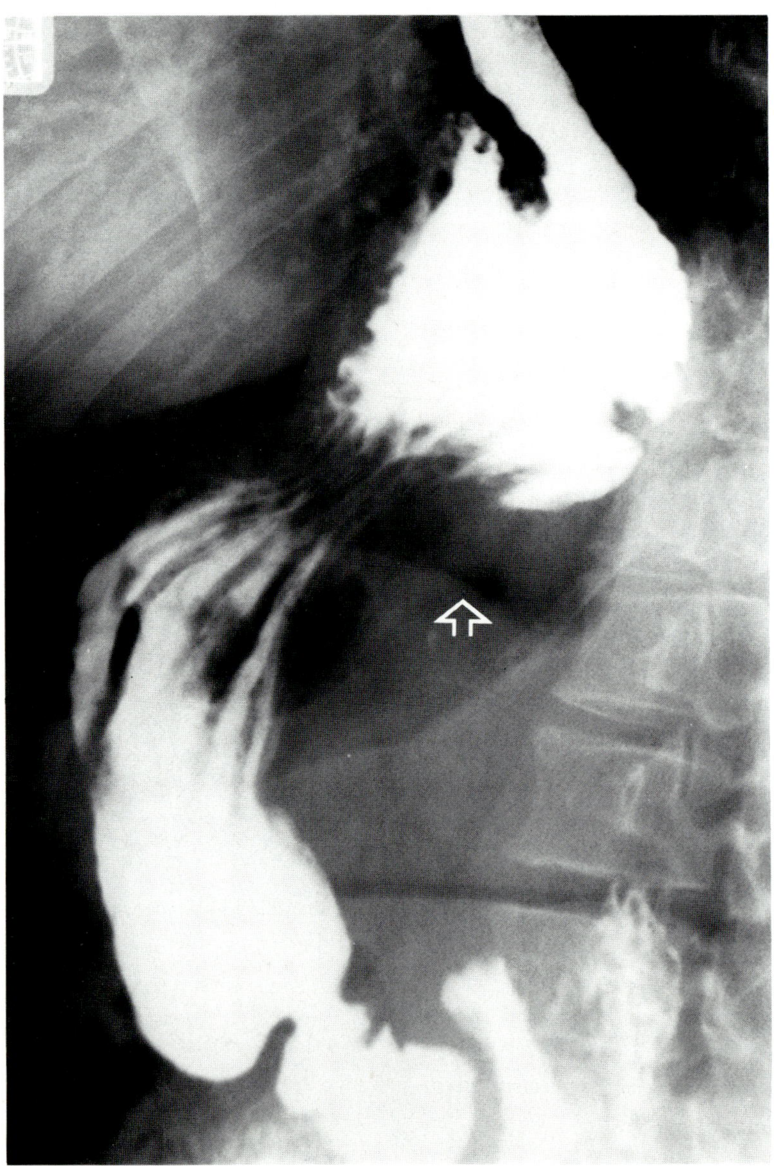

Figure 4.88. Hiatus hernia—mixed type; paraoesophageal component alongside lower oesophagus. Diaphragm is indicated by open arrow

unrelated conditions. The hernia is produced most readily when the X-ray table on which the patient is lying is tilted so that his head lies below the level of his feet, and the hernia commonly reduces again when the patient is brought upright. This finding is of no clinical significance in the absence of symptoms.

A paraoesophageal hernia occurs when part of the stomach passes through the oesophageal hiatus and rolls up alongside the lower oesophagus within the chest. Patients with this type of hernia are often asymptomatic, and the hernia may be found incidentally during barium examination for some unrelated cause, or on a chest X-ray. In the latter situation a rounded gas shadow lying above a fluid level is visible behind the heart. In some patients there is considerable bleeding from a paraoesophageal hernia, so that the presenting features may be haematemesis or melaena, or tiredness and dyspnoea from chronic anaemia. It is very rare for a para-oesophageal hernia to be present on its own: there is usually a sliding element as well, giving rise to a hernia of mixed type (*Figure 4.88*).

As has been mentioned, reflux oesophagitis may lead to ulceration and stricture formation in the lower oesophagus. In contrast to the appearances of a malignant stricture, the walls of a benign stricture are usually smooth and the lumen tapers gradually from the healthy to the strictured segment (*see Figure 4.87*). A stricture arising from gastro-oesophageal reflux lies at the gastro-oesophageal junction. The rare exception to this occurs when the oesophagus is lined by, or contains pockets of, gastric mucosa. In these circumstances the stricture may develop at a higher level.

While a smooth, concentric narrowing is typical of a benign stricture, a carcinoma of the oesophagus can sometimes produce a similar appearance. At other times, a stricture may show no special distinguishing features, and this is particularly the case when distortion produced by ulceration is present. For these reasons patients with radiologically demonstrated oesophageal strictures should in general be investigated further by oesophagoscopy.

A long, benign, fibrous stricture of the oesophagus may follow the swallowing of a caustic solution. As with benign strictures at the cardia resulting from gastro-oesophageal reflux, the narrowing tends to be more centrally placed and smoother in outline (*Figure 4.89*) than is typically seen in carcinoma. The relevant history of ingestion of a caustic may of course be obtained.

Achalasia

In the advanced stages of achalasia widening of the entire length of the mediastinum by the enormously dilated oesophagus may be visible on a chest X-ray (*Figure 4.90*). A fluid level can usually be seen in the dilated oesophagus, and the food, fluid and air retained above the cardia give rise to an opacity of non-homogeneous density. These features enable a widened oesophagus to be distinguished from other conditions that can cause broadening of the mediastinal

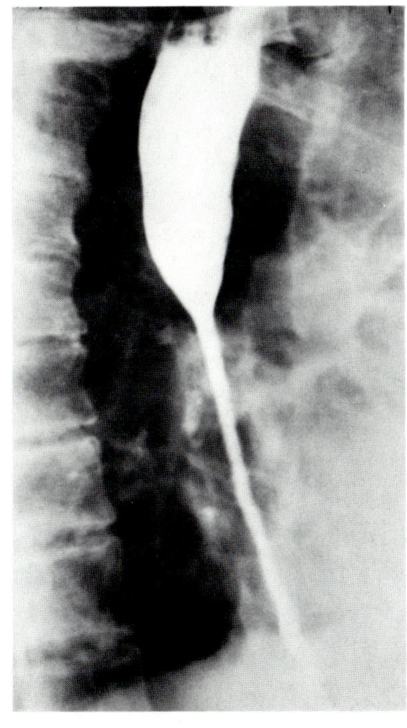

Figure 4.89. Benign stricture of the oesophagus caused by accidentally swallowed corrosive: smooth, narrow, centrally placed lumen; stricture commences just below aortic arch

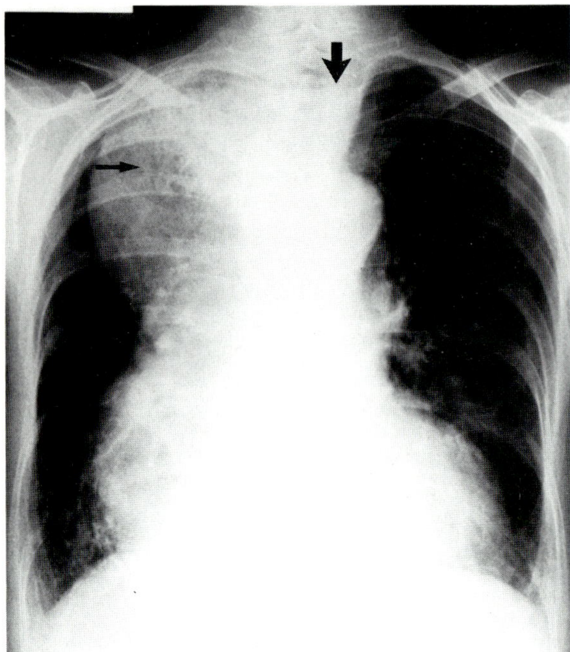

Figure 4.90. Achalasia in a patient with dysphagia for 20 years: mediastinum widened by grossly dilated oesophagus; non-homogeneous density of swallowed food, fluid and air within oesophagus (horizontal arrow); fluid level at upper end of opacity (vertical arrow); absent gastric air bubble

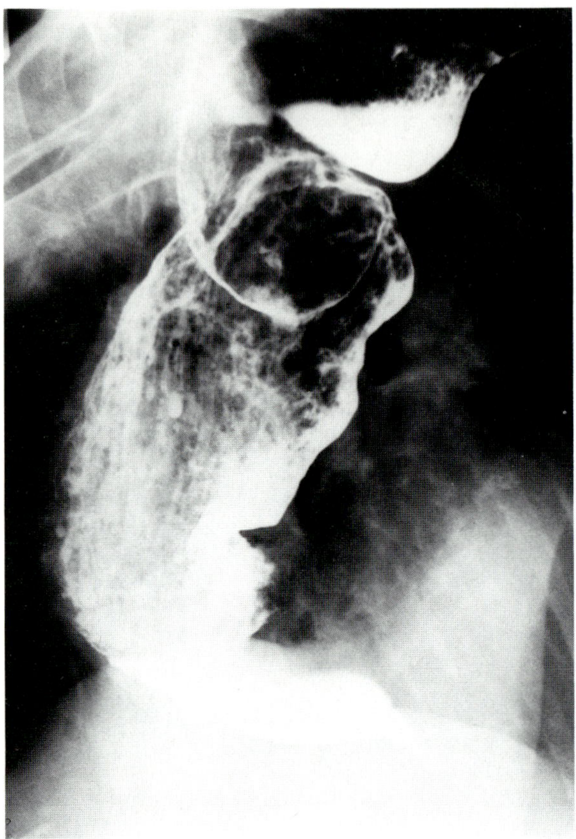

Figure 4.91. Achalasia. Same patient as in *Figure 4.90*; barium swallow: grossly dilated, elongated and kinked oesophagus; almost horizontal lower oesophagus, tapering smoothly to the cardia

shadow. The partially filled oesophagus acts as a reservoir, and typically there is no air in the gastric fundus in achalasia.

Dilatation of the oesophagus is readily confirmed on barium examination. The oesophagus is elongated as well as dilated, and the lower portion may run an almost horizontal course across the midline to the cardia. Characteristically, the distal portion of the oesophagus shows smooth, progressive tapering (*Figure 4.91*). On fluoroscopy small quantities of barium are seen to pass intermittently through the cardia during brief periods of muscular relaxation. Weak incoordinated contractions are visible in the oesophagus.

Hold-up of barium at the cardia may be the only radiographic abnormality in the early stages of the disease. In this situation relaxation of the cardia with partial relief of the obstruction can be seen on fluoroscopy after intravenous injection of Buscopan (hyoscine n-butylbromide).

Carcinoma is the main condition from which achalasia needs to be differentiated. The appearances of a carcinoma of the cardia can on occasion closely resemble those of achalasia, and there is an increased incidence of carcinoma of the oesophagus in patients with achalasia. Patients suspected on radiological grounds of having

achalasia should therefore be investigated further by oesophagoscopy.

Oesophageal varices

On a normal barium swallow examination, three or four mucosal
folds coated with barium can be seen running the length of the
oesophagus. In the presence of varices these folds lose their parallel
arrangement and are displaced and stretched in a random manner
by the varicosities in the underlying submucosa (*Figure 4.92*). If the
varices extend into the stomach they can produce multiple rounded
filling defects, resembling a bunch of small grapes, in the vicinity of
the cardia (*Figure 4.92*).

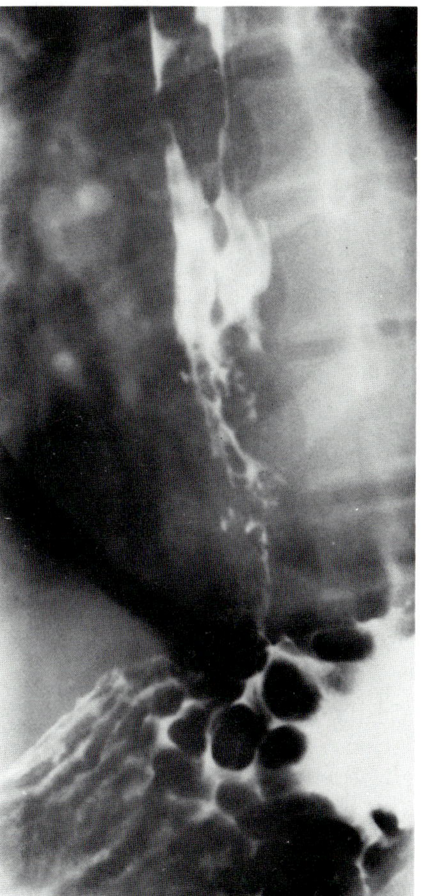

Figure 4.92. Oesophageal varices: irregularity of the normally parallel oesophageal
mucosal folds, produced by submucosal
varices; rounded filling defects below the
cardia due to gastric varices

Either barium swallow examination or portal venography (*see*
page 144) will show the presence of varices in most patients with this
condition. At times one technique may show varices not demonstrable by the other. Since barium examination is simple and non-
invasive, it should be the initial radiological investigation for
suspected varices.

5 Radiology of the head and neck

Arthur J.A. Wightman and G.H. du Boulay

The bones of the skull

There are three main indications for radiology of the skull:
1. When the clinical findings suggest a local bone condition, such as a fracture or a lump on the head.
2. When some general condition is present that is likely to be associated with changes in the bones of the cranium.
3. When an intracranial lesion is suspected.

The uses of radiology in head injuries have been described in the section on Trauma (*see* page 27).

The size of the head

The size of the head is so easily measured by direct means that radiographs are not necessary for this purpose except in the case of the fetus. On the other hand, radiology is often useful in elucidating the cause of the enlargement, as in acromegaly (*see* page 282) or Paget's disease (*see* page 90).

Peculiarities of shape

Radiological examination may be of use in demonstrating whether peculiarities of shape are confined to the vault or are associated with abnormal development of the base. Some peculiarities are the result of premature closure of one of the sutures; if, for instance, the coronal suture closes prematurely the skull will be short in the anteroposterior diameter, and some compensation for this will be gained by an increase in height, producing oxycephaly or tower skull.

Infections of the vault

Infections of the vault are rarely of haematogenous origin. More commonly they arise by direct spread from an infected frontal sinus or mastoid, or they may follow a scalp wound, a penetrating bone injury, or an operation on the bone. The X-ray changes tend to understate the actual degree of infection; after penetrating injuries or operations on the vault there are often no X-ray changes of osteomyelitis although the bone edge is known to be infected.

The principal radiographic feature of acute infection of the skull vault is of one or more areas of translucency with ill-defined margins. Subperiosteal new bone formation, which is commonly seen in infection of long bones, is rare in osteomyelitis of the skull vault, and sequestra are seldom present. As elsewhere in the skeleton the poorly demarcated translucencies of osteomyelitis may be indistinguishable radiologically from malignant bone deposits, although differentiation is usually obvious clinically.

Chronic osteomyelitis of the skull may show as an area of sclerosis, resulting from an osteoblastic bone reaction. This is sometimes seen in the frontal bones adjacent to chronically infected frontal sinuses. Low-grade infections such as tuberculosis or syphilis usually produce areas of lytic destruction of the skull, but very occasionally a sclerotic reaction is found.

Developmental defects and tumours of the skull vault

An underlying meningioma is one of the most important causes of a palpable lump on the head. Occasionally there are no other clinical manifestations, except perhaps persistent headache. The tumour may induce a boss of sclerotic bone which can reach 10 cm or so in size. A bony lump without other clinical manifestations is, however, more commonly due to primary bone disease, e.g. fibrous dysplasia.

An exostosis may produce a small lump, usually in the posterior temporal region behind the mastoid process, and can often be diagnosed by its trabecular structure, although sometimes the lesion is more solid and homogeneous. A cyst-like area with a stellate pattern of strands of bone across it suggests a haemangioma, while a local, transradiant, blister-like expanding lesion of the diploë suggests fibrous dysplasia. A sarcoma can occur in the vault but is uncommon: it may accompany Paget's disease.

Many lesions arise in the vault without a palpable lump, although in some a local area of softening may be felt. In a child a 2–3 cm area of bone erosion, or several erosions over a large area, suggests eosinophilic granuloma or deposits from a malignant tumour of childhood, such as a neuroblastoma. In an elderly person a single erosion or multiple 5 mm erosions lacking any reactive sclerosis at the margins would suggest secondary deposits or myelomatosis. Typically, myeloma deposits have sharply defined, rounded margins, giving the impression of defects created with a mechanical punch (*see Figure 2.89*), while the borders of secondary deposits are less clearly demarcated. Although these distinguishing features may be useful in making a presumptive diagnosis, overlap in the appearances of the two conditions does occur, and confident differentiation should not be made from the radiological examination alone.

As mentioned above, lytic defects due to acute osteomyelitis may resemble those of malignant bone disease. Translucencies due to local bone thinning of the skull can occur as a normal finding at the site of Pacchionian (arachnoid) granulations. These are most commonly situated in the parasagittal region (where they can be confidently recognized by their symmetrical distribution close to the midline) or beside the transverse sinuses. When they occur elsewhere in the skull they may sometimes be mistaken for metastases.

A well-defined transradiant area in the skull vault may be caused by a developmental defect such as a meningocele, by parietal foramina (small defects of no clinical significance situated close to the midline in one or both parietal bones), or by an intradiploic dermoid. The latter produces obvious bone expansion.

Chronic swelling of the face over several years may be the result of leontiasis ossea, a disorder in which the facial bones on one or both sides are enlarged and very dense. This condition is usually due to fibrous dysplasia of the facial bones but can be a manifestation of Paget's disease.

The central nervous system

Intracranial lesions

The skull X-ray

The following, suggesting an intracranial lesion, will call for radiographs of the skull: headache, especially if severe and persistent; vomiting and papilloedema; recent disorders of speech, vision or memory; cranial nerve palsies and other neurological signs; epilepsy of late onset; and character changes or lowering of the level of consciousness. Traditionally four views are taken initially; a true lateral, a posteroanterior, an anteroposterior half axial (Towne's) and a submentovertical. It is important that the radiographs are of high quality and free from blurring due to movement by the patient. In more than a fifth of cases of cerebral tumour, some abnormality can be seen in the radiograph.

The introduction of computed tomography (CT) has relegated plain skull X-rays to a less important place, except in patients suspected of lesions in or around the pituitary fossa. In centres where CT is available the initial plain X-ray examination may consist of a single lateral view. This must often be supplemented to give more information when either the plain lateral X-ray or CT shows an abnormality.

Direct evidence of an intracranial lesion

1. Calcification within the lesion.
2. Local bone erosion.
3. Local bone sclerosis.
4. Enlargement of the basal foramina, an optic foramen, the internal auditory meatus, or ballooning of the pituitary fossa (*Figure 5.7*).

Calcification   Calcification can be seen within many pathological lesions arising within the cranium. Consideration of the position and pattern of the calcification is useful in deducing the possible nature of the lesion: thus a cluster of dense specks of calcification lying in the midline directly above the pituitary fossa is most likely to indicate a craniopharyngioma. The pattern of calcification is most simply classified as comprising one or more curved lines, or an area of speckled or amorphous density, or opacities disseminated widely within the cranium.

As elsewhere in the body, fine curvilinear calcification within the cranium commonly represents calcification within blood vessels (either in atheromatous major arteries or in an angioma). While a complete or partial ring of calcification may form within the wall of an aneurysm of the carotid or basilar artery, this is rarely seen. Visible calcification due to degenerative change in undilated intracranial vessels is almost invariably restricted to the carotid siphon, situated on either side of the pituitary fossa. Characteristic wavy bands of calcification may be found, usually in the occipital region, in Sturge–Weber syndrome. These represent calcification arising in the occipital cortex and occur in conjunction with the clinically obvious port-wine naevus on the face and skull.

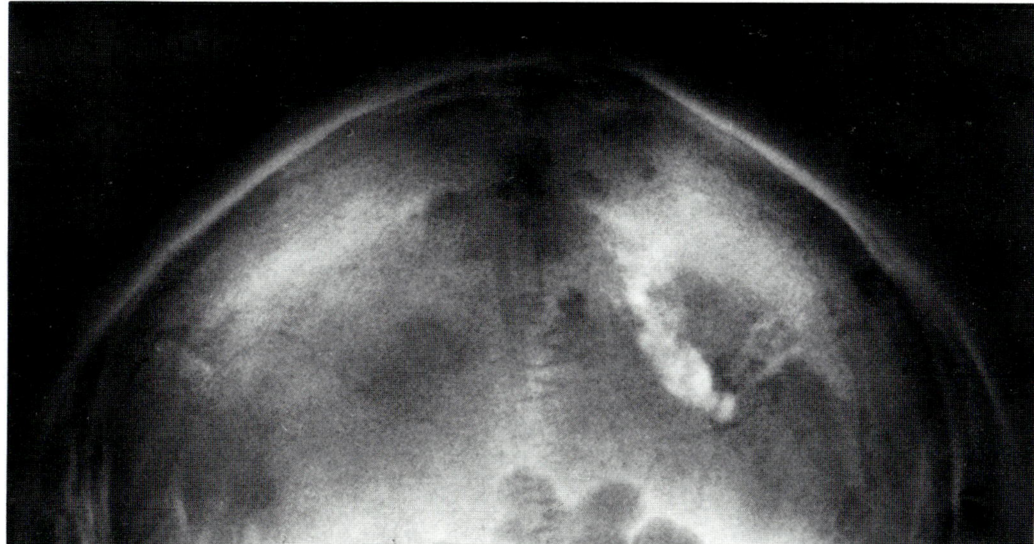

Figure 5.1. Skull, PA view showing amorphous calcification in a glioma

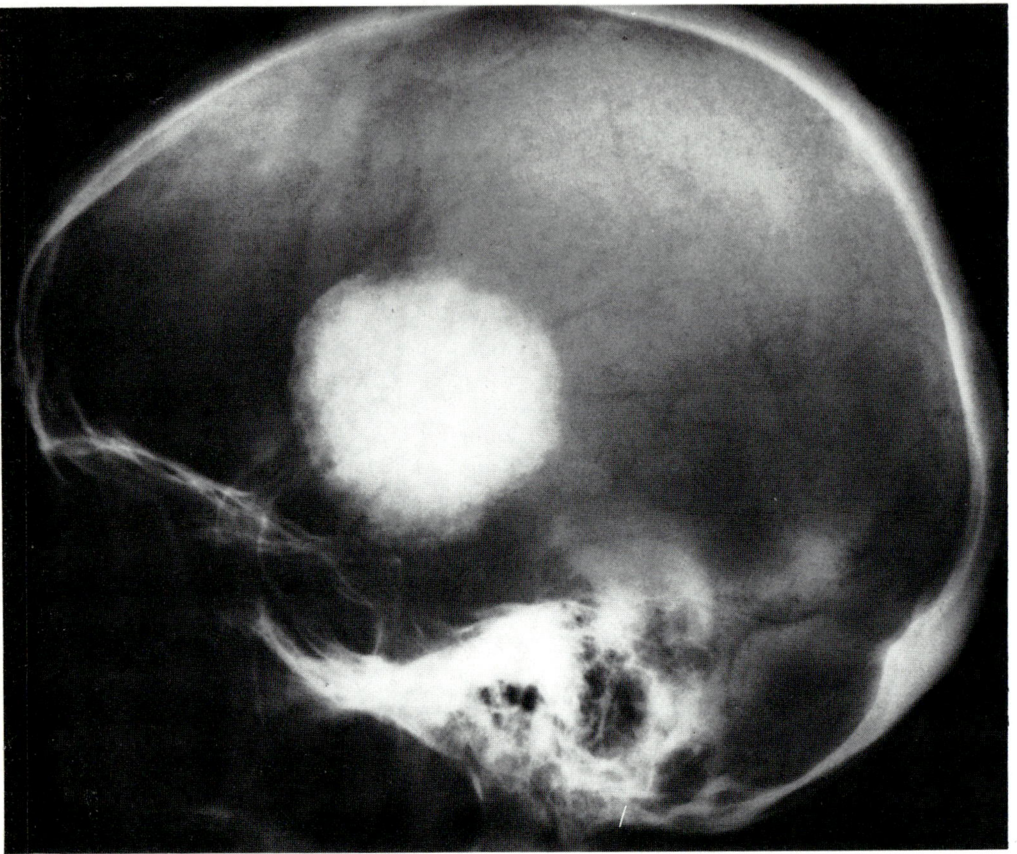

(a)

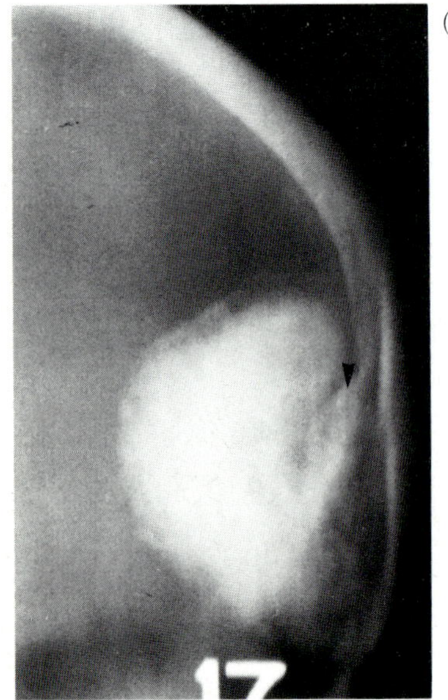

(b)

Figure 5.2. (a) Skull, lateral view: showing well-circumscribed, dense, amorphous calcification in a meningioma.(b) Skull, AP tomogram: showing the relationship of the calcification to the inner table of the vault; an enostosis protrudes into the centre of the calcified mass

The most common cause of a localized area of speckled or amorphous intracranial calcification is a glioma (*Figure 5.1*): band-like calcification is sometimes seen in astrocytomas and oligodendrogliomas. Calcification also occurs in meningiomas and craniopharyngiomas. A meningioma will be suggested if the calcification, which tends to be homogeneous, is adjacent to the vault or floor of the cranium (*Figure 5.2*); if the adjacent bone shows lytic destruction or reactive sclerosis or thickening; or if the vascular grooves running towards the abnormal area on the inner table of the skull are enlarged. The features of a craniopharyngioma have been described above. Multiple flecks of calcification may also be seen in angiomas, and calcification at the base of the brain may develop after tuberculous meningitis.

Small nodules of calcification disseminated widely within the brain can be a manifestation of tuberose sclerosis and of certain infections, including toxoplasmosis and cysticercosis.

The presence of intracranial calcification does not necessarily indicate disease. There are four sites where calcification (or ossification) is a normal and common occurrence. These are in the pineal (*see* below), the choroid plexus, the falx cerebri (and less commonly the tentorium), and the interclinoid and petroclinoid ligaments. The usual site of choroid plexus calcification is in the trigone of the lateral ventricles; on the lateral skull film this is seen behind and above the normal position of the pineal, and on the posteroanterior film above and lateral to the pineal (*Figures 5.3* and *5.4*). The most distinctive features of choroid plexus calcification are

(a)

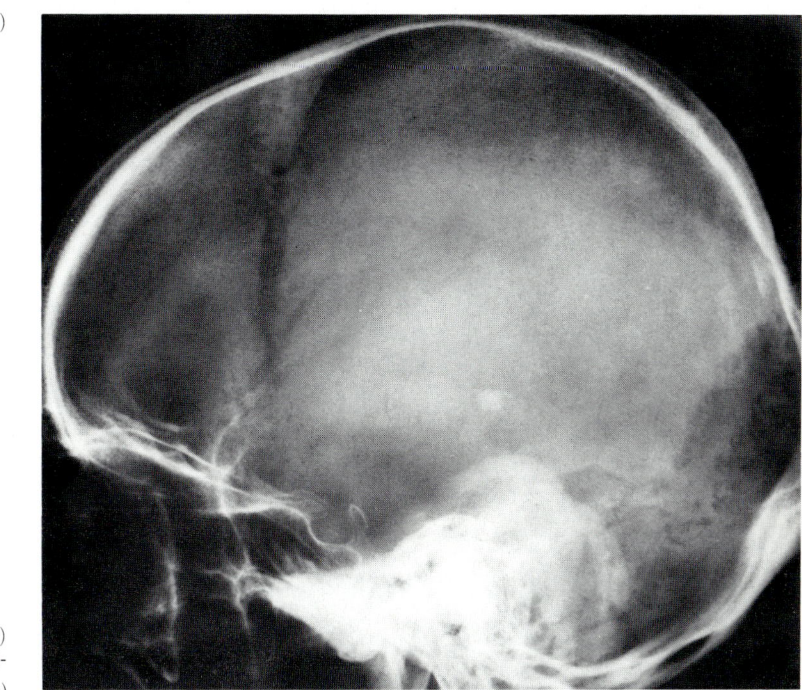

(b)

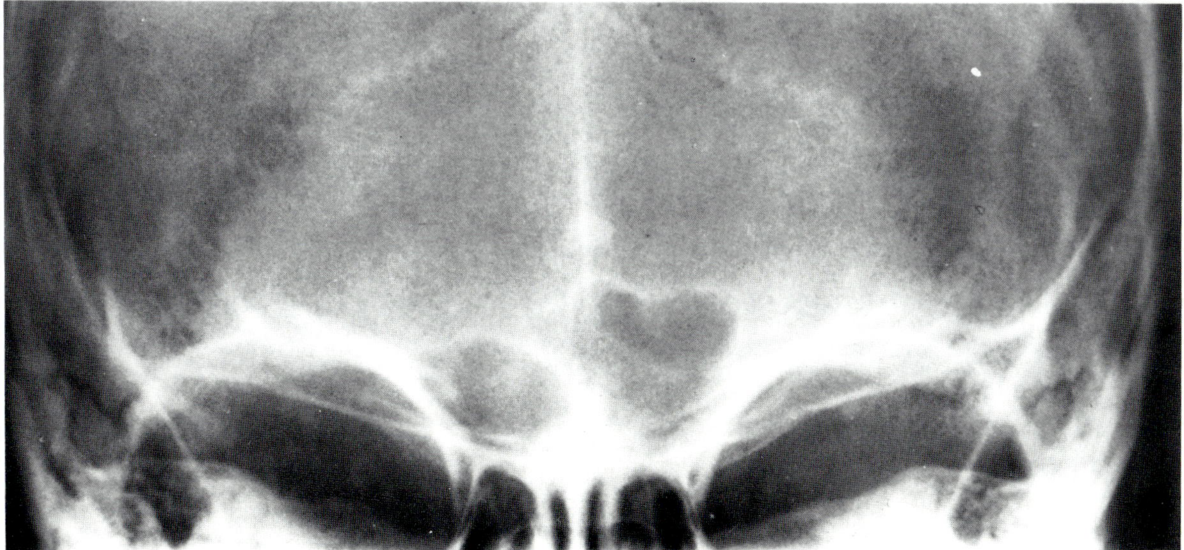

Figure 5.3. Skull, lateral (a) and AP (b) views: showing a normally situated, calcified pineal

(a)

(b)

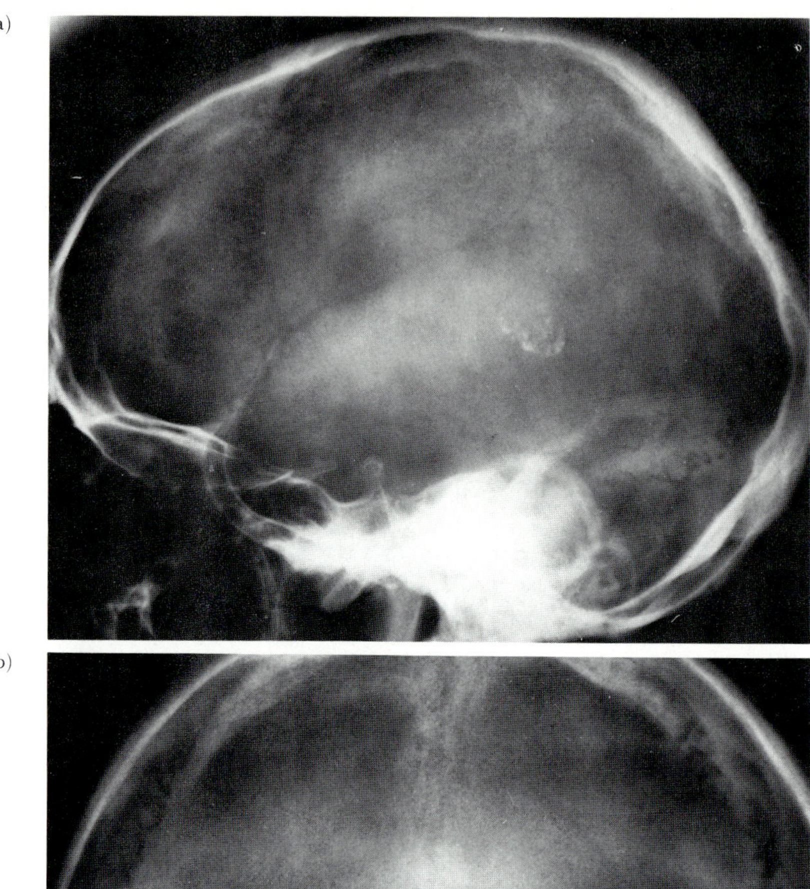

Figure 5.4. Skull, lateral (a) and Towne's (b) views: showing calcification bilaterally in the choroid plexuses

the characteristic position and the fact that the calcification is usually seen on the posteroanterior view to be symmetrically distributed on the two sides: this symmetry essentially excludes a pathological process. Ossification in the falx shows as a plaque with its flat surface in the median plane, and ossification in the interclinoid ligaments as a linear density between the anterior and posterior clinoid processes. The petroclinoid ligaments lie behind the dorsum sellae in the lateral view.

Indirect evidence of an intracranial lesion

Displacement of the calcified pineal away from the side of the lesion. The pineal gland is a midline structure and is sufficiently calcified to be localized on plain X-ray in over 50 per cent of adults. Displacement of the calcified pineal to one side of the midline provides simple evidence of a contralateral space-occupying intracranial lesion. When the pineal is visible on the posteroanterior or Towne's view, the distance in millimetres between it and the inner (or outer) tables of the skull can be measured on each side (*Figure 5.3b*). It is important that the film is taken with the patient's head straight, and if more than slight rotation is present the film should be repeated.

A discrepancy of up to 2 mm in the measurements of the two sides can be regarded as acceptable and not in itself signifying disease, but a difference greater than this should be regarded as strong evidence for the presence of a unilateral space-occupying lesion. The pineal may be central when bilateral intracranial lesions, such as bilateral subdural haematomas, are present.

The calcified pineal is also visible on the lateral skull film, and normally lies about 5 cm above the level of the external auditory meatus. No simple measurements can be applied to detect displacement on this view, so that recognition of displacement requires considerable experience.

Changes in the sella turcica   Characteristic changes may develop in the sella turcica in response to raised intracranial pressure of at least 6 weeks' duration, providing important evidence of this condition. Papilloedema is usually, but not invariably, present. The commonest early radiographic abnormality is loss of the sharp white line of the lamina dura (cortex) of the anterior aspect of the dorsum sellae and adjacent floor of the pituitary fossa (*Figures 5.5 and 5.6*). This does not occur as an age change and if present is highly significant and indicates raised intracranial pressure. It is found in less than 20 per cent of patients subsequently shown to have intracranial tumours. Its recognition demands first-class technique and much experience. The pituitary fossa usually remains normal in size in the presence of raised pressure but can enlarge slightly whilst retaining its shape in the 'empty sella syndrome' which is sometimes associated with long-standing slightly raised pressure.

Hydrocephalus, due to obstruction of the ventricular pathway, can lead to erosion of the top of the dorsum sellae by the dilated third ventricle. This lesion can be indistinguishable from erosion due to a local tumour. Finally, in severe chronic raised intracranial pressure, usually from frontal tumours, the whole of the sella floor and adjacent planum sphenoidale may become so deossified and weakened that they collapse downwards into the sphenoid sinus.

In contrast, an intrinsic pituitary tumour (e.g. in acromegaly) causing moderate or gross enlargement of the fossa results in backwards displacement of the dorsum sellae, ballooning down of the floor, and undercutting of the anterior clinoids without downward displacement of the planum sphenoidale (*see Figure 5.7*).

Changes in the vault in children   Raised intracranial pressure in

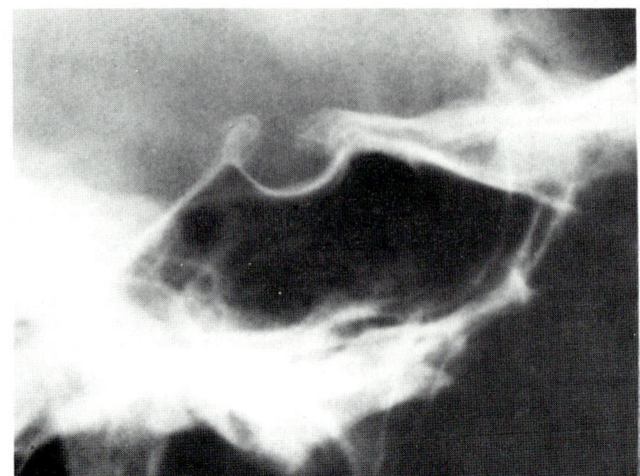

Figure 5.5. Normal pituitary fossa and sphenoid sinuses. Lateral view: patient facing to right. The anterior and posterior clinoid processes are clearly shown

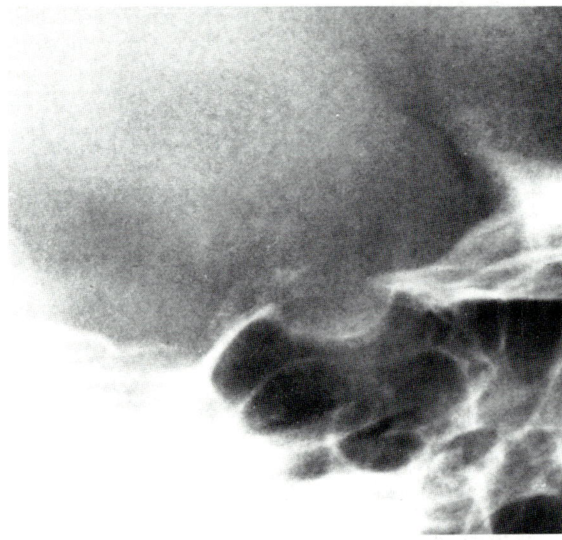

Figure 5.6. Skull, coned view of pituitary fossa: showing obliteration of parts of the lamina dura and sellar floor and erosion of the top of the dorsum sellae, due to raised intracranial pressure resulting from a left temporal cystic glioma

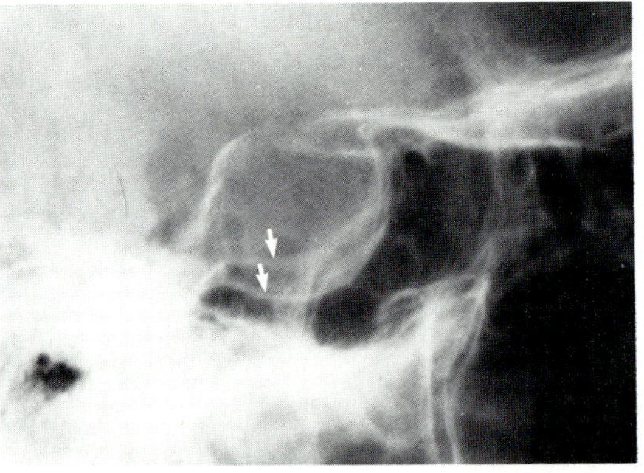

Figure 5.7. Acromegaly. 'Ballooning' of the pituitary fossa produced by an intrasellar tumour. Asymmetrical tumour enlargement has created uneven depression of the floor of the fossa on the two sides (arrows)

children may cause enlargement of the head, widening of the sutures, and the milder forms of sella change described above. Widening of the sutures is usually the most obvious feature. Raised intracranial pressure of more than 3 months' duration can also cause an increase in the convolutional markings on the inner table of the skull over the top of the head (giving an exaggerated appearance of beaten copper), and thinning of the vault. A copper-beaten appearance is sometimes seen in normal children, although not at the vertex, and great care should be exercised in interpreting this finding in the absence of other features of raised intracranial pressure.

Abnormal vascular grooves   The presence of abnormal vascular grooves may indicate abnormal vessels supplying a tumour, most commonly a meningioma.

Special neuroradiological investigations

Significant changes can be seen on routine plain radiographs in only about 20 per cent of cases of cerebral tumour (with the exception of those in the region of the pituitary fossa), and these changes are rarely sufficiently specific and informative for treatment to be initiated. Even the bone changes due to meningioma are often equivocal or overlooked.

Computed tomography

Computed tomography (CT), developed in the early 1970s, plays an immensely valuable role in the investigation of intracranial disease and has revolutionized neuroradiological practice. The method is sensitive and accurate in the detection and localization of intracranial lesions, and in many instances the information obtained is sufficient for patient management without the need for other radiological tests. In addition to this, the technique is non-invasive, not uncomfortable for the patient, and in itself (if intravenous organic iodine contrast enhancement is not required) carries no morbidity. The principles have been outlined in Chapter 1. CT is of overall diagnostic superiority to radioisotope scanning and is therefore the preferred primary special investigation in centres equipped with this facility, as are virtually all neuroscience centres in developed countries.

CT is extremely valuable when investigating head injuries. The accuracy in detecting and localizing acute traumatic intracranial haemorrhage approaches 100 per cent. Cerebral haemorrhage can be distinguished from contusion or oedema, and subdural and extradural haematomas can be demonstrated (*Figures 5.8 and 5.9*).

The examination result is abnormal in about two-thirds of patients presenting with subarachnoid haemorrhage. If CT is carried out within the first 4 or 5 days, blood is nearly always visible and its distribution helps to determine the probable site of bleeding. Angiography is of course necessary to reveal the cause and precise anatomical details, such as the exact origin of an aneurysm or the vascular supply and drainage of an angioma. In other stroke cases CT is invaluable in distinguishing cerebral haemorrhage from infarction.

CT is the investigation of choice in the detection of suspected

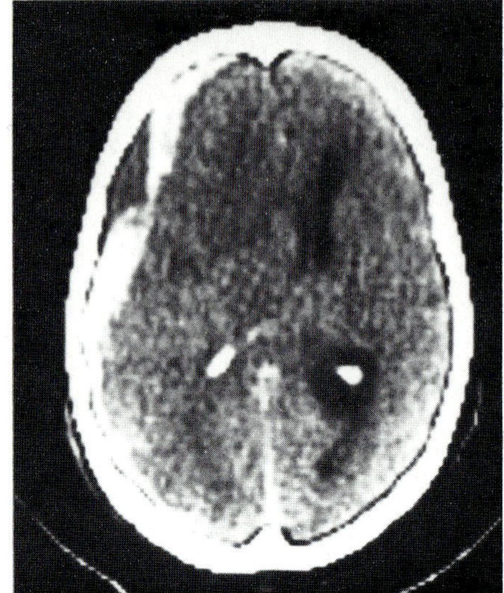

Figure 5.8. CT scan: showing a large left-sided extracerebral (chiefly subdural) haematoma. Much of this is of high attenuation, being of recent origin. There is extreme displacement of the ventricular system towards the right, due partly to the haematoma and partly to the underlying brain swelling

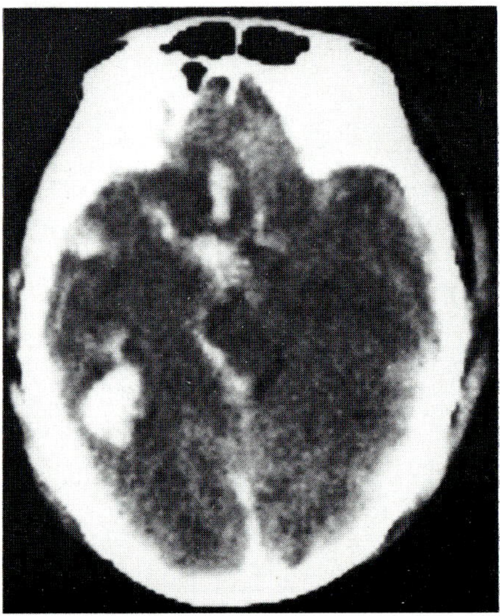

Figure 5.9. CT scan: showing intracerebral and subarachnoid haemorrhage following a road traffic accident

intracranial tumours (*Figure 5.10*), the accuracy exceeding 90 per cent. The information obtained can sometimes be rendered even more specific by intravenous organic iodine enhancement. This adds a degree of discomfort and a slight risk to the procedure. Notwithstanding these and the small radiation dose the procedure can be repeated to monitor tumour response to radiotherapy or chemotherapy, or to assess suspected tumour recurrence after surgery or therapy.

Cerebral abscesses are very reliably detected by CT, the accuracy approaching 100 per cent. The prognosis has been markedly improved as a result of this diagnostic accuracy and the precision with which cerebral abscesses can now be drained.

Hydrocephalus is simply diagnosed and some help can be obtained in determining the cause. CT is always used in monitoring this condition after surgical treatment in children and adults.

(a)

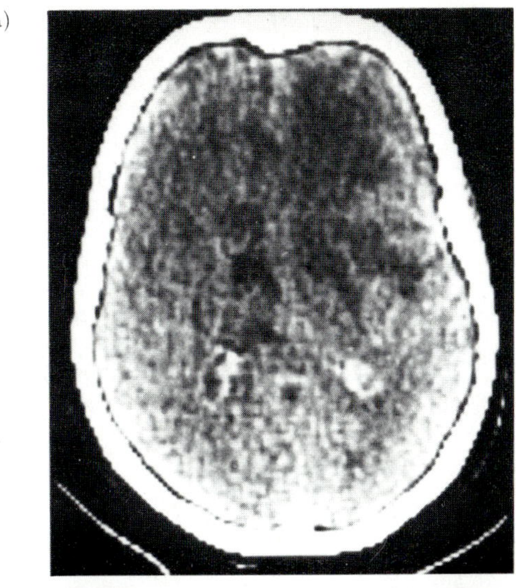

(b)

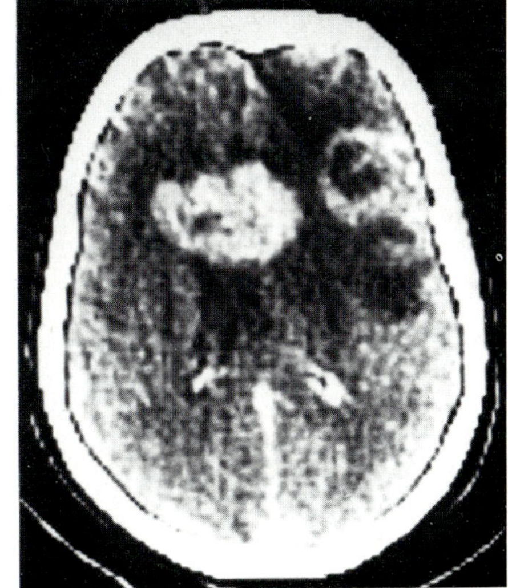

Figure 5.10. CT scan, unenhanced (a) and enhanced (b): showing a partly necrotic glioma involving the right frontal lobe and corpus callosum; there is a great deal of surrounding oedema. On biopsy, part of the tumour was found to be necrotic, which presumably coincides with the central area that failed to enhance with intravenous organic iodine

CT has brought many neurological diseases that were 'invisible' to radiology, such as multiple sclerosis and white-matter degenerations, within the compass of the neuroradiologist.

Radioisotope scanning

Radioisotope scanning entails recording with a gamma camera or rectilinear scanner the distribution in the head of a radiopharmaceutical, usually technetium-99m injected intravenously (*see* Chapter 1). Normally very little isotope is taken up in the brain, but considerable isotope concentration occurs in the scalp, dural sinuses and soft tissues of the face and neck: this has the effect of silhouetting the brain on the scan. Intracranial disease may cause a breakdown of the normal mechanisms that prevent isotope entering

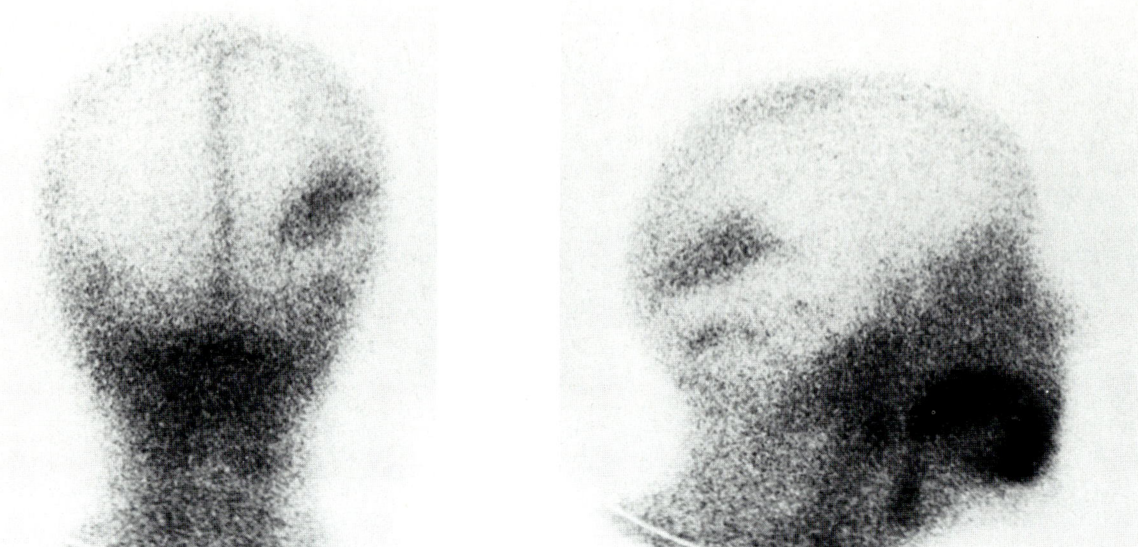

Figure 5.11. Cerebral infarct. Radioisotope scan: posterior and right lateral views. Isotope concentration in infarct in right posterior parietal–occipital region

the substance of the brain, resulting in uptake of isotope in the pathological lesion. This will appear as a 'hot spot' on the scan (*Figure 5.11*). 'Hot spots' of similar appearance are produced by tumours, abscesses, infarcts, etc., so that in general it is impossible to make a pathological diagnosis from the scan. This drawback, together with a slightly reduced sensitivity of radioisotope scanning compared with CT, its poor spacial resolution, and its failure to show anatomical structure have led to the establishment of CT as the primary non-invasive special investigation of intracranial disease. Despite this, radioisotope scanning is a valuable investigation for the initial detection of lesions when CT is unavailable.

Radioisotope scanning, for example, is very sensitive in confirming the presence of suspected malignant tumours, meningiomas and abscesses in the cerebrum and at a distance from the skull base. The technique continues to fulfil a common clinical requirement when CT is not readily available by providing a reliable means of showing suspected cerebral metastases: if two or more separate 'hot' areas are present in the brain and there is a known primary tumour, metastases are the most likely diagnosis. (It should be remembered, however, that abscesses and encephalitic processes may also cause multiple 'hot spots', as may a single large glioma). With meticulous technique over 90 per cent of malignant tumours exceeding 3 cm diameter can be detected in the cerebral hemispheres, and tumours as small as 1.5 cm diameter can sometimes be seen if they are near the surface. Radioisotope scanning is less sensitive in detecting masses in the posterior cranial fossa and is extremely unreliable in the perisellar region.

Cerebral infarcts may show as localized 'hot spots' on an isotope scan. If it is possible to wait, they can sometimes be distinguished from cerebral tumours by repeating the scan after an interval of 2–3 weeks: a reduction in size will indicate a resolving lesion. Radioisotope scanning is of little practical value after acute cerebral trauma, although a 'hot' area adjacent to the skull vault due to a subdural or extradural haematoma can sometimes be seen. A large chronic subdural haematoma is nearly always visible.

In many instances CT (and less often the radioisotope scan) taken in conjunction with the clinical findings provides sufficient information, enabling a diagnosis to be made and appropriate management instituted. At other times, and particularly if neuro-surgery is contemplated, more complex radiological investigations are needed to define the precise site and character of a lesion. Further investigation will usually be by arteriography. Air encephalography and ventriculography are rarely required when CT is available (*see* below). Cisternography (opacification of the basal cisterns with modern water-soluble contrast medium or air) can also be undertaken, and air cisternography combined with CT is the best method for excluding the presence of very small acoustic neuromas. These procedures are not without their own difficulties of execution and interpretation; they should be undertaken only after full consultation between the neurologist, neurosurgeon and neuroradiologist, so that the method of introduction of the contrast medium suitable for each patient and the views most helpful for the diagnosis can be selected. The preliminary CT or radioisotope scan can often be of great value by enabling complex invasive examinations to be modified and shortened.

Arteriography

Cerebral angiography is indicated in the following situations: in subarachnoid haemorrhage (to define and precisely localize an

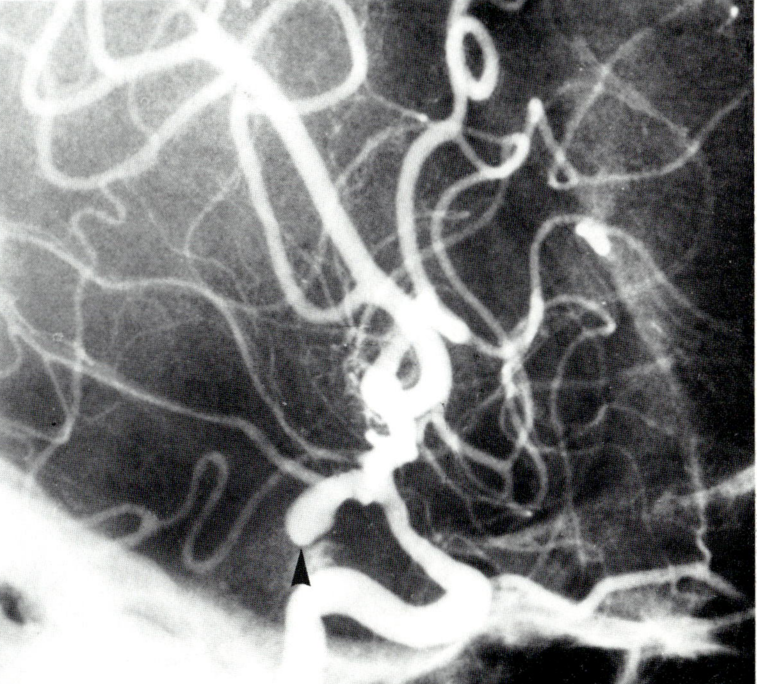

Figure 5.12. Carotid angiogram, lateral view: showing an aneurysm arising just behind the carotid origin of the posterior communicating artery. There is moderate narrowing of the termination of the carotid, probably due to spasm

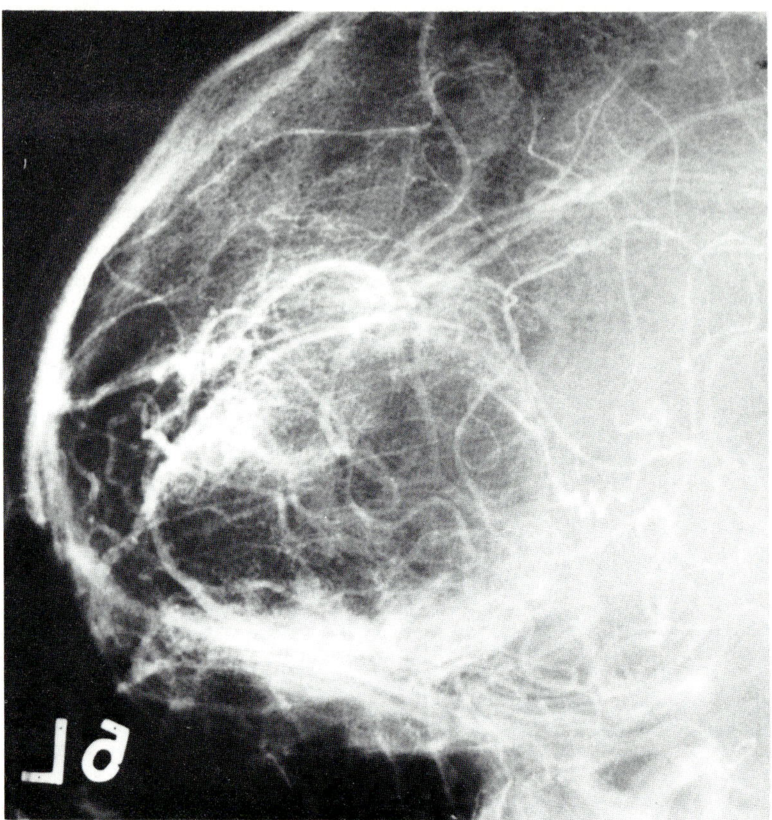

Figure 5.13. Carotid angiogram, lateral view. A malignant glioma with extensive, irregular tumour circulation and a rapid filling vein

aneurysm or other source of bleeding; *Figure 5.12*); when an arteriovenous malformation is suspected (for full characterization before surgery); in possible extracerebral haemorrhage (when this has not been confirmed by scanning); and in those patients with transient ischaemic attacks or minor strokes who might benefit from surgery (to show the extent of disease of the cerebral and neck vessels).

Arteriography may also be required to show the precise vascularity of a cerebral tumour when surgery is contemplated. A tumour is manifest in two ways: the cerebral vessels may be displaced by the mass, and abnormal vessels may be seen within it (*Figure 5.13*). If the tumour has many capillaries it will be outlined more or less homogeneously by the contrast medium, which produces a blush as it circulates through it.

Air encephalography and ventriculography

Air encephalography entails the injection of air into the subarachnoid space, usually by lumbar puncture. With the patient sitting upright, the air rises to the subarachnoid cisterns, passes over the surface of the cerebral hemispheres, and enters the ventricular system through the foramina of Magendie and Luschka. By appropriate positioning of the patient's head the air can be made to enter any part of the ventricles. The brain is outlined on radiographs by this air (*Figure 5.14*).

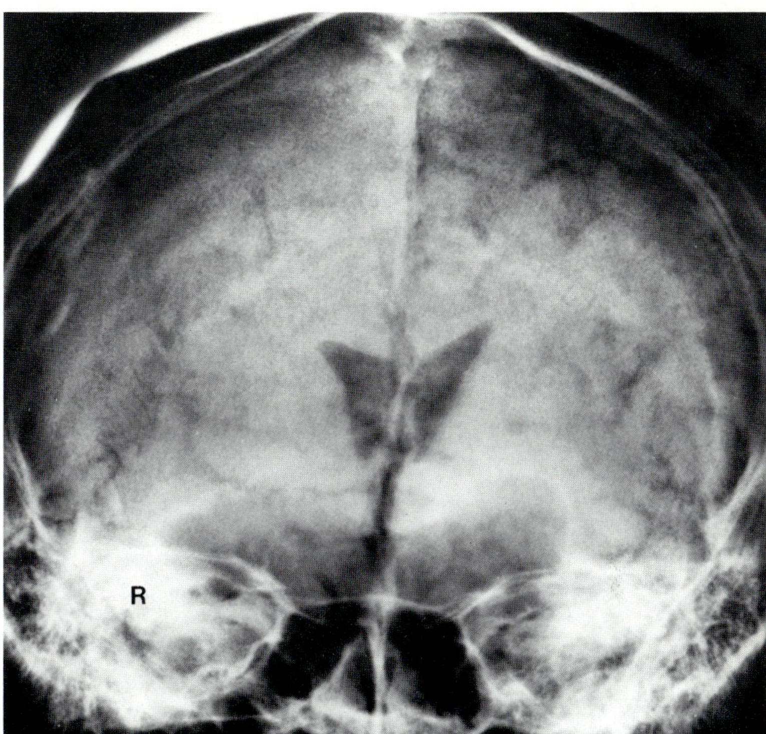

Figure 5.14. Air encephalogram, AP (brow-up). The right frontal horn is depressed and the midline structures are displaced towards the left, due to a right frontal, high convexity space-occupying lesion

Air encephalography is extremely sensitive in detecting displacements or deformities of the ventricles and basal cisterns produced by intracranial masses—such as tumours, abscesses, and especially suprasellar lesions—and will usually show the lower level of obstruction in obstructive hydrocephalus. The examination is, however, unpleasant for the patient and often induces severe headache and sickness: in many departments it is carried out only under general anaesthesia. It is contraindicated when the intracranial pressure is raised, because of the serious risk of inducing tentorial or tonsillar herniation. The advent of CT has greatly lessened the need for air encephalography, which is now primarily reserved for the detailed demonstration of suprasellar masses and lesions in the lower part of the posterior fossa in departments where the more up-to-date CT scanners have not yet replaced the earlier models.

Ventriculography involves the injection of contrast (either air or an organic iodine preparation) directly into the ventricles through a needle introduced into the brain through a burr hole. By appropriate positioning of the head the contrast can be made to outline the upper level of obstruction in obstructive hydrocephalus, or small masses indenting or displacing the ventricles. Even more than is the case with air encephalography, CT has reduced the need for this invasive procedure.

Where CT is completely unavailable air encephalography and ventriculography retain their former importance, ventriculography being reserved for patients with significant, known or suspected raised intracranial pressure.

The spinal cord

When there are symptoms or signs of spinal-cord compression it is usually possible to localize the level of the lesion on clinical examination, so that detailed radiography can be confined to a limited area of the vertebral column. If a tumour is present radiographs may reveal erosion of a pedicle or of the posterior part of the vertebral body, enlargement of an intervertebral foramen, or an area of calcification in the tumour. Sometimes the tumour mass spreads out beyond the immediate vicinity of the spine, and it will then cast a paravertebral shadow similar to that of an abscess (*see Figure 2.57*).

In only a proportion of cases will changes be seen in routine radiographs, and myelography may be indicated. This requires the injection of contrast medium into the subarachnoid space, most commonly by lumbar puncture but sometimes by cisternal puncture at the base of the skull or by lateral cervical puncture. The contrast medium is then made to flow under fluoroscopic guidance to the region of interest by appropriate tilting of the patient. The water-soluble contrast agent metrizamide (Amipaque) is gradually replacing in use the traditional oily iodine preparation iodophenyl-undicylic acid (Pantopaque, marketed in Britain as Myodil). The opacified subarachnoid space can be seen in finer detail with metrizamide. The use of Pantopaque is sometimes followed by chronic low backache and almost always by mild, symptomless arachnoiditis. Metrizamide does not have long-term complications but often causes headache, nausea and changes in awareness for a few days. In sensitive individuals and when inadvertently allowed to reach the head in high concentration or when the recommended quantity of injection is exceeded it may cause convulsions, muscle spasms and other neurological complications. Metrizamide is a far superior contrast medium in skilled hands but should not be used by the untrained.

Tumours occurring in the spinal canal are classified as extradural (of which the commonest are malignant secondary deposits spreading from adjacent bone), intradural, extramedullary (meningiomas and neurofibromas), and intramedullary (gliomas and other tumours of the spinal cord). The group to which the tumour belongs as well as the precise level can usually be determined by myelography.

An intervertebral disc may prolapse posteriorly, causing nerve-root or cord compression, or posterolaterally, producing nerve-root compression. Disc-space narrowing is usually shown on plain films after an acute prolapse of more than 15 per cent of the disc material, but sometimes the appearances are completely normal. Disc degeneration without significant protrusion also causes disc-space narrowing. Features of spondylosis, as described in Chapter 2, are present when the herniation is long-standing. Myelography is sometimes required to confirm the diagnosis of disc prolapse, especially before surgery to show the exact spinal level of the herniated disc. The prolapsed disc produces an anterior or anterolateral filling defect in the column of contrast (*Figure 5.15*), or occasionally hold-up of contrast due to complete spinal block.

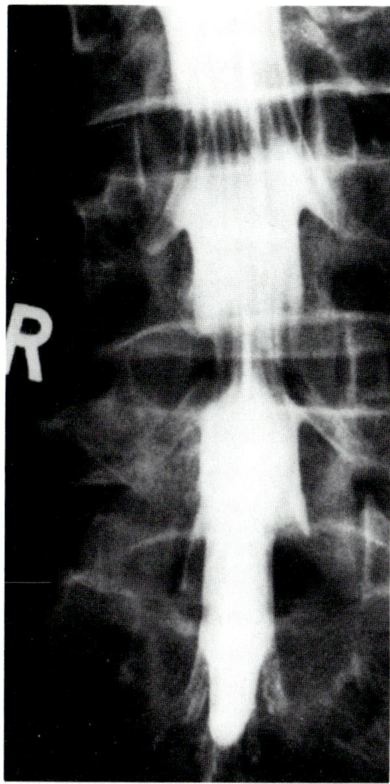

(a)

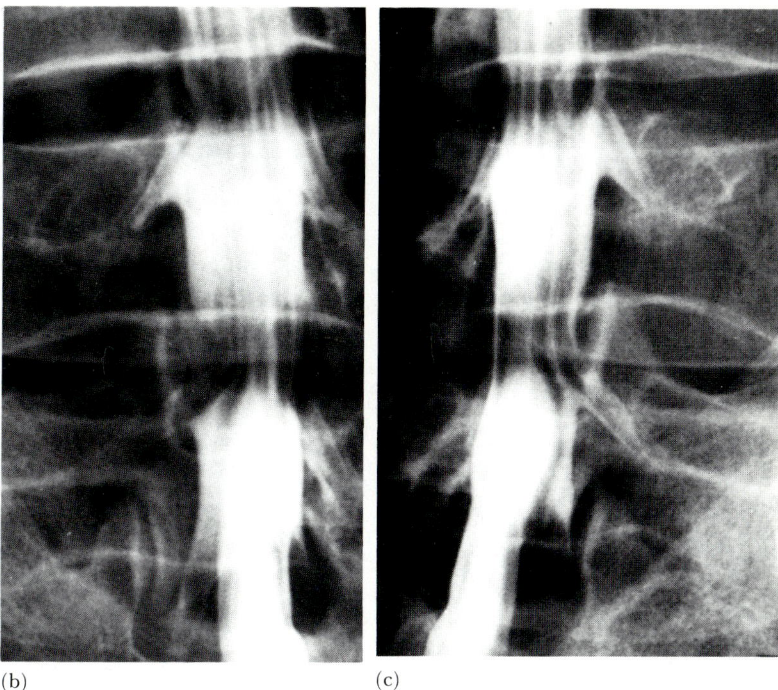

(b)   (c)

Figure 5.15. Myelogram, AP (a) and oblique (b and c): showing displacement of the contrast column, which is thinned from front to back due to a central and right-sided L4–5 disc protrusion which has obliterated the right L5 nerve root sheath (arrows)

Myelography is useful in showing the precise level of obstruction before emergency decompression of the cord in patients developing rapid paraplegia from cord compression by spinal metastases, pyogenic abscesses, etc.

The paranasal sinuses

X-ray examination of the paranasal sinuses is often indicated to confirm a clinical diagnosis of sinus disease, or to investigate unexplained facial pain or headache. Plain film views usually suffice, and tomography is reserved mainly for demonstration of fractures that have not been detected on plain films, and for estimation of the extent of bone destruction in sinus neoplasms.

Sinus disease is manifest by partial or complete opacification of one or more of the sinuses, which are normally aerated. It is often difficult to decide whether the degree of sinus translucency is normal. The most specific and reliable indicator of sinus disease is the presence of a soft-tissue shadow partly filling the sinus, the inner edge of which is outlined by some air remaining within the sinus (*Figure 5.16*). Sometimes a characteristic edge is not visible, and the following general observations may be useful. First, the antra are normally of fairly equal translucency, so that an opaque antrum on one side compared with the other is usually indicative of disease unless the overlying cheek is swollen. Secondly, the blackening of the antra is usually the same as, or greater than, that of the frontal

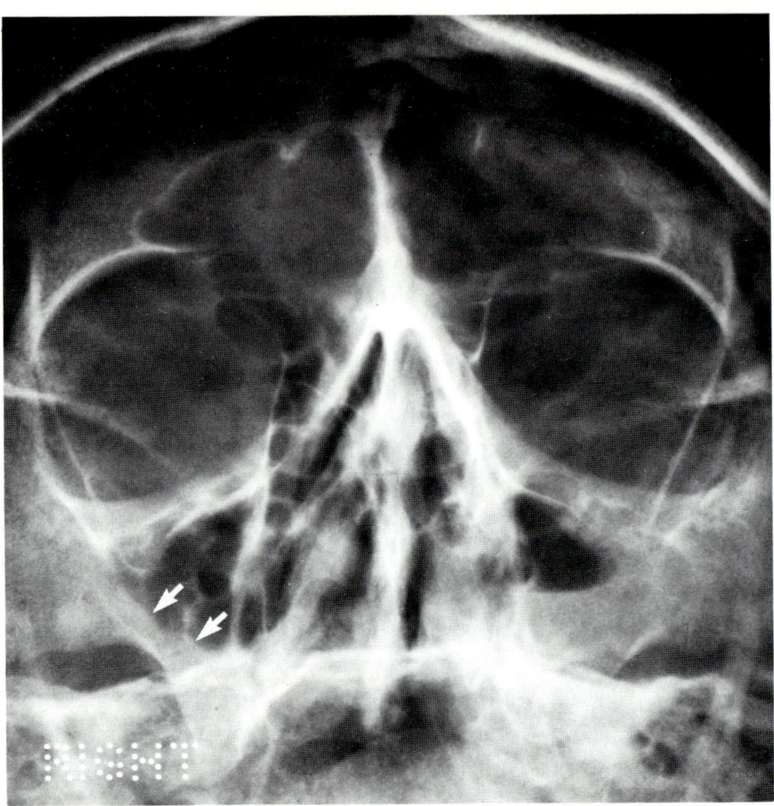

Figure 5.16. Infection of the maxillary antra: there is moderate mucosal thickening in the right antrum (arrows) and gross mucosal thickening and a fluid level in the left antrum

sinuses; so if both antra are equally opaque, and more so than the frontal sinuses, they are most probably diseased.

Infection and allergy are the commonest causes of mucosal swelling and in general give a similar radiographic appearance. One or more sinus groups may be involved. The edges of the swollen mucosa may be seen (*Figure 5.16*) or the sinuses may be totally opaque. Uneven mucosal thickening, with rounded shadows projecting from it, indicates the presence of polyps. A fluid level is sometimes present. Mucosal thickening often occurs during a common cold, and subsides rapidly as the cold clears. In order not to mistake this swelling for the more serious persistent swelling of chronic sinusitis, an X-ray investigation of the sinuses should be delayed for 2 or 3 weeks after an acute infection of the upper respiratory tract.

Several conditions produce a rounded shadow partially filling an otherwise aerated sinus. The commonest of these is a large single polyp, which gives rise to a spherical shadow about 1 cm in size, usually occupying the lower part of the antrum. A very dense, well-defined 1 cm circular shadow due to an osteoma may be seen in the frontal sinus. This is often asymptomatic, but if large may block the ostium causing retention of mucus and pain. A blow-out fracture of the orbit gives rise to a characteristic 'teardrop' shadow suspended from the roof of the antrum (*Figure 5.17*). This represents herniation of orbital contents through the fractured floor of the orbit. It is important to recognize this condition, since surgery may be required to prevent persisting diplopia. The fracture itself is sometimes not seen on plain films, and tomography may be required for its demonstration. CT gives clearer indication of entrapment of individual extraocular muscles in fractures either of the floor or medial wall of the orbit.

Primary carcinoma usually causes total opacification of the affected sinus. Destruction of the bony sinus wall may be present,

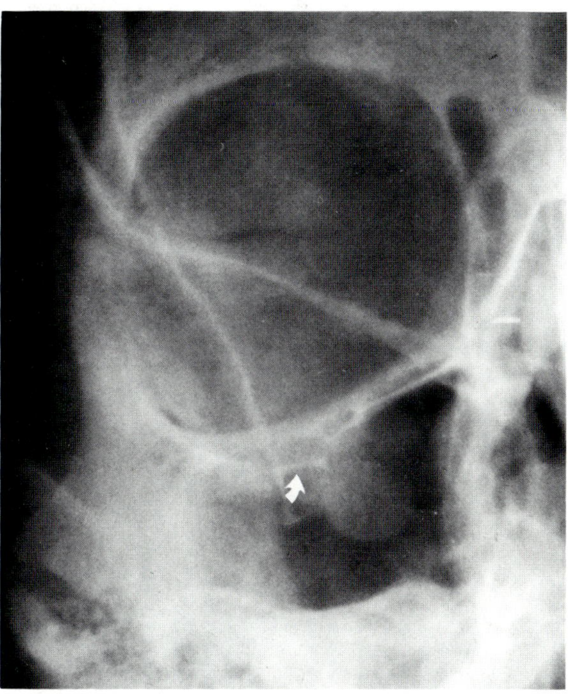

Figure 5.17. Blow-out fracture of orbit. Rounded 'teardrop' shadow representing herniated orbital contents arising from roof of antrum. A depressed fragment of the bony orbital floor can be seen (arrow)

and the extent of tumour spread into the surrounding tissues can be shown very accurately by CT.

The sinuses are not pneumatized at birth, and it is some years before the air spaces become sufficiently well developed for the purposes of X-ray diagnosis. The antra are sometimes fairly well pneumatized by the age of 2 years, but radiological investigation is often unhelpful before the age of 5.

The teeth and jaws

The teeth

Radiology is a useful addition to clinical investigation in revealing the site and extent of disease of the teeth and surrounding structures. Radiographs of the crown occasionally disclose a carious area that is not obvious on clinical inspection (*Figure 5.18*), while localized destruction of the lamina dura (the white line of dense bone lining

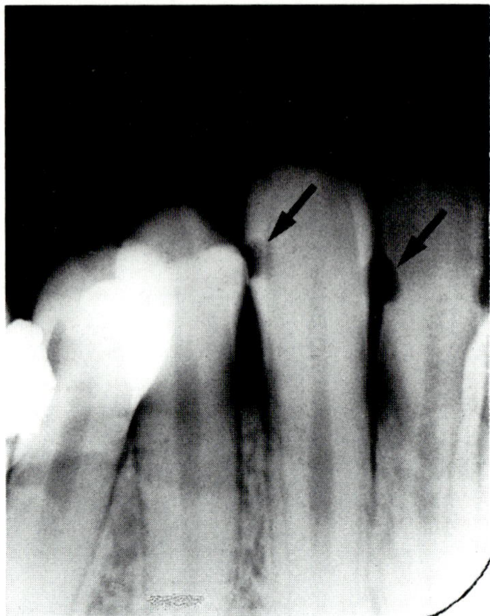

Figure 5.18. Dental caries: small erosions of the enamel and dentine (arrows)

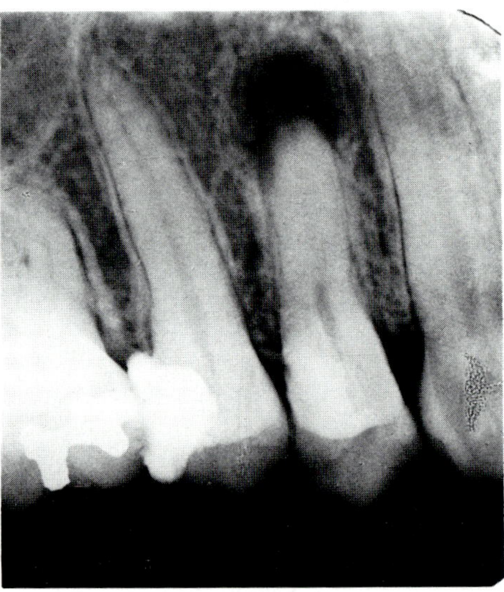

Figure 5.19. Apical abscess: bone destruction around the apex of the upper right 4; no reactive sclerosis

the socket, separated from the root by the narrow translucent periodontal membrane) or the adjacent alveolar bone may be seen in an apical abscess (*Figure 5.19*).

Radiographs are taken by many dental surgeons as part of the routine investigation of the teeth. They are also taken to show: the position and state of development of unerupted teeth; when the cause of toothache cannot be discovered from clinical examination; when there is a possibility that subacute bacterial endocarditis is being aggravated by focal dental sepsis; or when healing is unsatisfactory after the extraction of a tooth. Unsatisfactory healing may be caused by a retained root remnant, a sequestrum or chronic osteitis of the alveolus. The presence of these is usually readily detected on the radiograph.

The jaws

Fractures of the mandible and maxilla have been discussed in the section on Trauma (*see* page 27).

The causes and general X-ray appearances of acute osteomyelitis are described on page 49. In the jaws, the source of infection is frequently a diseased tooth. Acute swelling of the jaw is an indication for radiology, but it is often more valuable in the early stages to radiograph the teeth in the affected area rather than the bone of the mandible beyond the immediate vicinity of the teeth. X-ray changes in the tooth or the lamina dura are often present by the time the general bone infection has become obvious clinically, but the changes of osteomyelitis in the jaw will not be apparent in radiographs for at least a fortnight after the onset of infection. Demonstration of an apical abscess will suggest a local cause for the osteomyelitis.

A cystic neoplasm of the jaw will produce a palpable swelling or pain, or may be found accidentally on X-ray examination for some other purpose. Most of the cysts and tumours that have been described in Chapter 2 as affecting the skeleton generally can also involve the jaws. Most cysts of the jaws are, however, dental in origin; one tumour in particular, an adamantinoma, is rarely found in sites other than the mandible or tibia. This tumour most commonly shows on X-rays as a multiloculated, cystic lesion producing considerable local expansion of the bone.

The ear

Mastoid infections

Radiology is unnecessary during the first few days of acute infection of the middle ear and mastoid air cells, except in the rare event of inspection of the drum not being feasible. Although a loss of transradiancy of the cells will be seen due to oedema or infection of the mucosa, it is not possible to tell from this change whether there will be rapid resolution or whether the infection will progress and involve the bone.

Radiographs of the mastoid region are indicated if the infection is not controlled. These will show the presence or absence of bone destruction and the anatomy of the cells. It is rare to see bone destruction in an acute mastoid infection treated with antibiotics, but this is not uncommon in chronic mastoiditis. Radiographs may show coalescence of the air cells due to destruction of the cell walls, or erosion of the tegmen tympani or lateral sinus plate. Urgent surgical drainage may be required.

The mastoid may fail to pneumatize normally if chronic mastoiditis develops during childhood. X-rays will reveal a small mastoid with sclerotic bone and absent air cells. A cholesteatoma may form in the epitympanic recess and mastoid antrum in a patient with chronic mastoid infection. This may eventually be seen as a ½–1 cm diameter, rounded, smooth-margined, very sharply defined defect in the bone; but at operation in many cases of chronic mastoiditis a mixture of cholesteatomatous material, granulations and secretion is found within the mastoid antrum, tympanic cavity and air cells. Preoperative radiographs in these patients usually show opaque air spaces with some bone destruction.

Deafness

Detailed radiological examination of the anatomy of the ear is essential in congenital deafness for a decision to be made on the feasibility of surgery. The investigation may disclose, for example, an uncorrectable condition such as absence of the inner ear, or a treatable middle-ear anomaly.

Radiological investigation of the internal auditory meatuses is required when an eighth-nerve tumour (acoustic neuroma) is suspected. This usually presents with unilateral deafness, but sometimes vertigo or unilateral tinnitus may be the only manifestation. Larger tumours cause other neurological deficits. Expansion or erosion of the internal auditory meatus may be seen on the affected side (*Figure 5.20*). This is shown more reliably on tomography than

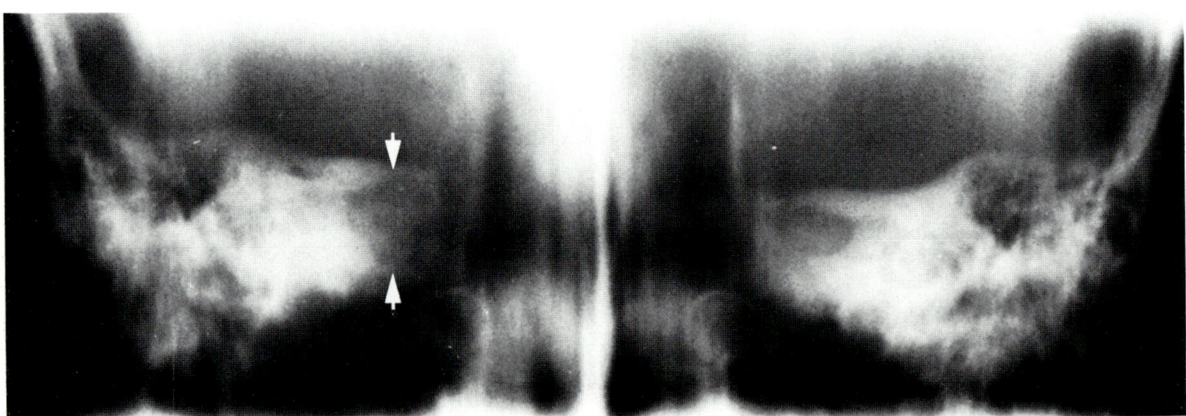

Figure 5.20. Small right acoustic neuroma. The internal auditory meatus is expanded on the right (arrows); compare with normal meatus on the left

on plain films when the petrous bone is very extensively pneumatized. If there is a serious clinical or otological suspicion of an acoustic neuroma, plain films with or without tomography may not be sufficient. They are frequently equivocal. CT (to show tumours greater than 1.5 cm diameter) or cisternography with or without CT (to show smaller tumours) will then be required.

Radiology is seldom useful in diagosing other causes of acquired deafness. Radiographs to exclude an underlying sinusitis may sometimes be indicated. Changes can be demonstrated in otosclerosis, but their significance as a guide to treatment is unproven.

The neck, pharynx, larynx and salivary glands

The neck

The soft-tissue structures of the neck are largely obscured on the anterior view by the spine, and are best seen on the lateral view. One of the uses of the anterior view is to show on which side of the neck an abnormality visible on the lateral view is situated, and films in both projections are taken routinely.

The air column of the oropharynx, larynx and trachea is readily identified on the lateral projection (*Figure 5.21*). The soft tissues between this air column and the spine may be swollen by disease, so that it is important to be familiar with the normal appearances. In health the soft-tissue shadow between the back of the oropharynx and front of the spine measures approximately 3 mm, while the width of the shadow between the back of the trachea and the front of

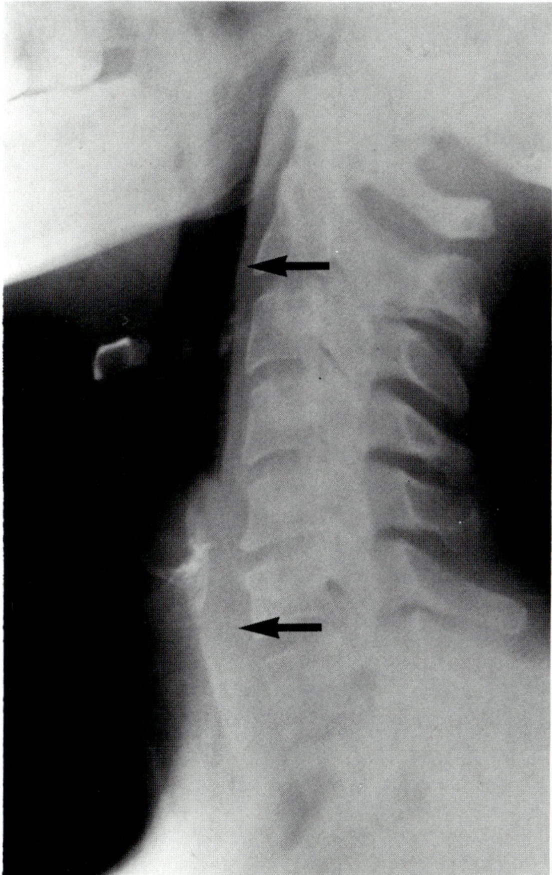

Figure 5.21. Normal lateral view of neck. Note the normal retropharyngeal and retrotracheal soft-tissue shadows (arrows)

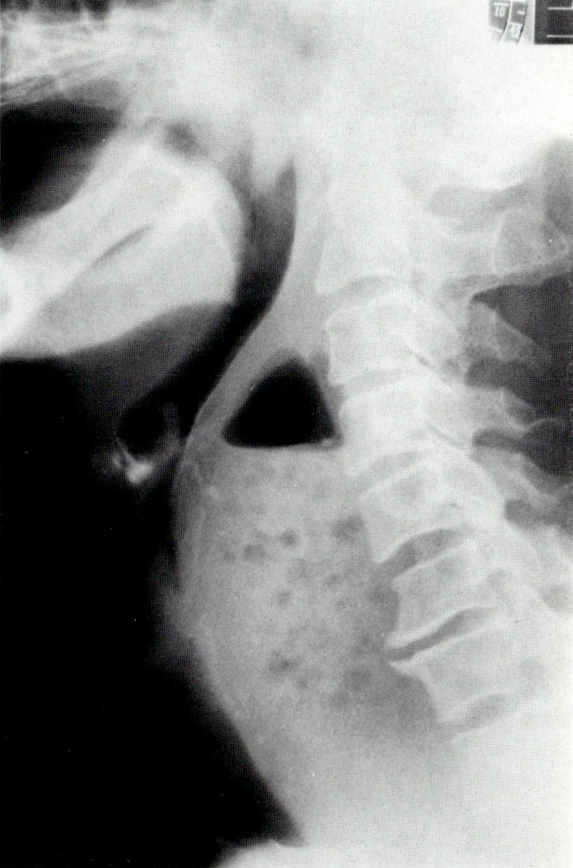

Figure 5.22. Retropharyngeal abscess. The abscess contains numerous small air pockets and a fluid level and is displacing the hypopharynx and trachea forwards

the spine does not exceed the diameter of one of the adjacent vertebral bodies. Retropharyngeal abscesses and tumours will cause a moderate or gross increase of these shadows (*Figure 5.22*). Both conditions may produce a swelling of soft-tissue density and so be indistinguishable radiologically, although the diagnosis is usually obvious clinically. However, pockets of air or a fluid level within the mass will indicate the presence of an abscess in communication with the pharynx.

Two short parallel lines or amorphous flakes of calcification are commonly seen in the necks of elderly patients indicating calcification in the carotid artery, most commonly at the carotid bifurcation. Areas of amorphous calcification in tuberculous glands are also commonly found. A goitre may produce a soft-tissue shadow anteriorly and laterally in the neck, and sometimes this becomes extensively calcified.

Diseases of the spine have been described in Chapter 2. It is important to check for possible atlantoaxial subluxation on the lateral view of the neck, particularly if there is a history of infection or trauma in this region. Normally the slit between the posterior surface of the anterior arch of the atlas and the front of the odontoid peg does not exceed 2 or 3 mm. The causes of atlantoaxial subluxation (*see Figure 2.60*) are trauma, pyogenic infection, tuberculosis, rheumatoid arthritis and ankylosing spondylitis.

The pharynx

Soft-tissue swellings arising in the nasopharynx are most commonly due to adenoid hyperplasia in children and to tumours (carcinoma, sarcoma or lymphoma) in adults. A mass in the nasopharynx can usually be seen on inspection with a mirror in the back of the mouth, but a lateral film is useful to confirm adenoid hyperplasia in children who cannot co-operate with the clinical inspection. When the possibility of tumour arises a submentovertical view to assess for invasion with destruction of the base of the skull is required in addition to the lateral view. Computed tomography determines with great accuracy the extent of invasion of the base of the skull by tumours of the nasopharynx.

The air-filled oropharynx is visible on the lateral plain film and on clinical inspection. Barium swallow examination is required for detailed assessment of the hypopharynx and cervical oesophagus. Filling defects due to tumours, hold-up due to impacted swallowed meat or fishbones, and other lesions are well shown on this examination.

A pharyngeal pouch may arise from the posterior aspect of the gullet at the pharyngo-oesophageal junction, developing at a site of weakness between the horizontal and oblique fibres of the inferior constrictor muscle. As the pouch enlarges it descends into the lower neck or upper mediastinum, where it usually comes to lie on the left side of the oesophagus. Patients with this condition may experience dysphagia, a sensation of fullness in the neck after eating, and regurgitation of undigested food several hours after a meal; or they may suffer from episodes of aspiration pneumonia. The size and position of the pouch can be demonstrated readily by barium swallow examination (*Figure 5.23*).

Perforation of an unsuspected pharyngeal pouch by the oesophagoscope is a well-recognized hazard of oesophagoscopy. The

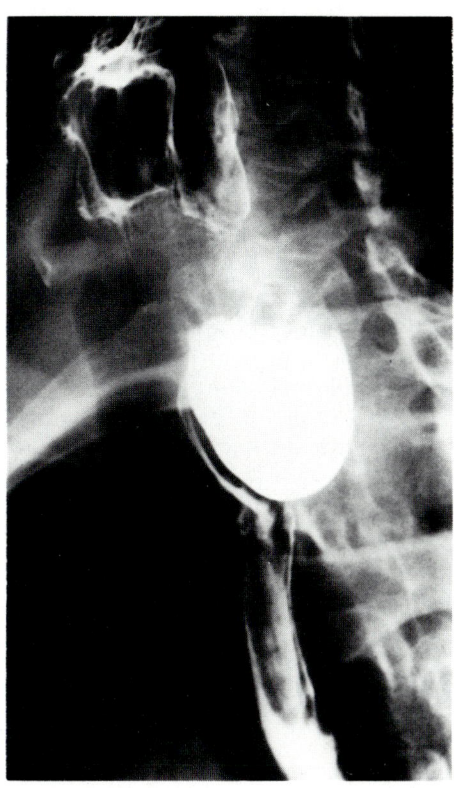

Figure 5.23. Pharyngeal pouch. Large, barium-filled sac adjacent to oesophagus at thoracic inlet

surgeon can be warned of the presence of a pouch, and the incidence of this serious complication largely reduced, if barium swallow examination is carried out routinely before oesophagoscopy.

The larynx

A large tumour of the larynx is usually visible on the lateral view of the neck as a soft-tissue mass encroaching on the laryngeal air column. The extent of the tumour is not clearly defined, however, and a small tumour can be overlooked altogether. Tomography shows the encroachment on the air column more clearly and is useful in demonstrating the lower limit of the tumour when this is obscured by the main tumour mass on endoscopy. Laryngography provides a further method for examining the larynx. This entails coating the anaesthetized laryngeal mucosa with oily contrast medium which is usually injected through a nasogastric tube positioned with its tip in the oropharynx. The procedure is clearly less comfortable for the patient than tomography, and the simpler examination suffices in most cases of tumour.

Since the opacified laryngeal and upper tracheal mucosa can be seen clearly on fluoroscopy, laryngography furnishes an excellent means for examining the calibre of strictures and other sequelae of trauma during different phases of respiration and speech.

The salivary glands

Pain and swelling of the parotid or submaxillary salivary gland, felt soon after eating, suggests the presence of a calculus. This is usually radio-opaque and can be demonstrated on plain films.

The duct system of the parotid and submandibular glands can be opacified with contrast agent injected through a cannula or fine catheter positioned with its tip in the gland orifice. This procedure—sialography—is used to demonstrate the internal structure of a diseased gland. Sialectasis (dilatation of the ducts, somewhat similar to the appearances of dilated bronchi in bronchiectasis) is seen in chronic salivary gland suppuration. In a mixed parotid tumour the ducts are typically stretched and displaced, while they can be frankly destroyed by a salivary-gland carcinoma.

Index